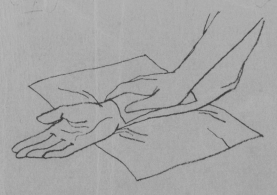

HEAVY BLEEDING

If a large blood vessel is cut, blood loss may be enough to cost the patient his life within minutes. With heavy bleeding, prompt attention is a necessity.

- Apply pressure directly over the wound using a clean cloth or your hand, if necessary.
- Add additional layers of cloth and fasten with a snug bandage.
- If blood saturates the dressing, do not remove it but apply more layers of cloth.
- If bones are not broken, elevate the bleeding extremity until it is higher than the rest of the body.
- Give the patient water as tolerated provided there is no stomach or lower chest wound.
- Don't use a tourniquet.

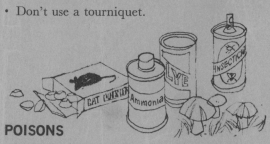

POISONS

Poisoning ranks third as a cause of accidental death among children and can best be prevented by keeping medicines, household supplies and chemicals locked away securely.

Signs and Symptoms

The symptoms of poisoning vary depending on the type of poison and how long ago it was taken. Some poisons cause immediate symptoms such as burns in the mouth and throat and others give no sign until the substance enters the blood stream. Visual difficulty, nausea, headache, deep sleep and convulsions can result.

Treatment

1. Call a doctor or poison control center.
2. Dilute the poison by giving the patient water or milk.
3. Provided the poison is not a strong corrosive like lye or a petroleum distillate such as gasoline or kerosene, induce vomiting by tickling the patient's throat after administering a large glass of water containing suds of a strong laundry soap or one tablespoon of mustard.
4. Be sure the patient's head is lower than his hips to prevent vomitus from entering lungs.
5. After emptying the stomach, give the patient a glass of water containing a teaspoon consisting of one part powdered burnt toast, one part strong tea and one part milk of magnesia. Induce vomiting after each dose and repeat several times.
6. Acid poisoning—give strong solution of bicarbonate of soda and water.
7. Overdose of sleeping pills—empty stomach and give stimulant such as strong coffee.
8. Phosphorus poisoning (matches, rat or roach paste)—empty stomach and give solution of one part hydrogen peroxide or oil of turpentine to 10 parts water.
9. Food poisoning—empty stomach and give castor oil or epsom salts.
10. Always save poison container to show to physician.

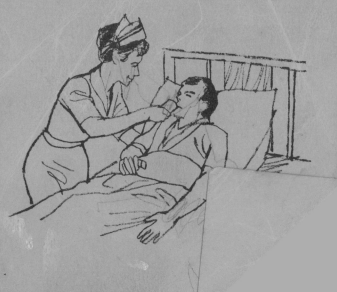

The Home Medical
Encyclopedia

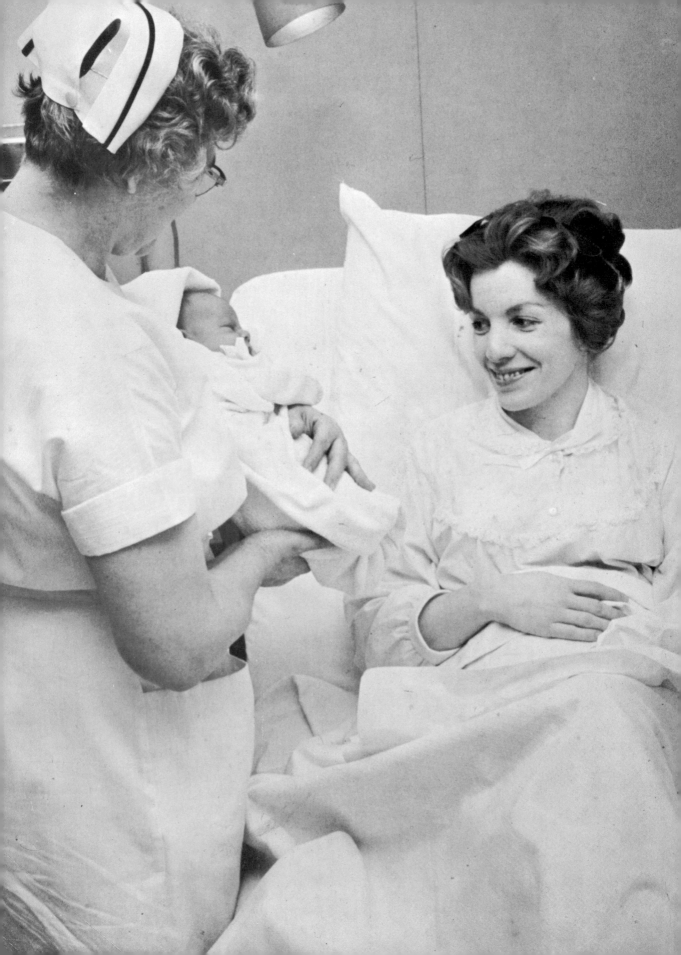

The Home Medical Encyclopedia

*Your guide to good health
for you and your family*

W. B. McKnight, M.D.

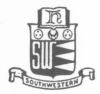

THE SOUTHWESTERN COMPANY
Nashville, Tennessee

Meet the Author

THE AUTHOR was born in Murfreesboro, Tennessee in 1896 where he spent the first seventeen years of his life. He attended the Middle Tennessee State University, then Middle Tennessee Normal School where he was captain of the school's first football team. In 1915 he entered the Normal School of Physical education in Battle Creek, Michigan and graduated in the fall of 1917.

Dr. McKnight taught physical education in the schools of Helena, Arkansas for one year and while there enlisted in the Air Force of the United States Army. He earned his wings as a pilot and was separated from the Army, March 19, 1919 as a Second Lieutenant.

He entered the University of California at Berkeley in the fall of 1919 and achieved his BA degree in 1921. He commuted to San Francisco for four years where he taught physical education in the high schools of that city while he was completing his premedical requirements at Berkeley.

In 1926 he was admitted to the University of California Medical School in San Francisco and interned at the Highland Hospital in Oakland, California County, 1930-1931. He served as Resident at the Fairmont Hospital of Alameda County, California, 1931-1932. In the fall of 1932 he accepted a position at the Western Pacific Hospital in Portola, California. He became the Division Surgeon and Medical Director of this hospital in 1934 and held this position for 12 years engaging in private practice during the same period.

Dr. McKnight married Ida Beckwith of Palo Alto, California in 1922 and their first son, who is now practicing law in Sacramento, California, was born in 1928. Their second son, born in 1936, is now practicing medicine as a General Practitioner in San Rafael, California.

In 1946 the family moved to Berkeley, California to permit their sons to attend college while living at home. The author was engaged in private practice in Berkeley until the fall of 1952. During this period he served on the staff of Cowell Memorial Hospital, which is the Students Medical Center at the University of California. He was also a member of the staffs of Alta Bates, Herrick Memorial, and Providence Hospitals.

From 1953 until 1966 Dr. McKnight served in the capacities of Plumas County Physician and Health Officer, Quincy, California. He was the Autopsy Surgeon for the Coroner's office, the Hospital Administrator, the County Registrar, and during the last few years was the Director of the Plumas County Mental Services which were furnished by a team composed of a psychiatrist, a clinical psychologist, and a psychiatric social worker.

This Mental Health Clinic is growing rapidly and performing many much needed services for the county. The implementation of this clinic is in line with the policy of the State Department of Mental Hygiene to treat mental illness in the local hospitals rather than sending patients to state mental hospitals which are overcrowded.

While in medical school the author was a member of the medical fraternity Alpha Kappa Kappa, and upon graduation was elected to Alpha Omega Alpha, a medical honor society.

In 1966 when Dr. McKnight reached the age of retirement as a public servant he returned to the private practice of medicine.

He is a member of the California Academy of Medicine, the American Academy of General Practice, the Quad County Medical Society, the California Public Health League, the California Medical Association, and the American Medical Association.

Preface

IN COMPILING information of the nature and scope found within *The Home Medical Encyclopedia,* I studied and made extensive notes from literally hundreds of medical textbooks, medical magazines, and pamphlets, as well as many articles written by outstanding medical authorities.

Using the experience gained in thirty-five years of working as a family doctor, I have tried to assemble these medical facts in such a way as to make it possible for anyone to read and understand them. It is to be hoped that the contents of this book will help ease suffering, prevent disease, and improve health in many homes.

I wish to express my sincere thanks to those who have helped in making this work possible. To my wife, who typed most of the original manuscript and gave valuable assistance throughout, I am especially indebted.

Mrs. Helen Cavaille, who typed the entire manuscript, is mentioned because, without her very efficient labors the book would have remained unpublished. Mrs. Jean McCleave, who typed the first part of the manuscript, has earned my lasting gratitude. Mrs. Lasswell, Mrs. Bar, Mrs. Strang, Mrs. Walker, Mrs. Robison, Mrs. Bennetts, Mrs. Gillespie, Mrs. Stevens, and Adrienne Robison contributed timely and appreciated help in proof reading, editing, and preparing the glossaries. To the Illinois College of Optometry for use of picture on page 332.

The publishers and I are grateful to Willard Nelson for his technical advice and tireless effort in creating this book; and to Michael Stancik as designer and art director.

To these, and all others who helped, I express my thanks.

W. B. McKNIGHT, M.D.

Quincy, California

Table of Contents

Part 2   DISEASES OF MANKIND

Part 5 ACCIDENTS AND FIRST AID

Part 6   EMOTIONAL DISORDERS AND MENTAL DISEASES

Appendices

Index

Introduction

WHEN I THINK OF the science of medicine, I like to picture it as a living thing which is as old as the pyramids and yet as new as tomorrow's newspaper. Almost since the beginning of time men have studied the human body and have tried to find ways to cure and prevent disease. This knowledge has been passed on from generation to generation and since it is ever changing and always growing, a vast amount of material has accumulated.

In writing this book, my objective has been to choose from this mass of knowledge the simple, fundamental truths which have been proven by the test of time, and to combine them with the wonderful modern discoveries in medicine. It has been my purpose to bring forth a guide written in simple words, to be used in any home to help prevent and cure sickness and suffering. Indeed, some of these facts, if properly used, might be the means by which lives may be saved.

This does not mean that self treatment, if serious illness is present, is advocated. On the contrary, these procedures are to be used when simple sickness or accidents are encountered—never forgetting that in some cases the further advice of a doctor should be sought as quickly as possible.

A patient can only be treated adequately by a doctor of medicine who is in a position to examine him and have the indicated laboratory tests performed and X rays taken as needed. He can also get other doctors to consult with him if he feels that this should be done.

This book, *The Home Medical Encyclopedia* is not intended in anyway to encourage the patient to try and treat himself. It is hoped that the person who uses this book will go and see his family doctor when the need arises. The recent numerous advances in medical science make it more important than it has been in the past for the patient to consult his doctor.

W. B. McKNIGHT, M.D.

PART 1

Reproduction of Life

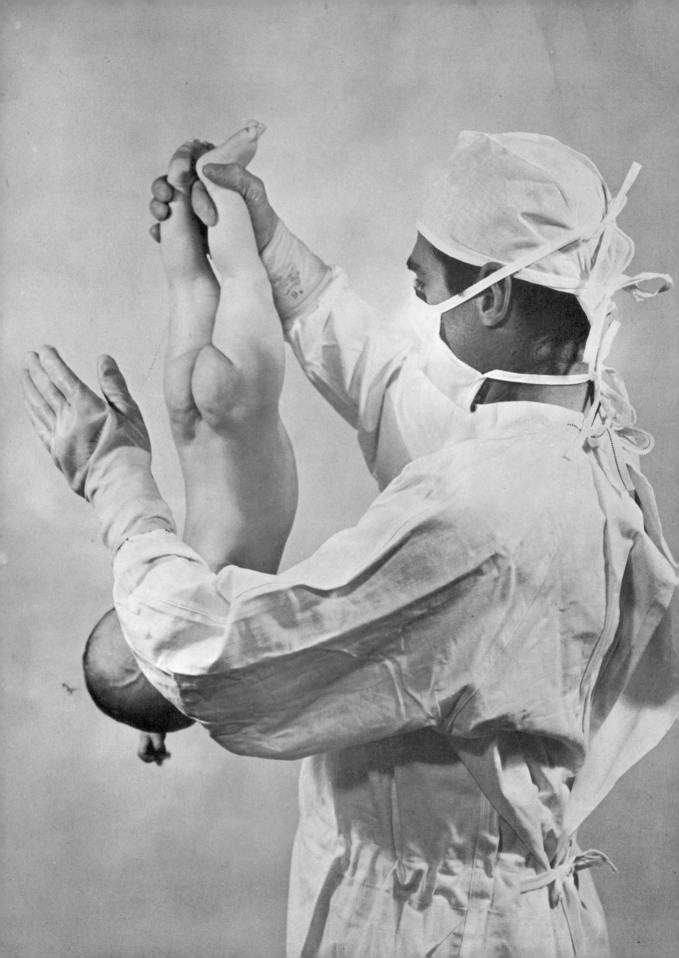

Chapter 1

Pre-natal Care

THE HUMAN BODY is the most wonderfully complicated machine in the whole world—and like all machines, it should be properly cared for and maintained.

CONCEPTION

A good place to start is with the baby, and in protecting the baby's health, we should not wait until the baby is born, but should begin at the very time of conception, when life is initiated. Conception is the moment when the spermatozoon from the male meets and enters the ovum or egg of the female. This meeting usually occurs in one of the Fallopian tubes, and the fertilized egg then becomes embedded in the lining of the womb or uterus, where it begins to grow. (See illustration on the next page.)

The mother should begin at this time to protect and improve the health of her baby and herself. She will suspect that she is pregnant when her monthly period fails to occur. After two or three periods are missed, she should consult her doctor.

VISITS TO THE DOCTOR

The doctor, after confirming the fact that she is pregnant, will advise her to live a normal life. He will probably ask her to come in for examinations about once a month until the baby is born, and on these monthly visits he will examine her blood pressure, her urine, and her weight. This is done because one of the first indications of abnormality during pregnancy is often noted by damage to the kidneys. This will be detected by albumin in the urine and an elevation of blood pressure. Then, appropriate steps can be taken.

The expectant mother should realize that her condition is a normal one. Babies have been coming into the world since the beginning of time and there is no cause for fear. There is also no need for drastic change in the mother's life. She should proceed with her customary routine—only leaving out the more violent exercises, such as horseback riding.

Every prospective mother can have thorough and sometimes life-saving prenatal care, simply by going to the doctor early in

3

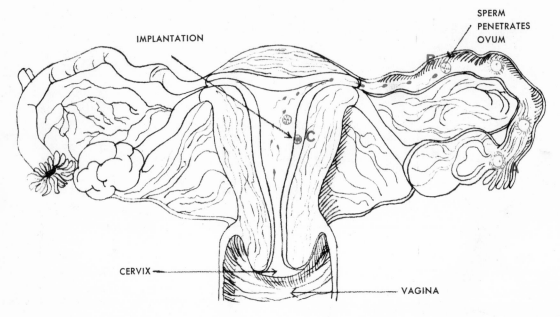

Life begins: A. Egg enters tube from ovary. B. Spermatozoa penetrates egg in tube. C. Fertilized egg enters uterus and is imbedded in wall where it begins to develope into baby.

her pregnancy. The cost is just the same, because a doctor usually charges the same fee whether he just delivers the baby or whether he sees the patient eight or ten times before the delivery.

When the doctor sees the patient early in the course of her pregnancy he can help straighten out certain emotional problems that some pregnant women have.

Some women have needless fears that their baby will be abnormal and because of this suffer a great deal mentally during the pregnancy. Others are afraid without cause and will have a feeling of guilt because they do not want the baby. The doctor can explain all these things to the patient, and even have her visit the delivery room in order to know what to expect at the time of delivery. She may be shown the nursery where her baby will be kept for the first few days and in this way, the fear of the unknown can be overcome.

In addition to helping out with the emotional aspects of pregnancy, the doctor will take the patient's pelvic measurements and assure her that she is large enough to have her baby; and he will watch her weight to see that she doesn't gain too much. Early in the pregnancy he will take a blood test to see if she has syphilis. This is important because if syphilis is detected the mother may be treated during pregnancy and the baby will be perfectly normal. If, on the other hand, the mother has syphilis, which she may have without knowing it, and is not treated, the baby may be born with congenital syphilis. This cannot be cured and the baby will be handicapped for its entire life.

The mother's heart, lungs, and teeth will be watched during pregnancy. The size and position of the baby will be checked often to see if the development is progressing as it should. The mother's blood pressure will be watched closely; this is a very important test because a change in blood pressure is often the first sign of an abnormality which may lead to convulsions. This is called the toxemia of pregnancy or eclampsia. If the blood pressure starts going up, the doctor may take the proper steps to prevent this very dangerous condition from developing. If the ankles start to swell it is possible, by changing the diet and eliminating salt, to prevent this, or at least lessen it.

Anemia which may be present can be corrected by taking iron, and the mother's teeth can be protected by taking calcium. This preventive measure changes the old saying, "For every baby a tooth." The baby needs calcium for its bones, and the mother's teeth used to suffer.

When first examining the patient the doctor may take a "Pap" smear from the cervix and early cancer of the cervix is sometimes detected. It can be treated early by conization of the cervix even though the mother is pregnant and thereby save her life without affecting the pregnancy.

The blood type of the mother is taken to determine the Rh factor. If the mother is Rh positive, there is no need for further study, but if she is Rh negative—meaning she has no Rh factor in her blood—then her husband's blood should be tested. If he is Rh positive and she is Rh negative, then the baby should be watched closely. A blood test can be taken from his cord when he is born and if necessary an exchange transfusion can be done to save the baby's life.

These are some of the many steps which make it important for the mother to see her doctor early in the pregnancy and to continue to go to him regularly throughout the pregnancy. An easier and safer delivery can then be expected.

Not many years ago the mortality rate or deaths among mothers at childbirth was fifty out of every ten thousand live births. Today, because of improved prenatal care the number of deaths among the mothers has been decreased to only three for every ten thousand live births.

GLOSSARY

Anemia   a blood condition in which the blood is deficient in quantity or quality
Congenital   born with
Conization   surgical removal of diseased tissue
Convulsion   an involuntary muscle contraction
Cervix   mouth of the womb
Eclampsia   convulsions and coma in pregnant women
Fallopian tubes   tubes that conduct the egg from the ovary to the uterus
Pap test   a painless method in which the cervix is scraped and checked for cancer
Pelvis   bony structure containing female organs
Prenatal   before birth
Rh factor   concerns blood types of both parents
Syphilis   venereal disease
Toxemia   a general intoxication due to the absorption of poisons or toxins

ECLAMPSIA

(A Complication of Pregnancy)

Cause and Nature

The true cause of eclampsia is not known and this condition is one of the dangerous complications of pregnancy. Fortunately the severe cases are seldom seen any more, especially if the patient has gone to the doctor and received proper prenatal care.

The condition has been classified in two forms: pre-eclampsia, which never develops into true eclampsia because of proper treatment, and eclampsia which is a serious complication.

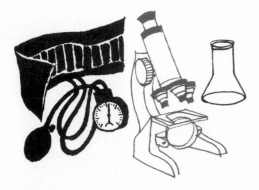

Indispensable tools for doctor and laboratory technician.

Signs and Symptoms

This disease is seen most often in women who are pregnant for the first time and begins, as a rule, after the sixth month. The first symptoms are loss of appetite, headache, and excessive gain in weight. The doctor will detect a gradual rise in blood pressure and there will be albumin in the urine—this being one of the reasons a urine specimen is requested from the pregnant woman on each visit to the doctor.

As the condition progresses there are visual disturbances which may lead to blindness. This clears up after the pregnancy has been terminated.

The most dramatic and feared of the symptoms of eclampsia are convulsions and coma. These may lead to death if the pregnancy is not promptly terminated. In cases where the baby is not delivered spontaneously, a Caesarean section is performed.

When a woman is over thirty-five and previously has had severe eclampsia, she should not become pregnant again. This is one of the cases in which an operation to tie the tubes is justified and may be lifesaving. Younger women with mild preeclampsia may have other babies if followed carefully by the doctor. The word "pre-eclampsia" is most often used to indicate these cases which do not have severe symptoms such as convulsions.

Treatment

The treatment should be dictated by a doctor. He will restrict the use of salt at the very first sign of edema (swelling of the legs) which is accompanied by a rise in blood pressure. (This does not apply to the common swelling of the legs often seen late in pregnancy because of pressure of the baby on the blood vessels. In other words, a swelling of the legs late in pregnancy is common and does not mean that the patient has eclampsia.) A proper diet is important to further restrict the intake of salt or sodium, and drugs to lower blood pressure are helpful. Diuretics, such as Hydrodiuril, are often used by a doctor to help prevent the development of eclampsia.

Some doctors use large doses of penicillin which for some unknown reason seem to lessen the toxicity of the condition. If loss of vision, convulsions, or coma appear, the pregnancy should be terminated at once, by operation if necessary.

The outlook in these cases is good for the mother if proper steps are taken. When the pregnancy is terminated the mother regains her vision, the blood pressure goes down, and she returns to the same state of health which she enjoyed before becoming pregnant.

GLOSSARY

Caesarean operation to remove baby from womb through the walls of the abdomen
Coma a "sleeplike" state with no response to sound, touch, etc.
Convulsion twitching of voluntary muscles
Edema swelling
Spontaneously without help
Terminate pregnancy to end pregnancy

Chapter 2

The Baby Is Born

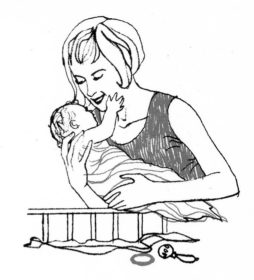

THE FIRST THING that every mother wants to know is whether the baby is perfectly normal. Then she wants to know whether it is a boy or a girl.

The young mother should always keep in mind that the chances of her baby being abnormal are extremely rare; and she should remember that in this modern day, many abnormalities can be corrected.

Today it is almost impossible to find a young person with a club foot because this condition can be corrected soon after birth, and the child may never know that he was born with something wrong with his foot. So it is vitally important to have hope, and to know that many conditions can be corrected by modern medical science.

The preceding paragraphs have been written to give the mother and father a feeling of confidence. This is of great value in taking care of a newborn baby. If the baby is born in a hospital, a nurse will take care of him for the first three or four days, and the mother has a chance to rest and become acquainted with her offspring. If the baby is born at home, it should be wrapped in a clean, light cotton blanket and placed in a safe place until the mother is taken care of. If the baby has difficulty breathing, the phlegm should be cleansed from his throat by suction, using a rubber ear syringe, which is a rubber ball with a long tip. This should be sterile. The baby should be cleaned and bathed after a short time, if he is strong and healthy. It is better to let a small, weak baby lie warm and quiet until his breathing is good before attempting to clean or bathe him. Care should be taken not to allow the baby to be touched by one whose hands are not scrupulously clean.

About twelve hours after the baby is born, he should be allowed to nurse at his mother's breast every three hours the first day, then every four hours after that. For the first few days the milk he gets from his mother will not be very good, but this gives him exercise, teaches him to suck, and encourages the production of milk in the mother's breast. The baby may have supplementary feedings while the mother's milk is coming in. This is usually a formula of:

16 ounces of water
8 ounces milk (evaporated)
2 tablespoons Karo syrup

7

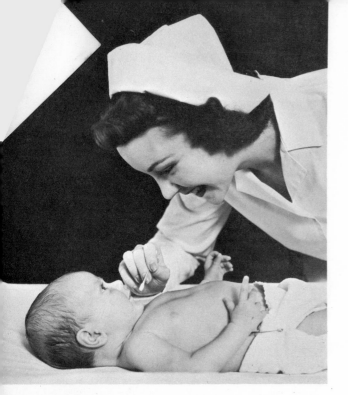

The baby appreciates attention and love. Especially love.

This is boiled, and placed in sterile bottles in equal portions. The above formula should be enough for one day. If possible, the mother should try to nurse her child, as this has long been proven to be the best food for the baby.

From the very first, it is of extreme importance to let the baby know that he is loved and really wanted. If he is fed by bottle, he should be held in his mother's arms and cuddled while being fed. Often babies swallow air while feeding, so two or three times during each feeding he should be held on his stomach over the mother's shoulder in order to let him "burp" or expel the air.

If the baby has difficulty in getting the nipple into his mouth, do not attempt to hold his head and force his mouth to the nipple, or to try to make him open his mouth by pressing on the cheeks with thumb and forefinger. This only makes the baby mad, and he will take longer than ever getting started.

Nursing a baby by breast is also good for the mother. It gives her a feeling of being close to her child and doing something for him that no one else can do. The most important of all the things noted above is to make the baby feel that he is loved.

THINGS TO HAVE READY WHEN YOU BRING THE BABY HOME FROM THE HOSPITAL

The following list of equipment should be accumulated before the baby is born:

1. Diapers—gauze or birds eye; three dozen, if washed often
2. Shirts—cotton, without buttons, long sleeves, size one year; six
3. Nightgowns—stockinette, long, size one year; four
4. Receiving blankets—cotton; four
5. Sweaters—with large opening for head
6. Wool cap—for cold weather, when baby is taken out

Equipment You Will Need

1. Something in which to bathe the baby. A folding tub is good because it is high and easy on the mother. The baby should be bathed at the same time every day, before the second feeding in the morning.
2. Some place to sleep. A bassinette is nice, but a clothes basket will do just as well if the sides are covered with soft material so the baby will not hurt his hands.
3. Mattress. Sometimes one can be made by folding a blanket. Do not use a pillow for a mattress.
4. Waterproof sheeting to cover mattress. Plastic materials are good and you should have at least two. Do not use plastic bags brought in by the cleaner or used to pack-

age vegetables. These thin plastic bags are dangerous and may suffocate the baby.

5. Pads. You should have four pads to place over waterproof sheeting. These should be washed and dried.
6. Cotton sheets, about six; diapers may be used as sheets
7. Four cotton blankets
8. One dozen medium-sized rubber nipples. Nine round or octagonal eight ounce nursing bottles.
9. Nine bottle caps to cover the bottles while being stored in the refrigerator.
10. Measuring tablespoon and teaspoon
11. Bottle brush
12. Strainer
13. Jar with wide mouth in which to sterilize nipples
14. Funnel that can be sterilized
15. Quart measure with ounce markings
16. Sterilizer (a pail ten inches high with cover will do)
17. Tongs to remove bottles, etc., from sterilizer. Tongs must also be sterilized
18. Rectal thermometer
19. Baby oil
20. Absorbent cotton
21. Cotton swabs
22. Baby powder
23. Soap. Use only a mild soap
24. Electric bottle warmer
25. Balance scales to weigh baby
26. Two diaper containers with cover; one for wet and one for soiled diapers
27. Zinc oxide ointment
28. Baby buggy

The above items may be varied and many of these articles may be improvised for the sake of economy. For instance, you can make your own cotton swabs from toothpicks and absorbent cotton.

CIRCUMCISION

It is my opinion that all male babies should be circumcised before they leave the hospital. At this early age, no anesthetic is needed, and the infants apparently do not feel too much pain. They often go to sleep during the procedure.

The reasons for circumcision are to make cleansing the penis easier, to avoid irritation, and to prevent its being done at a later age when it can be quite an unpleasant experience to an older child.

Some doctors advise simple retraction of the foreskin after the baby is several months old, and others advise doing nothing at all. If retraction of the foreskin is practiced, it is important that it be pulled back to its original position immediately or it may become stuck behind the head of the penis, interfere with circulation, and become a surgical emergency.

FEEDING YOUR BABY

The mother should breast feed her baby if possible. This is the best and easiest way to take care of his needs. However, if you are going to feed him from a bottle your doctor will give you a formula to start with, and will change it from time to time as the baby grows.

The most important thing in feeding your baby is to let him decide how much he wants and when he wants it. Formerly, we stuck to a four or three hour feeding schedule, and it had to be right on the minute. Now we let the baby have something to say about it. This is called a demand feeding schedule.

The fact is that as your baby gradually hits his stride in the eating department he will fall into a habit of his own, eating regularly every three or four hours. Do not try to make him take the whole bottle. Sometimes he will stop eating because of an air bubble in the stomach. When this is let out, he will eat again. But, if he does not seem interested in food, do not force him, for that will make him think of eating time as a time when he is forced to do something, and when he doesn't enjoy it he will not eat enough.

A well-baby clinic in your community or your family doctor will give you an idea of the proper feeding formula which you can use according to the baby's weight and age. Remember at all times that your baby is an individual, and may not eat exactly the same amount recommended by your doctor. He may want more or less. If, however, he seems to be happy, contented, and is gaining weight, the chances are that he is well satisfied.

Use evaporated milk, as we believe that it is one of the safest and most economical to use. Do not use the so-called sweetened milks.

The preparation of the formula is a time consuming job at first, but gradually, as you get a system worked out, it will take less and less time.

The bottles should be washed out with warm water and soap, and rinsed thoroughly, as should the nipples and bottle caps. The nipples are placed in the nipple bottle and the bottles in the sterilizer rack. These are all placed in the sterilizer along with the tongs, funnel, spoons, etc., and water is placed in the sterilizer pail to cover. It should be allowed to boil for five minutes. Sometimes it is easier to boil the nipples in a saucepan by themselves. Drop them into the boiling water and allow to boil for three minutes.

PREPARING THE FORMULA

As an example, place eighteen ounces of water in a double boiler. If your formula calls for sixteen ounces, allow about two ounces for evaporation. Then, to eighteen ounces of water in the upper part of double boiler, add two tablespoons of granulated sugar (leveling it off with a sterilized knife), or add the Karo syrup. Allow sugar to dissolve in water, then add seven ounces of evaporated milk.

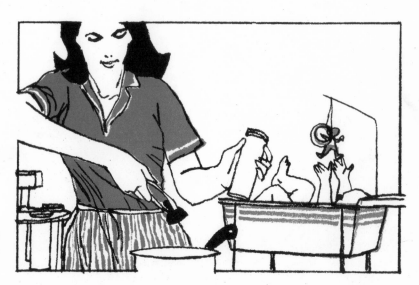

Mother preparing baby's feeding formula recommended by her Doctor.

Permit the whole mixture to boil for five minutes, then allow to cool. After cooling, pour through sterilized strainer and funnel into sterilized bottles, putting an equal amount in each bottle. Place your bottle caps (rubber) or nipples with nipple covers on each bottle, and after the bottles have cooled off, place them in the refrigerator. Before giving the baby a bottle, warm it in warm water until it is just about skin temperature. You can judge whether it is too hot by shaking a few drops on the skin of the inner surface of your wrist.

ADDITIONAL VITAMINS

Vitamin D

The baby should have a good supply of vitamin D, starting at about two weeks, to help his bone growth. The easiest way to give it is in concentrated fish oil form. Drisdal is a good product. Give fish oil drops daily. Do not place them in milk, as some will be left in the bottle. Let the baby lick them from a spoon or place them in the corner of his mouth while he is nursing water. Use a medicine dropper. Another form of vitamin D is cod liver oil, U.S.P. Give one teaspoon daily if this is used, instead of drops.

This vitamin D should be given daily until the baby is at least two years old. Preferably, it should be given until he reaches his full growth.

Vitamin C

This is another vitamin that should be added to the baby's diet as heat kills what little vitamin C there is in milk. If you use ascorbic acid tablets, 25 mg. each, the baby should have 50 mg. daily. You may add this to the bottle after boiling. Start this a few days after the vitamin D.

The easiest way to give vitamin C is orange juice. It is best to dilute the orange juice with water at first—one-half teaspoon of orange juice to one-half teaspoon boiled water. Then one teaspoon of each, until the baby is getting about two ounces of orange juice daily. Most babies like orange juice and it seldom disagrees with them.

SOLID FOODS

Begin feeding solid foods at about three or three and one-half months, adding one thing at a time. First, a cereal such as Pablum, then baby food vegetables, then baby food fruits.

Now you have your baby at home, and you are well started on the fascinating experience of watching him develop and change from day to day.

Because the baby seems so small and delicate, the father may be a little afraid to handle him at first. Actually your baby is pound for pound the toughest and most durable person in the house. He must be, to survive the beating he takes coming through the birth canal.

So again, let us emphasize—have confidence in yourself. Give the baby a great deal of love, but also use common sense and do not try to be too demanding or domineering. In other words, try to realize that if a baby does something, there is usually a good reason for it.

Diseases of the baby will be discussed under the general heading of "Diseases," as they are usually similar in children and in adults. However, a few special mile posts will be discussed before going on.

PROTRUDING NAVEL

Sometimes the place where the blood vessels from the mother to the baby were attached does not close over promptly, and the navel will protrude when the baby cries or strains. Do not be alarmed by this, for it practically always closes over. Sometimes your doctor will show you how to tape the navel to hold it in, on the theory that it will heal more quickly this way. When the baby is old enough, give him exercise to strengthen his stomach muscles. This will hasten the healing. Do not try to keep the baby from crying so that his navel will not protrude, because no harm ever comes of this protrusion and nearly always it corrects itself in time.

THUMB SUCKING

When a very young baby starts sucking his thumb, at six months or before, this usually means that he does not get enough sucking exercise from his bottle. The holes in the nipple may be too large. He should have to suck at least twenty minutes to get all the milk in the bottle or breast.

If, after the age of one or two, he continues to suck his thumb, that usually means that the child is bored or frustrated, and not satisfied with life. He is using this thumb sucking as a comfort to himself, perhaps when he becomes too tired. Do not attempt to restrain him by placing splints on his arm, or by nagging at him to remove his thumb from his mouth. This does no good and may even make him worse. Try to remove any reason the child might have to need to comfort himself, and eventually he will stop sucking the thumb or finger spon-

taneously. Bribing will sometimes help older children stop the habit; but at any rate, they nearly always stop before their permanent teeth come in. There is no need to worry about spoiling the looks of their teeth.

HYDROCELE

Cause and Nature

A hydrocele is a collection of serous fluid in the tunica vaginalis or portion of the peritoneum which has been pushed ahead of the testes as they descend into the scrotum from their place of formation up in the peritoneal cavity.

In a young male infant this failure to close may represent an opening into the peritoneal cavity through which peritoneal contents can descend and the baby has a hernia as well as a hydrocele.

Signs and Symptoms

There is a soft mass in the scrotum usually on one side which feels like fluid in a cyst. A light can be passed through it (transillumination) in a dark room, showing the mass to be fluid and showing the testicle. There is no pain and in a young child no discomfort.

In a grown man there may be some discomfort if this sac of fluid is large and it does sometimes occur in grown men.

Treatment

In a baby the hydrocele may go away within a year without any treatment if there is no connection to the peritoneal cavity and no hernia present. If it does not disappear it is best to operate to remove the cyst and at the same time repair the hernia.

In a grown man the fluid can be removed by a needle and syringe. If one or two removals in this manner do not result in disappearance, the hydrocele should be operated upon.

Peritoneum lining of the abdominal cavity
Scrotum sac containing testes
Serous pertaining to serum
Testes male reproductive organs
Testicles male sex glands
Transillumination passing of light through cavity

CROUP

This is one condition which may be very upsetting and alarming. A young baby or child may have a slight cold and seem perfectly happy during the day. When night comes, he may awaken with a brassy, croupy cough and seem to have great difficulty in breathing. The treatment consists of keeping the air in the room warm and moist. Sometimes a severe attack can be relieved by placing a sheet over the baby's crib and allowing steam from a steam kettle or vaporizer to enter the tent. If this does not help, call a doctor.

IMMUNIZATION

All infants should receive as many immunizations against disease as it is possible for them to have before they are one year of age.

If injections are given early, baby does not remember and is not afraid of doctors. Early protection is important. There is little pain.

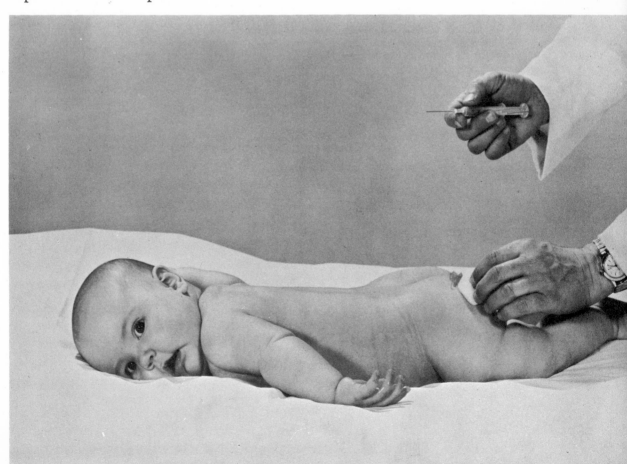

The reason is that as a child grows older he develops an imagination which makes him fear shots and in some cases the abnormal fear may last throughout his life.

The immunization practices throughout the United States have been improved greatly and there is no excuse for any child to suffer from some of the preventable diseases simply because his parents would not take advantage of the many immunization clinics which are nearly always available at no cost. Or the family doctor will provide all of the immunizations in his office.

At three months of age the child should have his first shot or injection. The first series is usually called D.P.T., that is protection against diptheria, whooping cough (pertussis) and tetanus. He will receive three of these injections at monthly intervals. (One year after the third D.P.T. injection the child should have a booster injection.)

When he is six months old, the polio drops should be started. Immunization against poliomyelitis is given in liquid form by mouth now. It is called the Sabin vaccine, is very little trouble to give, and produces almost 100 percent protection against this crippling disease.

Somewhere along the line the infant should have the smallpox vaccination which is described in detail below.

Since we see so little smallpox in this country now, the vaccination against measles should come before the smallpox vaccination if there is any question or conflict in the two immunizations.

Measles is a very dangerous disease. Cases of death from measles are reported every year and many cases of complications such as middle ear disease may handicap the child for life.

At nine months of age the baby should start his measles "shots." These injections have been given in two forms. The first and most commonly used is an injection of live measles vaccine in which the organisms have been weakened. The Schwartz strain is one example of this vaccine. In some cases a child will have a very mild reaction because the organisms are live, but by the same token he will have better protection against measles than he would receive from injections of dead organisms.

The second type of vaccine is one in which the organisms have been killed. This type is seldom used.

These reactions are characterized by a slight fever several days after the injection; in some cases a very mild rash may appear. These symptoms rapidly disappear and cause no lasting damage.

The reactions described above are rare and constitute no valid reason for the child to be denied protection against this serious disease.

This immunization is against rubeola or real measles, sometimes called red measles. To date there has been no vaccination perfected aginst German measles or three-day measles which is a much milder disease.

Work is being done on a vaccine to be used against mumps but no practical solution has been found.

GLOSSARY

Abnormality   not formed right
Absorbent   that which soaks up liquids
Anesthetic   drug used to produce unconscious state for surgery
Circulation   flow of blood through blood vessels
Circumcision   removal of part or all of the foreskin
Evaporated   milk with the water removed
Fertilized   when male seed has entered female egg

Foreskin   skin covering end of penis

Formula   milk mixed with water and sugar or syrup

Immunization   injection of medicine to prevent a disease

Inoculate   to induce mild form of disease to make person immune

Penis   male organ

Phlegm   thick, stringy material that collects in the throat

Scrupulously   exceptionally

Spermatozoa   male seeds

Sterile   free of germs

Supplementary   in addition to

Thermometer   instrument for recording body temperature

U.S.P.   United States Pharmacopoeia, the official standard reference book which specifies formulas to be used in preparing medicines and drugs

Vaccine   substance prepared for immunization and treatment

SMALLPOX VACCINATIONS

(Vaccinia)

Reason and Nature

Vaccination against smallpox is one of the immunizations that every child should have and it should be given during the first three or four months of life—certainly during the first year of life. This early vaccination prevents complications which sometimes occur and at the same time protects the child against smallpox which is, at times, a fatal disease and which is always a very serious disease. A successful vaccination—that is, one leaving a scar—will always protect a person against smallpox. The widespread use of vaccination has caused the dread disease of smallpox to become a rare disease whereas before vaccination this disease was a very common one. Smallpox vaccinations should be repeated every five to seven years in order to keep the protection at a high level. If there is immunity still present from the first vaccina-

tion the subsequent attempts at vaccination will be unsuccessful. Whenever there are one or more cases of smallpox in a neighborhood, everyone should be vaccinated or revaccinated at once. When traveling to a foreign country everyone should be vaccinated against smallpox within a year of the time that they begin their journey because in some countries smallpox is still quite common.

The smallpox vaccination is performed by introducing or pressing some fluid which contains live "cowpox" virus into the skin on the upper posterior portion of the child's left shoulder. This cowpox vaccine is obtained from pus in the lesions of cowpox which has been purposefully given to young calves. The virus is kept alive by storing it in small vials containing glycerol at a temperature of five to ten degrees centigrade, that is, keeping it refrigerated. If the vaccine is kept at room temperature for any length of time the virus dies and the vaccine becomes ineffective.

In nearly all cases in which the baby is vaccinated for the first time and does not get a "take" or scar, it means that the vaccine has not contained live virus, or that the medicine used to clean the site—ether or ethyl alcohol—has not been allowed to dry and has killed the virus. In all such cases the child should be revaccinated until a "take" is obtained for there is no such thing as natural immunity.

If possible, vaccination should be performed when the weather is not too hot. A child who is suffering from malnutrition or any other disease should not be vaccinated because there is a likelihood of complications. Any child who has eczema, impetigo, or dermatitis should not be vaccinated until the skin condition is cleared up, as this type of child is likely to have complications. One other word of caution: If there is a child in the family who suffers from eczema, dermatitis, or impetigo, his brother or sister should not be vaccinated while the two are living together as the child with the skin condition may come in contact with the vaccination and serious complications may occur.

Signs and Symptoms

The technique of vaccination has been improved in recent years so that only a small scar results.

The vaccination should not be covered and one should never use a shield. Most of the complications following vaccination result from secondary infection and therefore, the site should be kept clean. When the take is reaching its peak it may be wise to spot it gently with cotton saturated with alcohol two or three times a day.

A child should never be allowed to scratch the vaccination, first to prevent secondary infection, and second, to prevent spread of the vaccination to other parts of the body. If a child scratches a vaccination and then scratches his face, he will have ugly vaccination scars on his face or any other part of the body he happens to scratch. This means that for a whole month after a smallpox vaccination the child should wear a long-sleeved shirt day and night to prevent him from getting at the vaccination with his hands.

There are three kinds of results from smallpox vaccinations:

1. The immediate or "immune reaction" which results in a red pimple surrounded by an area of redness of the skin. This occurs within three days after the vaccination and disappears leaving no scar. It means that the person has recently been successfully vaccinated or that the vaccine contained an inactive virus. If the person has not been recently vaccinated, it should be done again because the inactive virus will not confer immunity.

2. The accelerated reaction or vaccinoid reaction which reaches its height in from three to five days and consists of a blister surrounded by red skin and perhaps accompanied by fever and generalized aching. It leaves no scar and confers but very little immunity. These people should be vaccinated again.

3. The typical "take" or primary vaccination reaction. This is the one to be desired. In the primary take nothing is seen around the site of the vaccination until the third or fourth day when a slight redness of the skin appears. On about the fifth day, a vesicle or blister appears and the redness increases, reaching its peak on about the ninth or tenth day when a hard black scab gradually appears. This scab must be protected until it falls off in a few weeks leaving a typical scar. It is during this period that the itching and irritation is the worst and the baby must be kept from scratching so he will not vaccinate himself on other parts of the body.

Also from the fifth to the tenth day, there may be a reaction with fever, generalized discomfort, and local tenderness around the vaccination. The arm may swell up and the lymph glands may be enlarged and tender under the arm. During this period the child may be given aspirin —one grain for every year of age—in order to try to relieve this distress. After the tenth day, the scab is formed and the child feels better. Such reactions do not occur in all children; some of them never seem to notice any discomfort.

Treatment

If fever and discomfort occur the child should be kept comfortable with aspirin as described above. The vaccination should be cared for by seeing that no tension or tight bandage or clothing is applied. It should be kept clean by dabbing it with alcohol and scratching should be guarded against.

There are a few complications which may follow vaccination and these should be treated. It must be emphasized that in properly cared for vaccinations these complications are very, very rare and in very young babies—four months or under—the complications are practically never seen. This is a good reason for having your baby vaccinated against smallpox early in his life.

The complications may result from secondary infections when there is dirt or scratching. There may be blood poisoning, erysipelas, or scarlet fever, which can be treated with antibiotics.

In very rare cases, gangrene sets in around the vaccination involving the skin only; it must be treated vigorously. Hyper-immune gamma globulin has been used to cure this complication, as in the very few cases seen the person is nearly always short on gamma globulin in his blood. If a child has eczema it may be wise to inject hyper-immune gamma globulin before vaccination.

In other countries so-called post vaccination encephalitis may be seen but this has hardly ever been reported in the United States. It can be treated effectively.

In spite of the very rare cases in which there are complications, all of which can be treated, every child should be vaccinated against smallpox as this may mean saving his life. Smallpox vaccinations with a good "take" or scar give absolutely certain protection. Never vaccinate a child who has eczema.

BABIES' COLIC

Cause and Nature

Most pediatricians or baby specialists will tell you that there is no such disease as "colic" in a baby. Yet down through the ages we have been told by our friends, neighbors, and relatives that the baby who cries often or who is irritable at night has "colic." All too often this diagnosis or label placed upon the irritability of the baby may even be called colic by the doctor who is in charge.

Dr. F. M. Smith, a well known pediatrician, has stated that in his opinion there is no such condition as colic in the infant. He correctly calls to our attention the fact that it would be impossible to find the diagnosis of "colic" written on the chart of a sick baby in any large children's hospital. Babies, while they are still in the hospital before being taken to their homes, never have colic, because the nurses know how to feed and take care of them properly.

What then is the cause of some babies crying at all hours of the night and day and why are some children so fretful and nervous? This is not a disease but is an attempt on the part of the baby to adapt itself to a new environment. Colic—so-called—is most usually seen in the first born child. It appears soon after the child is taken home from the hospital and usually is seen in babies with parents who are nervous, apprehensive, overindulgent, and inexperienced in taking care of a baby. They feel insecure and this is reflected in the actions of the baby.

Signs and Symptoms

First of all crying is about the only way babies can communicate with the outside world, so many things will make them cry. If they are wet, cold, or uncomfortable in any way they cry. If they are hungry they will cry, and if they are in real distress or pain they will cry. Experienced parents can tell by the tone of the baby's cry which one of these conditions is causing the crying. They will then confidently and expertly try to relieve the situation. Other parents will go into a panic and handle the baby with impatience, uncertainty, or fright, and this communicates itself to the baby. The parents then call their neighbors or members of the family who tell them that the baby has colic and all too often when they call the doctor, he will agree that this is probably the diagnosis.

At times a baby will be distended with gas and cry loudly only to be relieved when given an enema. This is not colic but simply an overabundance of air (most of which has been swallowed) in the baby's digestive tract. If the baby nurses through a proper nipple and is held over the shoulder to burp at frequent intervals, he will not swallow so much air. In other words, the formula does not need changing on account of an overabundance of gas. If there is too much gas, a small enema and mild heat to the abdomen will usually relieve it.

Treatment

High on the list in treating or preventing fretting and crying on the baby's part is the preparation of the mother and father for taking care of the baby. They should feel confident that they know how to take care of their offspring and should be able to detect from the actions of the child what the cause of the crying is. If it is a hungry cry, feed the child. If it is a cry of mild discomfort, put dry clothes on the baby, and if it is

a cry of real pain, find out the cause and correct it.

In former times parents were told to feed the baby at regular intervals and to stick rigidly to schedule. This is no longer considered good practice. The baby should be fed when it is hungry. This is the so-called demand feeding. Some babies may take three or four ounces of formula and go to sleep only to wake up crying lustily in about an hour. If they are then given a little more formula they will be perfectly satisfied and sleep for several hours.

The formula should resemble mother's milk as closely as possible since this is nature's way, and by far the best way to feed a baby is to breast feed it. If the formula is not like mother's milk it may be difficult for the baby to digest and cause discomfort. It does not necessarily cause gas.

The baby should not be given solid foods too soon as, again, this is not nature's way. A baby who is nursed at the breast does not need solid foods for several months.

The very first and most important step for a baby that is unduly restless or cries too much is to have an examination by a doctor who will be able to tell if there is anything physically wrong. If the baby is healthy then the mother must learn not to be nervous and not to become upset every time the baby cries. All babies cry at some time or another and even the ones who cry a great deal outgrow this as they become older.

Picking up the baby and holding it in your arms to let it know that you love it will do more to cure so-called colic than any medicine.

Occasionally there are excessively tense and nervous babies who cry a great deal. This is not because of colic but usually because they have inherited this trait. Both of the parents may have behaved similarly when they were babies. The infant will outgrow this if given intelligent care.

Changing the formula too often is not good. As mentioned above, mother's milk is the ideal food for a baby and it does not change from month to month. Hence it is wise to pick out a milk that is as nearly like mother's milk as possible and stick to this. Bottle fed babies will need additional vitamins, such as vitamin D and C. The first is found in cod liver oil and the second in orange juice. Sometimes restless babies are in need of vitamin B6 and the addition of this to the formula may help quiet them.

Many years ago the use of a pacifier was frowned upon but a great many doctors now feel that the sucking reaction is a normal one and the use of a pacifier does no harm but may help with some babies.

GLOSSARY

Apprehensive afraid of what might happen
Communicate to give or carry a disease to another
Digestive tract channels where food is made ready for body use
Distended sticking out
Enema putting water into lower bowel to force out waste
Irritable fretful
Pacifier nipple without a bottle to keep a child quiet

TEETH

The milk or deciduous teeth may appear at varying times in different families. The first two lower incisors appear from six to eight months, the four upper incisors from eight months to one year. Next come the lower lateral incisors and the first molars, at twelve to fifteen months. The four ca-

nines usually appear between the sixteenth and twentieth month, the four molars some time in the third year. When all of the milk teeth are in, there should be twenty.

Meanwhile, the permanent teeth are pushing against the roots of the milk teeth, and the roots are absorbed. The teeth become loose and fall out. The six-year molars appear back of the baby molars. The baby teeth are lost in the same order in which they came; the incisors, the molars, and the canines. The permanent teeth that take the place of the baby molars are called bicuspids.

The permanent teeth should be in about the twelfth or fourteenth year. Two twelve year molars appear behind the six year molars. The eighteen year molars, or wisdom teeth, come in during the eighteenth year, or later. (See page 173.)

When the teeth come in crooked, they sometimes straighten out later, but the child should be seen by a dentist regularly to determine if treatment is needed.

GLOSSARY

Bicuspids permanent teeth with two points; the fourth and fifth teeth counting from the center
Canines "eye" teeth next to the incisors
Deciduous temporary
Incisors front teeth
Lateral to the side
Molars back teeth

TOILET TRAINING

(Assistance in Bowel and Bladder Control)

If I were a mother with a young baby, my first effort would be to train myself and to realize that if I want my baby to learn how to use the toilet, I should let the child accomplish this by itself. The fact is, that if the mother makes little or no attempt to train the baby, he will soon learn what the urge to urinate or to have a bowel movement means, and will connect this with the act of going to the bathroom to perform this function.

If the mother really wants to help the baby, she will allow him to make his own decisions, thus teaching him self-reliance. The very biggest mistake she can make is to try and force the baby to have a bowel movement or to urinate when she wants him to. He will begin to rebel and let her know in many ways that this is his operation, and he will do it when and where he wants to.

I would watch my baby carefully, noting what times during the day he urinates or wets his pants, and what times he has a bowel movement. Some babies naturally fall into a more or less regular pattern. When the baby is ten to twelve months old, it may be possible to have him connect the urge to urinate with the proper place to do it. Trying to train him earlier than this is useless.

After the baby is a year old, he should be given the opportunity to use a pot at certain times, which may have been previously noted as his regular times.

The pot or potty should be a small one, his own, that allows him to rest his feet on the floor, and should have arms on it, so that he will feel comfortable and proud. This is suggested because a baby may be frightened by having to sit on a high toilet seat with his feet hanging down and may be frightened by the flushing of the toilet, so that he will withhold his movement.

The mother should maintain a friendly attitude while helping him use the potty. She should not overpraise him for having a movement and she should never, never scold him for having the movement in his diapers or pants.

Sometimes a baby's bowel movements become hard and painful so that he is afraid to have a movement and holds back. This should be detected, and the baby given more sugar in his formula. Brown sugar is good for this, or he should be given prune juice several times a day. This will usually make the stool softer. If these things do not soften the stool, a doctor should be consulted for some type of medicine.

After the baby is walking, training pants in the daytime and a diaper at night often help, as the pants are easier to get off when the baby has to go, and soon he can learn to take them down himself.

Different children show many variations in their bowel and bladder habits, and a mother should not become impatient with one child because he doesn't act the same way as her previous child or her neighbor's child.

Some children make a certain noise or assume a certain expression when they feel the urge to go. Watch for these things but never rush the child into the bathroom in order to be there in time, as this may frighten him.

After the child becomes a little older, try to get him to go under different conditions, that is, let him get on a small seat over the regular toilet from time to time. This will keep him from becoming too set in his habits, and will make it easier when you take him on a trip.

Never show anger or disgust when the baby soils or wets his pants as this is a normal function, and it is not wise to make the child have a guilty feeling about it.

In summing up, the important things to

be remembered in helping a baby to form the proper bowel and bladder habits are:

1. Do not try to train a baby before he is ten to twelve months old.
2. Be casual and friendly about it; never overemphasize.
3. Study the baby carefully before trying to help him.
4. Remember that being too strict or too ambitious about bowel training may have a lasting effect on the child's emotional stability.
5. Realize that if you do nothing at all, the baby will train himself just by watching the other members of the family.
6. Always keep in mind that this is the baby's function and that he resents your telling him when and where he is going to perform it.
7. Never scold a child for soiling or wetting his pants.
8. Do not use suppositories in trying to develop a certain time for the movement. Watch the child; he may automatically fall into the habit of having a movement at a certain time every day. Try in a friendly way to encourage this.

GLOSSARY

Automatically   without help
Bowel movement   to expel or pass waste products
Emotional stability   how well a person controls his feelings
Emphasize   to stress something as being important
Suppositories   objects made of soap, glycerine, etc.; placed in rectum to encourage a bowel movement
Urinate   to pass water from bladder

ENURESIS

(Bed-Wetting)

Cause and Nature

When a child is less than a year old he has no idea when his urinary bladder is full, and urinates without actually knowing that he is going to. Between the age of one and two a child can usually detect the fullness of his bladder and may, by his expression or activity, let you know that he wants to urinate.

Between the ages of two and four and one-half years, he automatically develops the ability to hold his urine and start and stop his stream. This is done by using the diaphragm and abdominal muscles to push down on a full bladder, at the same time relaxing his shutoff muscle which closes the bladder. No amount of training by the parent will teach a child to control these muscles. This is automatic, and time spent in trying to teach it is wasted. As the child grows older, the urinary bladder becomes larger, so that the bladder will hold about twice as much at the age of four as it did at the age of two. The child who wets the bed at night is one whose bladder has simply failed to grow enough, and remains too small to hold a night's output of urine. Hence he wets the bed. It has been estimated that about twelve percent of all children may continue to wet the bed for varying lengths of time after they are four and one-half years of age. They have not learned bladder control, and this is because their bladders have not grown in capacity as they should.

Signs and Symptoms

The emptying of the urinary bladder in babies is automatic—usually the child can learn to control this by the time he is four and one-half years of age. He learns this automatically, and no training will help him. This control is effected by the voluntary use of the abdominal muscles and diaphragm. When the bladder remains too small this control is lost at night and the child wets the bed.

Treatment

All of the old methods to correct this condition have proven to be of no value. The giving of prizes for not wetting the bed, and punishment when it is done, have no effect on the size of the bladder. Not allowing the child to have any fluids after four o'clock in the afternoon, and getting him up at frequent intervals at night do not correct the small bladder which simply cannot accommodate the night's output of urine. The most effective way to cure a child of wetting the bed after he is four and a half, is to stretch or enlarge his bladder to the size it should have attained. This is done by teamwork on the part of the mother and child. First, you prepare a "voiding chart" and get a glass measuring cup that will measure up to fourteen ounces. The child is trained to urinate into this cup and mark down how many ounces he voids each time. Mark the time and the amount on the chart. He should also keep track of how much fluid he drinks during the day by drinking from a glass that is marked in ounces. Explain to the child that his bladder is small and that is why he wets the bed. Tell him he can make his bladder grow large enough and stop the bedwetting by holding his urine as long as he can, and by finally being able to put up to twelve or fourteen ounces in the cup. Voiding of two, four, six, or eight ounces is not enough. He must be able to void at least twelve ounces at one time before he can feel that his bladder is large enough and he will be able to hold his urine all night.

By drinking more water than usual and holding his urine longer and longer, he will be able to achieve this goal and the bed wetting will cease. It usually takes about three months or more, but it is certainly worth the time and effort.

Sometimes drugs that relax the bladder, such as Probanthine will hasten the stretching process, but they must be prescribed by a doctor.

GLOSSARY

Abdomen belly
Capacity amount
Diaphragm muscular wall separating the belly from the chest
Urinate to pass water
Void to pass water

UNDESCENDED TESTICLE

Cause and Nature

In some male babies one or both of the testes (usually just one) may not move down into the scrotum. This is called an undescended testicle. The testicle is either in the groin or even up in the abdomen. There is always an indirect hernia with an undescended testicle, but the hernia may be so small as to not need treatment.

Signs and Symptoms

The presence of only one testicle in the scrotum proves that one is undescended. Sometimes the testicle may be there one day and up into the inguinal canal the next day. There is seldom any pain except when the testicle is in the groin where it may be easily struck or bumped.

Treatment

In almost fifty percent of these cases the undescended testicle will come down into the scrotum spontaneously. This usually occurs at puberty. If the testicle has not come down to its proper place by the age of ten or twelve, it should be brought down by surgery.

If there is a large hernia present it should be repaired and the testicle brought down at an early age. Some doctors think that injections of hormones will bring the testicle down and in a certain percentage of cases, ten or twenty percent, this treatment is successful. The injections of chorionic gonadotropin should be given about three times a week. If this injection treatment is not successful after a trial of six weeks, it should be stopped.

GLOSSARY

Chorionic gonadotropin gonadotrophic substance from human placenta (after birth); this stimulates certain cells of the testes
Groin space between the thigh and the main part of the body
Hernia rupture
Inguinal canal canal carrying male seed cord; the round ligament in the female
Puberty time when boys or girls are able to reproduce
Scrotum double pouch containing male organs (testes)
Testes testicles; male reproductive glands in the scrotum

PILONIDAL CYST

Cause and Nature

A pilonidal cyst or sinus is caused by a defect in the development of the baby, and is found on the back at the lower end of the spine.

As the name implies this cyst contains hair and is usually first noticed at puberty. If it does not become noticeable before the age of thirty it seldom needs treatment. The cyst may be fairly large, or may be just a dimple or small hole in the midline near the bottom of the spine.

Signs and Symptoms

If these cysts become infected there is an accumulation of pus, and they must be drained just as any other abscess. Riding horseback or riding in a rough car, like a jeep, may aggravate the condition.

Treatment

The treatment is surgical. If the cyst becomes infected, it should be incised and drained; and if these infections recur too frequently, the entire cyst should be removed by surgery. The time for removal should be after one of the acute flareups has subsided.

GLOSSARY

Abscess collection of pus in one area
Acute active
Aggravate stir up
Cyst sac containing liquid
Incise to cut into
Infection a diseased condition resulting from the presence of microorganisms or germs
Pilonidal containing hairs in a cyst

THE LEFT-HANDED CHILD

Cause and Nature

Although a great deal of investigation has been conducted over the years to determine the reason why one child is left-handed and his brothers or sisters are right-handed, there is still no absolute knowledge of the cause.

It is thought that in the left-handed person the centers in the brain which control the movements are located on the opposite or right side, while in right-handed people these centers are on the left side.

At any rate nearly everyone agrees that it is perfectly normal for some children to be left-handed, and there should be no

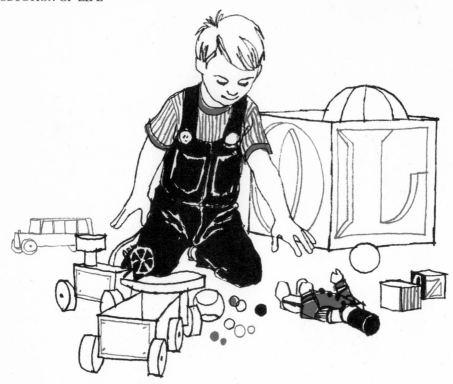

Young child shows tendency to use left hand.

stigma attached to it. In other words, if your child shows a tendency to use his left hand predominately, the most dangerous thing you can do is to try to force him to use his right hand. On the contrary, if you see that the child is left-handed, encourage him in every way to become a real lefty or a strong left-handed person.

There is enough pressure on him already when he sees that he is different from most people. Since most people use their right hands he may feel insecure in being left-handed. Parents and teachers should try to do away with this feeling of insecurity by encouraging him to be left-handed. It may be pointed out to him that many fine baseball players are left-handed; as a matter of fact, left-handed pitchers and first basemen are at a premium. Many famous men have been left-handed—Michelangelo, Leo-

nardo da Vinci, and Picasso. Doctors have found that trying to force a naturally left-handed child to become right-handed may have a very serious effect on his life.

Some children may become what is called mixed dominant. They may eat and write with their right hand and throw with their left hand. At times this is very hard on a child. This can be illustrated by a boy who was encouraged by his teachers to write with his right hand, when he had a left-handed tendency. This boy could not get beyond the third grade in reading until the mistake was noted and he was taught to write with his left hand. After this he developed into a normal reader. It may be well to realize that modern industry is recognizing the fact that many people are left-handed, and left-handed machines are being manufactured. There are left-handed baseball gloves, and golf clubs for left-handed players are common. The fact that being left-handed is not a handicap should be universally recognized. Mothers and fathers should recognize left-handedness in their child and encourage rather than discourage it.

Signs and Symptoms

When a child is just a few months old he may use either hand and reach first with the right and then with the left if a toy is handed to him. This is perfectly normal, but after the age of eighteen months, if your child shows a definite preference for his left hand, then it is decidedly harmful to force him to use the right.

Forcing a left-handed child to use his right hand may lead to poor muscle coordination, slowness in thinking, awkwardness, delayed ability to talk, stuttering, and difficulties in reading and writing.

The eternal conflict with your child in trying to force him to use a hand which he does not want to use may lead to a feeling of insecurity and inferiority. He may become restless, irritable, and unhappy. This sort of forcing may lead to bed wetting, the development of tics, or twitching muscles, or movements which are not natural; and as mentioned before, he may become awkward and retarded in learning to write and read. It has even been thought that seclusiveness, pugnacity, lying, theft, and tantrums may be corrected in a child by finding out which side is the dominant side and helping to develop that one even if it is the left side. In cases of mixed dominance, the child may write with his left hand and kick with his right foot. An attempt should be made by a doctor to find out which is the dominant side.

Treatment

In cases of mixed dominance—that is, a child or person who writes with his left hand and shoots with his right eye—a definite attempt should be made to teach him to do everything with the left side.

Sometimes an adult will persist in stuttering until he is taught to use the same eye, hand, and foot for doing everything. Then he stops stuttering. Usually this means teaching him over a period of years—in other words, converting him to a real lefty. When parents are reasonably sure that the child is a lefty they should train him with great care to do everything with his left hand; writing, throwing, buttoning, and eating. If this is not done, some children will be influenced by the fact that all of their playmates throw with the right hand and try to do the same.

The people who are truly ambidextrous are rare, and it is a mistake to try to teach your child to use either hand equally as well as the other. It is perfectly normal for some children to be left-handed and parents should do everything in their power to make a real good lefty out of the child who shows this preference.

GLOSSARY

Ambidextrous able to use both hands equally well

Coordination muscles and brain working together

Handicap a cause making normal actions difficult; a hindrance

Illustrate to picture or show

Inferiority lack of self-confidence

Insecurity not to be sure of things

Predominate rule over or use more readily

Preference choice

Retarded backward

Seclusiveness staying to oneself

Tantrum fit of anger

HERNIAS OR RUPTURES

There are two types of hernias most frequently seen in young babies and children—the inguinal hernia or rupture in the groin, and the umbilical hernia or protruding navel, which has been discussed briefly above.

The mother and father of the infant are always anxious about the treatment of these conditions and a clear understanding of the cause of such hernias along with the proper method of treatment in each case will do away with some of this worry.

GLOSSARY

Inguinal   groin
Umbilical   navel

THE INGUINAL HERNIA

Cause and Nature

The inguinal hernia or lump in the groin may be first noted by the mother when she is bathing the baby. She should call this to the doctor's attention.

This lump is called a congenital inguinal hernia. The baby is born with it and it can be either complete—that is, may extend all the way down to the scrotum in boys—or incomplete and only go as far as the groin. The lump can usually be pushed back into the abdominal cavity. That is, the hernia can be reduced, and most often it disappears at night or when the baby is asleep and quiet, only to reappear when the baby cries or strains. Many babies have been "spoiled" by mothers trying to prevent them from crying in order to keep this lump from appearing.

The congenital hernia is caused by a slight defect in the formation of the body.

When the male fetus begins to form in his mother's womb, the testicles are up inside the abdominal cavity. As the baby develops, these testicles travel down and finally come to rest in the scrotum where they belong. To get out of the abdominal cavity the testicles have to push ahead of them the fine membrane, called the peritoneum, which lines the abdominal cavity. This "pushed-out" part of the peritoneum is carried all the way down into the scrotum and is called the processus vaginalis. In nearly all boy babies this pouch closes off before they are born but in some the processus vaginalis or pouch of peritoneum fails to close, and they are born with an inguinal hernia. Since this is an opening into the abdominal cavity the small bowel slides down into the pouch and causes the lump which can be pushed back into the abdominal cavity. Sometimes this piece of small bowel goes all the way down into the scrotum. The baby does not get this hernia by straining his muscles but is born with this defect, and in spite of the advice of the grandparents, neighbors, and friends that he will outgrow it, the only way to correct it is by surgical repair. The mother and father like to put this off as long as possible, and some doctors will agree with them, but in a healthy boy the time to repair the inguinal hernia is soon after it is first noticed.

Although the inguinal hernia is most often seen in boys, it also is noticed in a small percentage of girl babies. In one large group of inguinal hernias which were repaired by surgery in a New York hospital, about ninety percent of the cases were boys and about ten percent were girls. This group consisted of 1,294 patients.

The lump or hernia may not be seen until the child is older and may appear at any

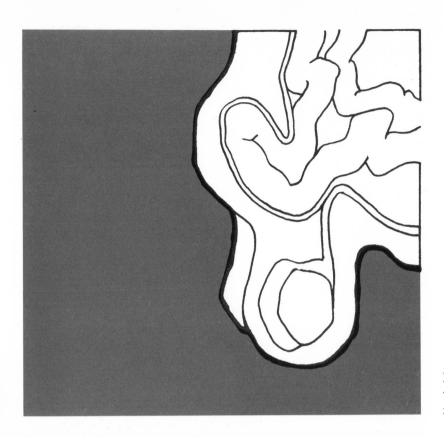

Inguinal hernia (side view) with small bowel in the scrotal sac.

time up to nine or ten years of age. Indeed, in some cases a congenital hernia may not be found until the person is fully grown.

For some unknown reason, over twice as many congenital hernias are on the right-hand side. Hernias on both sides are seen in about eight percent of the cases, which makes it important for the doctor to examine carefully the opposite side when a hernia is to be operated on. If the other side is found to be abnormal both sides can be repaired at the same time with very little more expense and trouble. If, however, the second side has to be repaired many years later, this means another anesthetic and operation.

As noted above, these inguinal hernias may be found in your children at any age, usually on the right side and sometimes on both sides. They are found more often in boys than in girls and should be repaired when they are discovered if the child is in good health and can stand the operation. This is not a very dangerous operation, and there are, as a rule, very few complications. If possible, a surgeon who has done many operations on young children should be chosen to repair the hernia, for even in expert hands the hernia may recur in a small percentage of cases.

Signs and Symptoms

The inguinal hernia appears as a small lump in the groin which usually can be pushed back and made to disappear, or it may disappear when the child is quiet only to come out again when he strains or cries. There is no pain nor is there any danger if the hole in the abdominal wall is large enough; but when a small opening exists the bowel may come out and later become filled with fecal matter or gas so that it cannot be reduced or pushed back. Then the hernia is said to be incarcerated or strangulated. The baby has real pain and may vomit. This is a true emergency and should be seen at once by a doctor. If the doctor cannot gently reduce or push back the hernia, he must operate at once for if the bowel is strangulated the circulation is cut off and part of the bowel may become gangrenous or die, and the baby may not survive.

Treatment

As soon as an inguinal hernia is noted, it should be repaired by surgery. It does no good to wear small trusses or delay the operation until the baby is older. This operation, while not particularly difficult or dangerous, should be in the hands of a competent surgeon, and especially it should be seen to by the surgeon that a good anesthetist gives the anesthesia.

Remember that the baby is never too young to have this repair work done and it does not help to delay until he is older, or to have him wear a truss, or to try and keep him happy so he will not cry. The only answer is an operation—and the danger of putting the operation off is that the piece of bowel that comes down into the hernial sac may get caught there or become strangulated. Then you have a real emergency on your hands.

GLOSSARY

Anesthetist   person giving anesthetic
Competent   qualified to perform task
Fecal   waste material—bowel movement
Fetus   child in the womb
Incarcerated   when rupture can't be pushed back through the opening
Peritoneum   lining of the abdominal walls
Strangulate   choke off blood supply

UMBILICAL HERNIA

(Protruding Navel)

Cause and Nature

This is quite a different problem from inguinal hernia and only in rare cases is surgical repair needed. The hernia usually heals by itself as the child grows older.

Everyone has an umbilical hernia before birth because the vessels which feed the unborn baby go from the mother through this opening to the baby. In most babies the hole or opening in the abdominal fascia is closed very soon after birth. In cases where there is a slight or even marked protrusion through this hole and the navel sticks out, it nearly always closes up as the baby grows older and begins to walk and develop strong stomach muscles. A good way to make these stomach muscles grow stronger is to give the baby exercises such as holding his feet down and asking him to sit up from a reclining position on his back. These exercises will strengthen the stomach muscles and the protrusion or sticking out of the navel will nearly always disappear.

When babies are very small and cannot be given exercises, it may be helpful to place adhesive tape over the navel. This is done by pushing in the hernia sac with the middle finger so it goes back through the ring of fascia which can be felt. Then with the thumb and index finger pull up a roll of skin from each side and fasten this skin by a wide piece of adhesive tape to hold the skin together. Some babies will have their skin irritated by the constant application of adhesive tape, and a better way to contain the offensive protrusion is to have the baby wear a circular two way stretch elastic belt. These are on the market now.

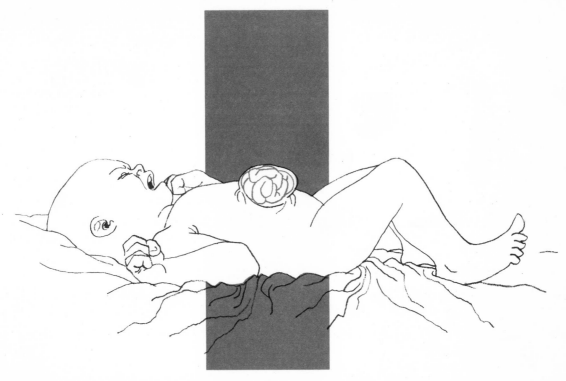

Protuding naval: Contents return to abdominal cavity when baby relaxes or is asleep—usually corrects itself.

It must always be kept in mind that in almost every case these umbilical hernias heal themselves as the child grows up and surgical repair should not be considered until the child is two or three years old. If the hard ring can be felt to grow larger after the child is two or three years old and a large protuberance is still present, then surgery should be considered. A case of incarceration or strangulation of a piece of bowel caught in the hernia is a surgical emergency, but this almost never happens.

Signs and Symptoms

There are, as a rule, no symptoms or any discomfort on the part of the baby. The parents, however, may suffer from worry or mental distress if they do not understand how insignificant this condition is. In most cases the navel will protrude when the baby cries or strains, and it does not do any good to try to keep the baby from crying in order to prevent the protrusion. Time will take care of that.

Treatment

Exercise and strengthening of the abdominal or stomach muscles will cause the hernia or opening to close over in time. When the baby is very young adhesive taping or wearing of a circular elastic belt may help. If after the baby is two or three years old the protrusion seems to be getting larger, surgical repair should be considered. When the repair is done by a surgeon it is important that he make his incision so that the umbilicus or navel is retained after the hole in the fascia underneath the skin is closed. This is important as it may embarrass the child later on when absence of a navel is noted by his schoolmates.

The important thing to remember about a protruding navel is that the parents should not worry about it as it nearly always goes away or closes up as the child grows older.

GLOSSARY

Fascia fibrous tissue
Incision opening made by sharp instrument
Insignificant not important
Reclining lying down
Umbilicus navel

CONGENITAL DEFORMITIES

The common deformities or abnormalities with which children are born will be discussed in this chapter. The very first thing a mother wants to know about her new baby is that it has a normal body and as the baby develops it is watched carefully for abnormal conditions which can usually be corrected by proper treatment.

Most of the crippling abnormalities caused by disease or injury to babies can be prevented or corrected, and there are some deformities present at birth which may cause the child great embarrassment, and disability as he grows older. Even though it is not always possible to prevent or completely correct these abnormalities, a better understanding of them may lead to early detection and the use of all corrective procedures.

When any abnormality in a baby is noticed the child should be taken to a doctor and corrective steps should begin as early as possible. The doctor will know what corrective procedures to take and when to begin them.

Congenital Dislocation of the Hip

Cause and Nature

Some babies are born with the head of the femur outside of the acetabulum or hip joint. This abnormality may be detected by X ray at an early age or it may first be noted when the child begins to walk. In either case it can be corrected by a good doctor, and in all instances it should be discovered and treated in order to save the child from a lifetime of limping.

Signs and Symptoms

When the child begins to walk a limp will be noted and this will make the doctor suspicious of a congenitally dislocated hip. By taking an X ray of both hips the diagnosis can be made.

Treatment

The baby is given an anesthetic and the top of the femur or thigh bone is manipulated so that the head rests in the acetabulum or hip joint. This does not require surgery and it may be held in place by a cast until the doctor feels that it will not slip out again. This reduction of congenitally dislocated hips can always be performed successfully.

GLOSSARY

Acetabulum cup-shaped hip socket
Congenital existing at birth
Manipulate to move
Femur thigh bone

Web Fingers or Toes

(*Syndactylism*)

Cause and Nature

Occasionally a baby that is perfectly normal in all other respects will be born

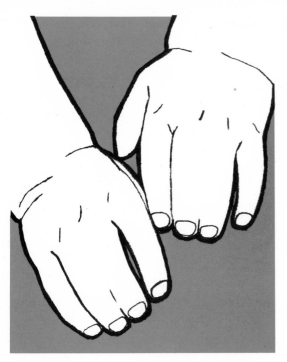

Web fingers: May be corrected by surgery.

with two fingers connected together by a flap of skin. This is called syndactylism, and it may be present on one or both hands. The same condition may occur in which the toes have a web between them. The web may be very small or it may cover the whole length of the fingers or toes.

Signs and Symptoms

There are no symptoms and the peculiar look of the hand with two fingers joined together is the only ill effect suffered. In the case of the toes there is very little inconvenience.

Treatment

The fingers of the hand should be operated on by a good surgeon when the child reaches the age of four or five. The age chosen for the operation should depend upon the judgment of the surgeon. Usually a flap

of skin is taken from the thigh to help heal the incision which is made when the web is cut. In all cases there should be no resultant disability when the child grows up. In the case of webbed toes no treatment is needed, as a rule.

Congenital Syphilis

Cause and Nature

Congenital syphilis or syphilis in a newborn infant is caused by a spirochete called "treponema pallidum." This spirochete is passed directly from the blood of the mother through the placenta or "afterbirth" into the blood stream of the unborn baby. Therefore the mother must have the disease in order for it to be passed on to the baby. There have been no cases reported in which the father alone had syphilis and the baby was born with it.

Since the introduction of penicillin and the other antibiotics syphilis has become less common and the general public has become more or less complacent about it. This is unfortunate because a great many cases of syphilis are still being diagnosed and treated every day. This is the reason why in some states every pregnant woman has a blood test made on her first visit to the doctor in order to determine whether or not she has syphilis.

It is possible to have syphilis and not know it, and that is why a blood test for syphilis is such a common procedure. On the other hand, syphilis can be one of the most terrible crippling diseases known to mankind. Many babies are born dead because of syphilis and those who do survive may die early or carry the marks of syphilis throughout their lives, if untreated. If a person is born with syphilis and is able to reproduce, this dread disease may be passed on to the next generation.

Fortunately if a mother is found to have syphilis early in pregnancy, prompt treatment with penicillin will prevent the disease from being passed on to her baby. This is another reason why every pregnant woman should see a doctor early and have a blood test taken. This is also the reason why every young person who is going to be married should first have a blood test for syphilis. If this disease is discovered before marriage it can be treated with penicillin and the person who has it may safely marry after one year.

Signs and Symptoms—Early Signs

As stated above many babies who have contracted syphilis from their mother are born dead. Those who survive very seldom thrive in the normal way unless treated. The signs of congenital syphilis may appear early—from the fourth to the eighth week. The baby may first develop the characteristic "sniffles." A pus-like, bloody discharge from the nose will appear and persist. This discharge may cause ulceration of the bones of the nose which results in a depression of the bridge of the nose and the characteristic deformity of congenital syphilis, sometimes called a "saddlenose." This condition may extend to the middle ear and cause permanent deafness.

The baby's skin will not have a healthy look, and a syphilitic rash may appear, which may be in the form of reddish-brown patches. The skin may have a wrinkled, old look, and lines will appear in the corner of the mouth. These lines are called "rhagades." Sometimes ulcerations around the lips and mouth appear and these ulcerations are very infective to other people.

The wet nurse or other member of the family may acquire syphilis from the baby. The hair of the head and eyebrows may fall out and enlargement of the lymph glands will be noted.

Late Signs

If newborn babies with syphilis recover their nutrition and lose the wasted appearance, they may go on in a perfectly normal way until they get their permanent teeth or until they reach the age of puberty, at which time the late signs of congenital syphilis will appear.

These children are retarded so that a boy of eighteen may appear to be about twelve years old. The forehead is usually prominent and the bridge of the nose has a depression in it. The upper central incisor teeth—that is, the permanent ones, may be pointed or peg shaped and may have a small notch in the cutting surface. These are called Hutchinson teeth. Lines may run from the corners of the mouth and at puberty the child may have trouble with the eyes. A slight steaminess of the cornea will first appear and this will go on into a condition known as "interstitial keratitis." This condition usually clears after a few months but may leave opacities which interfere with vision. Bone lesions occur frequently and one of the most common ones is the so-called "sabre shin" in which the front part of the shin bones becomes thickened and presents a sharp edge which sticks out.

In past years when congenital syphilis was seen more often than it is now, the three signs, saddle nose, sabre shin, and interstitial keratitis, were considered the triad of congenital syphilis signs. Syphilis is again increasing because the public is becoming careless since the advent of penicillin.

Treatment

The treatment is prevention by discovering syphilis early in the mother and treating it with penicillin. In the properly treated cases of syphilis a perfectly normal baby may result.

When the baby is found to have congenital syphilis, early treatment with penicillin will halt the progression of this dread disease.

GLOSSARY

Interstitial   space between tissues
Keratitis   inflammation of cornea of the eye
Lymph   liquid found in lymph glands
Placenta   afterbirth
Spirochete   germ causing syphilis
Ulceration   open sore

Club Foot

Cause and Nature

The cause of club foot is not known although babies are sometimes born with this condition. One or both feet on a newborn baby are turned inward and upward.

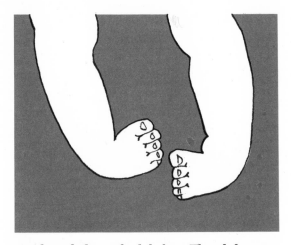

Newborn baby with club feet. This defect can be corrected by a doctor and should be done right after birth.

Signs and Symptoms

If this condition is not corrected the foot will remain turned in; and if it persists until the child walks, the side of the foot will be stepped on instead of the sole. Many years ago one would see adults with club feet but now that the method of correcting this deformity is so well understood, a case of congenital club foot in an adult is a very rare sight.

Treatment

Club foot should be detected by the doctor soon after birth and immediate steps should be taken to correct it. The deformed foot or feet may be placed in a plaster of Paris cast in an over-corrected position—that is, the foot will be turned outward and downward. These casts are changed on a young baby every few weeks to adjust to growth of the foot. The deformity may be completely corrected in this way and by having special shoes after the cast is removed.

Flatfoot

(Pes Planus)

Cause and Nature

There are many causes for flat feet and there are many degrees of this deformity. Sometimes it is so slight that it is barely noticeable and at other times it may be quite marked. The extreme degrees of flatfootedness are sometimes the result of a congenital malformation, but the lesser degrees may result from too much weight bearing on the foot when the muscles are in a weakened condition—as after a long illness.

In this condition the longitudinal arch of the foot is flattened out because the mus-

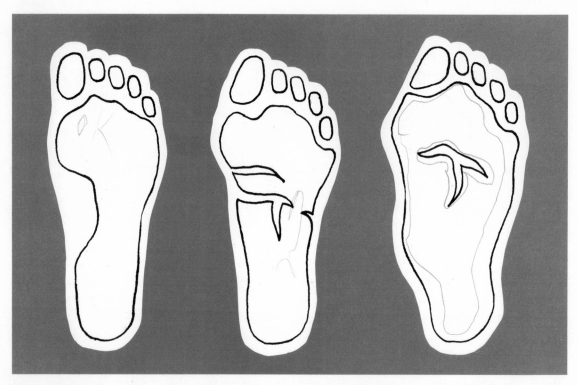

Foot prints shown above (from left to right) are from a normal foot, a moderately flat foot, and a markedly flat foot.

cles and tendons are too weak to support the arch, and the feet are usually turned outward in walking.

Many babies appear to have flat feet before they start to walk. This is often a needless source of worry to the mothers because as the baby starts to walk the muscles will be strengthened and the arch will assume its normal condition at the same time. The use and strengthening of the muscles will cause the feet to stop turning outward. In these cases no treatment is needed.

Signs and Symptoms

The longitudinal arch of the foot is flattened out or absent in this condition and the toes usually point out in walking.

People with flat feet usually suffer from pain in the feet or legs after walking for long periods of time because of the overuse of these weakened muscles.

Treatment

The most important part of the treatment is prevention. This is done by not allowing a child to be on his feet for long periods of time after he has been in bed for some time with a weakening disease. Get him up gradually, and strengthen the muscles gradually by exercises. Corrective shoes help to correct flatfootedness. These shoes are made to turn in and are built up slightly on the inner borders and may have arch supports built in the shoes.

The most important method of correcting flat feet in addition to protecting the arches when the feet are weak is to strengthen the muscles of the feet by special exercises after the child is old enough to cooperate. A doctor will explain these exercises.

Malformation   formed wrong
Tendons   cords attaching muscle to bone or other structure

Claw Foot

Cause and Nature

The cause of claw foot is not fully understood. This deformity is caused by the toes being bent or flexed at their tips and drawn up and back at their base. The transverse arch across the foot at the base of the toes is flattened out and the longitudinal arch is increased—the knuckles of the toes stick up.

Signs and Symptoms

The toes being raised, the knuckles usually press against shoes and very painful corns result. This condition can cause a great deal of discomfort and disability if not corrected.

Treatment

The claw foot or claw toes should be detected early and exercises and massage used to straighten out the toes. Proper shoes with an arch support for the transverse or metatarsal arch should be worn.

Extreme cases which do not respond to the above outlined treatment should be corrected by surgery.

Hammer Toe

Cause and Nature

The most likely cause of hammer toe is wearing shoes which are too short. The

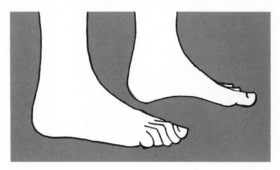

Hammer Toe: A painful deformity which may be prevented by wearing proper shoes. In severe cases surgery may be required.

longest toe will be constantly bent up and soon will become permanently bent. This is similar to claw foot, only in hammer toe only one toe is elevated.

Signs and Symptoms

The abnormally bent toe will press against the shoe and cause a tender, painful corn to develop.

Treatment

Prevention is the best treatment in these cases. That is, do not wear shoes that are too short.

If the deformity is present it should be corrected by splinting, exercise, wearing a transverse or metatarsal arch support. If these methods do not correct the deformity, orthopedic surgery should be performed.

German Measles as a Cause of Congenital Deformities

Cause and Nature

It has been well established that German measles (Rubella) when contracted by a woman in the first three months of pregnancy may cause many physical abnormalities in her offspring.

The exact rate of occurence of these abnormalities has not been accurately determined, but it is estimated that if a mother contracts German measles in the first three months of pregnancy there is a ninety percent chance of having a normal healthy baby and only a ten percent chance that the baby will have some abnormality. If she contracts German measles after the third month of pregnancy there is very little chance that the baby will be affected.

Signs and Symptoms

If the mother has german measles during her first three months of pregnancy, the fetus may die or as is most often the case, it may be quite small at birth. Such babies may show retardation of development, both physically and mentally, or they may show some definite physical abnormality.

The most common abnormalities noted in the small percentage of babies who are affected are:

1. Blindness
2. Deafness
3. Congenital heart disease

These defects may vary greatly in degree and it has also been noted that one of the less serious abnormalities resulting from German measles in the mother is a dental hypoplosia or retardation in the normal growth of the baby's teeth.

Treatment

Every pregnant woman who is exposed to German measles during the first three months of pregnancy should have injections of gamma globulin which has been especially prepared to protect against measles.

As one attack of German measles usually confers life-long immunity, the woman who has had German measles as a girl is not likely to contract the disease again. However, it is possible to have the disease twice. The real measles (rubeola) do not cause these deformities. Since German measles is usually a mild disease, it is considered wise to allow girls to go through this in childhood, so that they will be protected when they become pregnant.

Spina Bifida

Cause and Nature

Spina bifida is a term used to define a failure in the closing of the arch in the back part of one or more vertebrae. The condition is present at birth and may be seen in approximately one in every one thousand births.

If the defect is confined to the vertebrae, there are no symptoms or bad effects. This is called "spina bifida occulta" and may be discovered only by the presence of a dimple or some hair or a birth mark at the lower end of the spine. Later in life, the diagnosis may be confirmed by X rays showing a defect in a vertebra. This form of spina bifida causes no trouble and may not even be detected.

However, if the defect in the vertebra is large enough, there may be a herniation or bulging of the nervous tissue of the spinal cord through the hole and then symptoms will be noted.

Signs and Symptoms

If the defect or hole in the vertebra is large enough, the meninges or covering of the spinal cord may bulge through and be noted as a lump or a so-called meningocele and there may be no symptoms.

If part of the spinal cord is protruding in this lump, it is called a myelomeningocele and there may be symptoms such as weakness of the legs, difficulty in walking, a clumsy gait, and in some cases, shrinking of the leg muscles. Persons affected also may have trouble in controlling their bowels and bladder.

Treatment

If the nerves are involved, operative treatment aimed at closing the hole or defect is the treatment of choice. Physiotherapy and other symptomatic treatment will help the weakened legs.

GLOSSARY

Meningocele enlargement or cyst with fluid inside the meninges or lining of the spinal cord

Myelomeningocele a cyst containing part of the cord and fluid in a sac comprising the meninges or lining of the cord

Physiotherapy treatment of disease by physical means—heat, massage, and exercise

Vertebrae backbone or spine; each segment of the spinal column is a vertebra

CONGENITAL DEFORMITIES OF THE CHEST

Funnel Chest and Pigeon Breast

Cause and Nature

The cause of funnel chest and pigeon breast is not known. The baby is born with these deformities and no way of preventing them has been discovered. Fortunately, these abnormalities are quite rare. It has been estimated that only six babies in ten thousand are born with funnel chest and about one fourth of this number are born with pigeon breast.

Funnel chest or "pectus excavation" is characterized by a broad depression of the lower anterior chest. This depression usually involves the lower part of the breast bone or sternum and also the lower ribs. There are all degrees of funnel chest. The mild cases do not cause any disability, but usually the condition is a source of embarrassment as the child grows up. The severe depression may cause the heart and lungs to be affected and thereby limit the activity of the child as he grows older.

Pigeon breast or "pectus carinatum" is characterized by a sticking out or a ridge formation of the lower part of the breastbone. The lowest part of the breastbone, known as the xyphoid process, usually sticks out. This deformity is not as common as funnel chest and it may be either very slight or in some cases, quite marked. Pigeon breast does not, as a rule, cause as much physical disability as a marked funnel chest.

Signs and Symptoms

The slight depression or sticking out of the lower chest may be detected when the baby is quite young. As the child grows older the funnel chest is usually accompanied by a "pot belly" and in some cases a rounding of the upper back, or hunch back, appears as the child goes through puberty.

The greatest damage in most cases is caused by the fact that the growing boy is ashamed of his deformity and hesitates to appear in a locker room where his playmates will notice the abnormal chest. He may be reluctant to go swimming or to take part in athletic contests. The body usually adapts itself to this depression and actual physical disability is rare except in very marked cases.

In the case of pigeon breast there is seldom any physical handicap but the embarrassment caused by the sticking out of the lower chest may be as great as in the case of funnel chest.

Treatment

In mild cases no treatment is needed. Exercises which will develop the chest muscles may do much to hide the deformity.

When there is a marked depression a competent surgeon may correct the condition by an operation. Now that the art of giving anesthetics has developed so greatly and the antibiotics can be used to prevent post-operative infections, the risk involved in such an operation has greatly decreased.

The results with improved surgery have been good and it is thought that in the marked cases the best time to operate is between three and five years of age.

Again it must be emphasized that in the mild cases exercise to build up the chest muscles may be all that is needed and only in the cases of marked depression should surgery be performed.

CYSTIC FIBROSIS OF THE PANCREAS

Cause and Nature

The nature of this condition which is usually found in babies or young children is not entirely understood but much work is being done to determine its cause.

At the present time it is thought to be hereditary; that is, in some families the rate is about one in four children while in others it occurs less frequently. It has been seen about equally in the sexes. White people have it more often than the Negro and it has never been seen in an Oriental.

The principal trouble seems to be in the secretions of the mucous glands (so-called exocrine glands) in which the mucous becomes dried up thereby blocking the outlet of the gland and causing it to become swollen, finally destroyed, and then replaced by fibrous tissue—hence the name.

Since these glands are located in many parts of the body cystic fibrosis may affect many organs, such as the lungs, the liver, the gastrointestinal tract, and the gall bladder.

When these glands are not functioning properly, signs and symptoms occur which most frequently are seen in the pancreas and lungs.

Signs and Symptoms

In a few cases the disease is first detected in very young infants when they have a bowel obstruction caused by meconium; when this is operated upon the real disease is detected. This obstruction is called a "meconium ileus."

Other symptoms which appear later are large foul-smelling stools which contain a large amount of undigested fats and starches.

There may be many lung symptoms which may include a brassy cough that is difficult to cure and may recur time after time. One of the things noted in this disease is the presence of staphylococcus aureus which may be isolated from the bronchial secretions. Some of these cases are mistaken for asthma because of the frequent occurrence of the lung symptoms such as cough and wheezing. If this condition is not treated there may be parts of the lungs which collapse and cease to function. Then there will be cyanosis or blueness of the skin and a clubbing of the ends of the fingers. X rays of the lungs are helpful in making the diagnosis as is the examination of the stools for undigested fat and for an absence of certain enzymes that are manufactured by the normal pancreas.

Another characteristic of this disease is that the sweat glands put out more salt than usual and this can be detected by testing the sweat for sodium and for chloride. The patient does not sweat more than other people, but in the summer there may be so much salt in the sweat that serious salt depletion may cause illness which could be prevented by giving the patient salt tablets.

Treatment

This can be very successful in most cases if the diagnosis is made early. First of all the diet can be carefully arranged so that a low fat, low starch diet is used and pancreatic substances can be given by mouth to help make up for the deficiency in enzymes. Antibiotics such as penicillin, aureomycin, and terramycin can be given to prevent the staphylococcus infection. In some cases the use of these drugs is based on a preventive schedule, which means taking a certain amount every day to prevent infection, especially in the lungs and bronchial tubes.

The third treatment has been mentioned above—that is to give additional salt, especially in the summer.

In summary it may be said that this is not a very common disease. It is thought to run in families and it can be seen in varying degrees of intensity, from very mild cases to serious ones.

Cystic fibrosis has been recognized in most of its variations only recently. Therefore much work is being done in the treatment of the disease, and the chances for a normal life with proper treatment are increasing all the time.

GLOSSARY

Enzymes   chemical ferment formed by living cells
Fibrosis   formation of fiber tissue
Gastrointestinal   stomach and intestines
Hereditary   from the family
Ileus   loss of motility of the bowels; may be caused by mechanical obstruction or by disease such as peritonitis
Meconium   bowel movement of the newborn
Mucous Glands   glands secreting watery material

CELIAC DISEASE OR CELIAC SYNDROME

Cause and Nature

Celiac syndrome is a group of symptoms describing a chronic disturbance of the digestive function.

It is never seen in breast fed infants while they are on the breast but usually is detected in infancy or early childhood. This is a chronic disease which requires a long term of treatment and there may be many causes for the condition.

One of the most common causes is an allergy of the intestinal tract to certain forms of food. Other causes are infections of the intestinal tract and poor functioning of the pancreas. Sometimes it is caused by a congenital deformity of the bowel or intestinal tract.

Signs and Symptoms

The onset may be slow and insidious. There is a loss of appetite and a loss of weight. The child becomes irritable and the stomach may seem to protrude because of a loss of weight in the buttocks and legs.

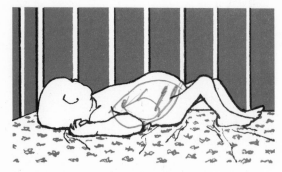

A baby afflicted with Celiac disease.

Growth seems to slow up and the child becomes apathetic, that is, it becomes less active. In addition to the above the child may pass many copious, ill-smelling abnormal stools.

Treatment

Once the diagnosis has been made and other conditions such as cystic fibrosis of the pancreas have been ruled out the treatment is mostly by watching the diet. There are many different variations of the diet depending upon how the child progresses and begins to eat more and put on weight.

Foods which the child cannot tolerate should be withheld. Sometimes there is an allergy to grain foods. Nearly always starches and fats are not well tolerated.

Therefore the diet should be high protein, low fat, and medium carbohydrate, using only simple sugars and no starches.

Ripe bananas are thought to be an excellent food to use in this condition and should be eaten daily.

The treatment of this condition usually lasts over a long period of time and will vary according to the change in the child, the gaining of weight, the change in the stools, and the regaining of appetite, etc.

This treatment must always be in the hands of a doctor and the parents should know that if properly treated, there is hardly ever a death caused by the celiac syndrome. The patient eventually gets well.

GLOSSARY

Apathetic   listless-no energy
Chronic   disease or condition of long standing
Congenital Deformity   present at birth
Cystic Fibrosis   tumors made up of cysts
Pancreas   internal gland
Protrude   stick out like a knot

HYALIN MEMBRANE DISEASE

Cause and Nature

This disease is seen in infants and is called hyalin membrane disease because a thin membrane which resembles a very thin plastic is found in the small air sacs in the baby's lung.

This membrane interferes with the exchange of gases in the lung, that is the oxygen going into the blood stream and the carbon dioxide being expelled from the body.

The cause for this condition is not known, but it is often connected with immaturity and is found in babies born some weeks ahead of the estimated date.

Signs and Symptoms

The first sign is difficulty in breathing. The baby has to struggle for breath and soon assumes a bluish or cyanotic color.

X rays of the chest will show that the lungs present a ground-glass appearance. If prompt measures are not taken at once the baby will not survive.

Treatment

This treatment is highly specialized and nearly always has to be taken care of in a large hospital, preferably in a hospital affiliated with a good medical school.

The baby should be given oxygen at once and this must be continued until he arrives at the hospital.

At the hospital a tube will be placed down the baby's throat and air will be forced in and drawn out by a mechanical respirator. A tube will be inserted into the umbilical vein through which blood transfusions can be given. A careful study of the child's blood will show what chemicals need to be introduced through intravenous tubes.

The baby will be placed in an isolette, that is a plastic cage which keeps out all infections.

It may be necessary to operate and put a tube into the baby's stomach, through which milk may be passed; the infant cannot be fed by mouth because the tube from the respirator is in his throat.

A doctor or nurse must be present at all times to watch the baby's progress. If given this kind of treatment, many infants survive this disease and live to be normal, healthy people.

In some hospitals a new substance is being used against hyalin membrane disease. This is an enzyme called plasmin.

It is felt that the hyalin membrane is found in some babies because of a disturbance in their enzyme production. Some premature infants do not have any plasminogen in their blood at all. The hyalin membrane is made up largely of fibrin, and plasmin is a proteolytic enzyme which causes the fibrin to melt away. Thus plasmin helps the respiratory distress in these babies.

If plasmin is given intravenously or by aerosol inhalation, up to eighty percent of the babies survive. Earlier, those treated with the conventional methods described above and no plasmin had a forty-five percent survival rate.

GLOSSARY

Enzyme   organic substance that can cause specific chemical changes
Umbilical   navel

ECZEMA

(In Infants and Young Children)

Cause and Nature

The term eczema is used by some doctors to classify many kinds of dermatitis or inflammation of the skin. For instance, contact dermatitis, which can be exemplified by poison oak is a form of eczema.

In this chapter the term eczema will be confined to dermatitis in young children and infants as this is a very common form of eczema and causes the parents of the affected child many hours of worry. The cause is not known in the type called idiopathic infantile eczema, although a history of some form of allergic reaction in the mother or father is often noted. These may vary from hay fever to asthma to extreme sensitivity to poison oak. If the eczema of a baby is of the contact type the cause can be determined by removing the irritating agent. The site of the eczema may be important. If it is confined to the scalp it may be seborrheic dermatitis, called dandruff in adults. This type is sometimes called "cradle cap."

Signs and Symptoms

The widespread or idiopathic type usually is most noticeable on the face, which becomes inflammed and swollen in places; scales will form and sometimes little blisters. There is itching and scratch marks will be seen. At times the baby's hands will have to be tied to keep it from scratching the face or other parts of the body. Patches of inflammation may be noted on the inside of the elbows. If the baby is allowed to scratch these itching places there will be secondary infection in the scratch marks.

Treatment

The first thing to remember is to stop using soap of any kind on the baby. Baby oil or mineral oil should be substituted for soap. A soothing local application such as Calamine lotion may be applied to stop the itching. If the baby is sensitive to some kind of food an elimination diet should be tried. This means to take one of the foods in the baby's diet away to see if the eczema improves, then begin giving this again and see if the rash gets worse. This will give the mother a good idea of what is causing the eczema and then that food can be strictly kept out of the diet.

One good thing to know is that most of these cases clear up even without treatment by the time the baby is one or two years old. If there is a strong history of allergy in the family it may take longer.

Sunlight is not good for these cases and should be avoided. In all instances the mother should go to her doctor for advice in taking care of these problems.

GLOSSARY

Allergic Reaction   abnormal reaction to food, drugs, material, etc.
Dermatitis   inflammation of skin
Idiopathic   without definite cause
Infection   gathering of pus in affected part
Inflammation   redness, pain, swelling of affected part
Sensitivity   degree of reaction to various products

Chapter 3

The Female Genital System

THE PRINCIPAL ORGANS which have to do with reproduction in the female are the vagina, the uterus or womb, the Fallopian tubes, and the ovaries. (See illustration on next page.) The normal operation of these organs will be discussed before various diseases and abnormalities are considered.

MENSTRUATION

This word is used to describe loss of blood out of the uterus through the vagina at the end of each ovarian cycle. In all normal women, menstruation usually begins about the age of eleven to fifteen. The time of the first menstrual period varies greatly with individuals and with the type of climate in which they live. Girls in warmer climates usually menstruate earlier than girls in colder climates. Once the periods have started, they are usually repeated at intervals of about twenty-eight days. The menstrual flow usually lasts from three to five days. This is an absolutely normal function and should occur without much pain, although there is often a feeling of fullness in the lower abdomen. Painful menstruation is called dysmenorrhea, and will be discussed later.

When a woman becomes pregnant her periods cease for the term of the pregnancy—nine months—and at about the age of forty-five most women start going through the menopause (change of life) or cessation of periods. The age at which this change occurs may vary—coming earlier in some women, and later in others. Again, this is a perfectly normal function and should not cause any appreciable amount of trouble. In some women, however, there is seen a chain of symptoms associated with the menopause and these will be discussed in more detail later.

The menstrual cycle can be best understood if thought of in the following way. Every month the inside lining of the uterus, or womb, prepares to receive a fertilized ovum or egg—that is, one which has been fused with a spermatozoon from the male. If this fertilized ovum arrives, it is embedded in the thick endometrium or

43

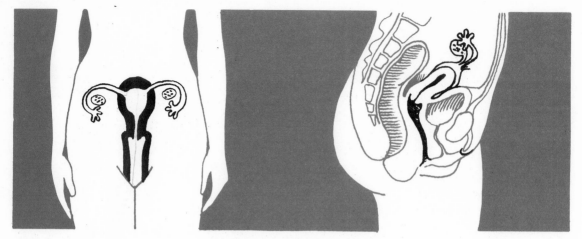

Female reproductive organs seen from front and side. Shown in side view are vagina, cervix, uterus and one ovary. Note fimbriated end of tubes to catch egg as it pops out of the ovary.

lining of the womb. The fertilized egg, or ovum, then begins to grow and this is the beginning of a baby or of a new life.

If, on the other hand, the egg or ovum that arrives is not fertilized, it passes out through the uterus, the lining of the uterus begins to bleed, or slough off, and the woman has a menstrual period. After the period of bleeding, in which the lining of the uterus shrinks back to normal, the endometrium, or lining, begins to build up again in anticipation of another egg. Hence, when a woman becomes pregnant, there is no bleeding because the prepared lining, or endometrium, remains to nourish the fertilized egg which changes into a fetus—the name for a baby in its earliest stage.

This process goes on month after month and somewhere between the two periods, usually about fourteen days before the beginning of a period, the process of ovulation occurs. This means that an egg or ovum pops out of one of the ovaries into the end of the Fallopian tube, and begins to travel down toward the uterus. It is during this journey down the tube that fertilization usually occurs. This means that one of many spermatozoa swimming up the tube meets the egg, and by striking it with its sharp head, penetrates the egg and fertilization has occurred.

Various abnormalities of the menstrual period will be discussed below. It must be remembered that a young girl first starting her periods may take several months or years to establish a regular cycle. These cases should be watched and, if possible, allowed to fall into the regular pattern without outside help in the form of medication.

GLOSSARY

Cessation stopping
Dysmenorrhea painful monthly periods
Endometrium lining of womb
Fallopian tubes tubes that conduct the egg from the ovary to the uterus
Fetus the baby in the womb after the third month until birth
Menopause change of life
Menstruation monthly periods
Ovaries female organs that secrete the egg
Ovum egg
Spermatozoon the male germ cell (*plural:* spermatozoa)
Uterus womb
Vagina birth canal
Womb where the baby develops

AMENORRHEA

Cause and Nature

Amenorrhea means the absence of monthly periods. The most common causes are:

1. Pre-adolescence (the female is too young)
2. Pregnancy
3. Menopause, or change of life

Also, very rarely, changes in climate or emotional disturbances may cause amenorrhea of short duration.

Signs and Symptoms

After the above normal causes have been ruled out, the physician will perform a careful examination to discover some cause, such as blockage, as in the case of an imperforate hymen. He then must seek to determine that a normal uterus is present, and that ovulation occurs. These causes, after they have been determined, may be treated successfully, as a rule.

Treatment

Such factors as obesity and emotional disturbances should be corrected, if present. Under-nutrition is also often found to be a factor.

Some endocrine substance, as thyroid, taken by mouth often helps to induce the period. If this fails, estrogen may be given and stopped each month, just before the period is due. This causes so-called withdrawal bleeding.

GLOSSARY

Endocrine   internal secretion
Estrogen   hormone
Hymen   membrane at the entrance of the vagina
Imperforate   not open
Ovulation   production and discharge of eggs
Uterus   womb

DYSMENORRHEA

Cause and Nature

Dysmenorrhea is a term used to describe painful periods. This may vary from slight discomfort to excruciating pain.

There are two types of dysmenorrhea:

1. Primary dysmenorrhea, which occurs without any disease of the pelvic organs
2. Secondary dysmenorrhea, which occurs in conjunction with some pelvic disorder or disease of the pelvic organs

In primary dysmenorrhea, there may be a strong psychological element. The girl may have been taught that this is a time of sickness, and that she must expect pain just as her mother suffered; when, as a matter of fact, this is an entirely normal procedure which should not require any pampering or reducing of activities. The girl should accept it as such, and proceed with her regular regime, just as if the period were not present. The old superstition that it is not healthy to take a bath during the period is one of the false conceptions which have been passed down from mother to daughter for generations. Primary dysmenorrhea usually ceases after marriage.

Signs and Symptoms

The primary type is usually characterized by sharp, cramp-like pains, which may be very severe. This type is not usually present when menses first start, but develops over a period of time. Such pains are often relieved by marriage, and more often cease after the woman has had a child.

The secondary type is more of a deep, dull ache, and is usually caused by pelvic congestion.

Treatment

Patients should be encouraged to continue with their normal activities. They should develop a proper mental attitude toward this normal phenomenon.

With the second type, some pelvic disease should be ruled out or treated. At times, the pelvic congestion which precedes menstruation may be alleviated by going on a salt-poor diet a week before the period is expected. The use of mild sedation and of analgesics such as aspirin and codeine helps relieve the more severe pain. A drug called Diuril has been effective in relieving pre-menstrual tension. This should be prescribed by a doctor.

GLOSSARY

Menses   monthly periods
Menstruation   monthly period
Pelvic   pertaining to the pelvis, the bony arch supporting the upper skeleton

LEUKORRHEA

Cause and Nature

Leukorrhea is a yellowish-white discharge from the vagina. It is one of the most common complaints of adult female patients, and has many causes.

There is a normal amount of moisture, or secretion, from the vagina in every woman, and this amount may vary from woman to woman, or may differ in the same woman under certain conditions.

Some of the causes of leukorrhea may be listed under two main headings:

1. Normal or physiological
2. Abnormal, of which there are two main types—pathological leukorrhea, and constitutional leukorrhea

The normal or physiologic causes may be menstruation, childbirth, ovulation, sexual excitement, or pregnancy. These all cause normal increases in the secretions of the cervical glands and mucous membranes of the vagina. The slight, clear discharge noted by many women about halfway between their menstrual periods may denote the fact that ovulation has taken place, and may be used as a guide for the best time for conception to take place if the parents are eager to have a child.

The abnormal types of leukorrhea, as stated above, are constitutional and pathological. Pathological leukorrhea is usually associated with disease of the genital organs. These are the vagina, cervix (or mouth of the uterus), the uterus itself, and the Fallopian tubes. Constitutional leukorrhea is caused by some systemic condition, such as fatigue, nervousness, or some other generalized illness.

These diseases or abnormalities can only be diagnosed and treated by a doctor.

Treatment

Treatment will depend upon what type of leukorrhea we are dealing with. The physiologic or normal type does not need treatment. The constitutional type may be corrected by curing the underlying cause such as fatigue, nervousness, or debility. The pathological type will require specific treatment, depending upon the pathology or cause.

In general, the non-specific treatment can be helped by using cleansing douches, alternating vinegar and soda bicarbonate in the water, one tablespoon of soda bicarbonate to a quart of warm water used for seven days, and then one tablespoon of vinegar in a quart of warm water used as a cleansing douche for the next seven days. More specific treatment than this should be under the direction of a physician.

Fallopian tubes   tubes that conduct the egg from the ovary to the uterus
Mucous membrane   moist lining of a body cavity, secreting mucus
Ovulation   production or discharge of eggs from the ovary
Vagina   external birth canal

TRICHOMONAS VAGINALIS

(Inflammation of the Vagina Caused by Trichomona)

Cause and Nature

Vaginitis or inflammation of the vagina may be due to many different causes. Among these causes are:

1. Monilia or one of the molds
2. Gonorrhea
3. Senile vaginitis
4. Nonspecific vaginitis
5. Trichomonas vaginitis

Trichomonas vaginitis is one of the common causes of irritation and is caused by a parasite that falls under the heading of protozoa. It may occur at any age but is most commonly seen in young females.

Signs and Symptoms

There are small red spots of hemorrhage beneath the mucosa of the vagina and the entire lining of the vagina and cervix is red. An abundant discharge is present and this is accompanied by itching with pain in the lower abdomen in some cases.

The diagnosis is easily confirmed by the doctor, who can take a drop of the vaginal discharge and look at it under a microscope. It is easy to identify the trichomonads that live and thrive.

Treatment

The most successful treatment in the hands of some doctors has been by using floraquin tablets or vaginal inserts. One or two of these floraquin tablets may be inserted high in the vagina before going to bed. The next morning the vagina is washed out with a mildly acid douche. This can be done by using one tablespoon of vinegar to a pint of water. After the douche, two more of the floraquin tables are inserted and a douche is taken again the following morning. This process should be carried out for about two weeks, or until the symptoms and signs have cleared up.

Sometimes the condition comes back and it must be treated for a longer period of time. When the condition returns, then the treatment should be carried out for the two weeks before each menstrual period. After the period ceases, the treatment should be carried on for one week. This should be repeated for about three months to completely eradicate stubborn infections. Also, a pill called Flagyl has proved extremely effective in treating stubborn cases of this disease.

Vaginitis should be treated under the direction of a doctor as different types of vaginitis require different treatment.

Cervix   opening into the womb
Hemorrhage   bleeding
Monilia   a fungus in the lower intestine or bowels
Mucosa   tissue lining cavities of body, i.e. mouth, nose, etc.
Parasite   an organism living on or within another (host) organism
Protozoa   one-celled organisms, often parasites
Vagina   external birth canal

VAGINITIS IN YOUNG CHILDREN

Cause and Nature

Usually vaginitis in young girls is caused by infection from the gonococcus. This is because the lining of the vagina in the young is immature and has practically no resistance to the gonococcus. It can be acquired by sleeping in the same bed with a parent who has gonorrhea, using the same towels, or the same toilet seat.

Signs and Symptoms

There is a discharge from the vagina which is usually profuse. This may be accompanied by signs of irritation such as burning and itching.

Treatment

Penicillin is specific for this condition, and vaginal suppositories containing estrogen may be used with the penicillin. Cleanliness is important and the hands should be washed often, taking great care not to transpose the infection to the eyes.

GLOSSARY

Estrogen   female hormone
Gonococcus   pus producing bacteria that causes gonorrhea
Gonorrhea   venereal disease
Transpose   carry to
Vagina   external birth canal
Vaginitis   inflammation of the vagina

SENILE VAGINITIS

Cause and Nature

This condition usually occurs after the menopause, or following removal of the ovaries by operation. Any condition which takes away the normal supply of estrogen may cause vaginitis.

Signs and Symptoms

There is usually some discharge and a persistent itching. The lining of the vagina is thin and pale, and there may be spots of ulceration. Symptoms which may accompany the itching are soreness and burning.

Treatment

The use of vaginal suppositories containing estrogen inserted every night for two and three weeks will usually relieve the symptoms. This can be aided by taking injections or estrogen by mouth for short periods of time. Taking estrogen by mouth or injections over too long a period may result in withdrawal bleeding when the estrogen is discontinued.

The vaginal suppositories may be followed by a mild vinegar douche.

GLOSSARY

Estrogen   female hormone
Senile   affected by the aging process
Suppository   a small medicated cone or cylinder which melts after insertion in the vagina

ABNORMAL VAGINAL BLEEDING

Cause and Nature

Any bleeding from the vagina which is not due to a regular menstrual period is abnormal. There are many causes, some of which are listed below:

1. Improper balance between the hormones that are manufactured by the ovaries—estrogen and progesterone
2. In some instances this bleeding is said to be of emotional origin
3. Tubal pregnancy
4. Infection of the tubes
5. Infection of the vagina

6. Infection and erosion of the cervix
7. After childbirth bleeding may be due to retention of a small piece of the placenta or afterbirth
8. Cancer of the cervix or uterus
9. Benign or harmless tumors such as polyps of the cervix, or fibroid tumors which are just under the lining of the uterus—so-called submucous fibroids

Signs and Symptoms

This abnormal bleeding can vary from occasional spotting in between periods to slight bleeding every day, to excessive bleeding. The causes can vary from very simple ones to dangerous conditions which should be corrected. In any event, a doctor should be consulted.

Treatment

Any abnormal vaginal bleeding which persists should be called to the attention of a doctor who, with the proper examination, can determine the cause and correct it.

GLOSSARY

Benign mild character
Cervix neck of uterus or womb
Erosion wearing away
Estrogen female hormone
Fibroid composed of fibers
Placenta acts as an organ of circulation and respiration for the unborn baby; afterbirth
Polyps a growth
Progesterone female sex hormone

DISCOMFORT AND PAIN IN THE PELVIC REGION

Cause and Nature

This symptom can vary from a dull, heavy feeling in the lower abdominal or pelvic region to sharp excruciating pain.

The causes are many. The most common, of course, is congestion just before a period, which in some women causes discomfort. The fact that the uterus or womb is retroverted, or tipped, was thought to cause backache or lower abdominal pain, but it has been proven that this condition, although abnormal, very seldom results in pain.

Injuries following childbirth often lead to discomfort or a bearing down feeling. This may cause nervousness, backache, and a general lack of energy. Among the most common of these injuries are those tears which result in a cystocele or rectocele.

The cystocele is a bulging of the urinary bladder into the upper part of the vagina, made possible by tearing of the muscle fibers in the roof of the vagina during childbirth.

The rectocele is a bulging of the rectum into the lower part of the vagina. It is due to a tearing of the muscles of the floor of the vagina.

These may be repaired by surgery; but, if possible, it may be well to wait until the woman has passed the childbearing age before the repair is performed.

Tumors of the genital organs may cause pain and discomfort. The most common tumor of the ovary is an ovarian cyst, which may be small or large, and may not cause any pain, unless it has a pedicle which happens to become twisted. In this case, the pain is sharp and severe.

Tubal pregnancy (when the fertilized egg remains in the tube, and continues to grow) will cause pain and vaginal bleeding. If not discovered, it may rupture the tube and cause dangerous hemorrhage into the abdominal cavity.

Infections of the genital organs such as salpingitis, or infection of the tube, may cause pain. Then the infection may go on to abscess formation, and in addition to pain there will be fever and other signs of infection.

Abnormalities or infections of the urinary tract may also cause pelvic pain which may be difficult to differentiate from pain caused by abnormalities in the reproductive organs.

GLOSSARY

Excruciating   extreme
Genital organs   reproductive organs
Pedicle   stalk or stem
Vagina   external birth canal

STERILITY

The inability of a young married couple to have children is fairly common and causes a great deal of heartache. When a couple have failed to achieve pregnancy after two years of trial without using any contraceptives, and if they sincerely wish to have children, both the husband and wife should be examined by a doctor. Often, simple changes will help them to a successful pregnancy. It is very important for the man as well as the woman to be examined, because in almost half the cases the trouble may lie in the husband.

The first thing the woman should do is to keep a temperature chart for several months. A sample chart is shown on the facing page. She should keep a thermometer by the bedside and every morning upon awakening, she should take her temperature and chart it immediately. This will show when she ovulates, and the egg or ovum starts down the tube. Intercourse should be practiced at this time, that is,

when the temperature goes up, for this is the best time to become pregnant. A record of intercourse, pain, period, etc., should be kept on the same chart.

If the above routine does not bring success, then a doctor should examine the patient to see if there is any abnormality of the genital organs, ascertaining if the tubes are open, etc. In many cases there is come slight abnormality which can be easily corrected. A basal metabolic rate should be taken to see if a little thyroid taken by mouth might make the difference between a normal ovulatory cycle and an abnormal one. Both the husband and wife should have a good diet, with additional vitamins.

The husband should submit to an examination and a spermatozoa count should be done. Motility and abnormality of the sperm should be noted. If all of these steps are taken, there is a reasonable chance for a pregnancy.

GLOSSARY

Basal metabolic   represents energy expended to maintain respiration, circulation, muscle tone, body temperatures, glandular activity, and other functions
Genital organs   reproductive organs
Motility   ability to move
Ovulates   produces or discharges egg from ovary or womb
Spermatozoa   male seeds

STERILITY IN THE MALE

Cause and Nature

In most cases when a couple is unable to have children everyone assumes that it must be the female who is at fault. This is far from the truth as we know that the sterility or inability to produce an offspring is often caused by some defect in the man.

TEMPERATURE CHART

Typical Waking Temperature Records in Various States of Ovarian Function

X = Intercourse   O = Ovulation

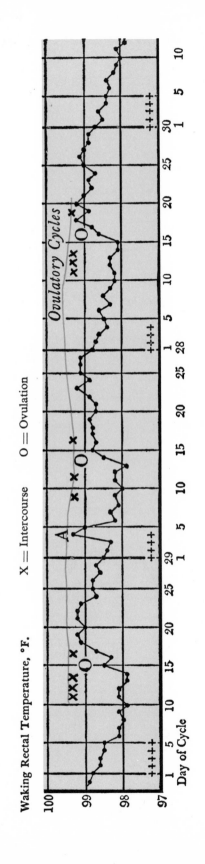

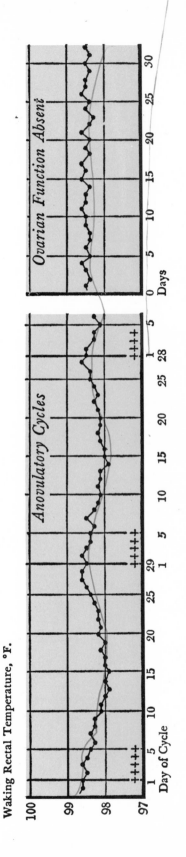

The most favorable time for conception to take place is just before and during the rise in temperature

There are many reasons why the spermatozoa of the male are not able to permeate the ovum of the female and thereby cause conception or the beginning of a new life.

These reasons may be physical and caused by some disease in the past or present. They may be due to improper or insufficient enzyme production, because enzymes do play an important part. First, the enzyme in the ejaculate must liquify it so the spermatozoon can swim freely and second, on the tip or the head of each spermatozoon there is an enzyme which melts or softens the membrane around the female egg in order to permit the spermatozoon to penetrate the egg. In every case of sterility the husband should undergo a careful examination.

Signs and Symptoms

There are very few symptoms connected with a man's inability to produce children because most of the conditions causing sterility do not have symptoms.

However, in a few cases painful ejaculation or premature ejaculation may have something to do with it and this will be considered by the doctor.

In most cases there is something wrong with the spermatozoa, such as:

1. Too few spermatozoa. It has been estimated the normal ejaculate will produce 80,000,000 sperm to one cubic centimeter. Anything below 60,000,000 is considered a low sperm count, although men with a much lower count than this have been known to produce children.
2. The spermatozoa may be abnormal in shape.
3. The spermatozoa may be lazy and not have the motility necessary to swim up through the uterus and into the tube.

Treatment

Your family doctor will examine the entire man, especially with regard to the genitourinary system. He will want a history of past illnesses and accidents. Most important of all he will want to do a sperm count. This is done by collecting the ejaculate in a clean glass jar with a screw top. If the speciman is collected in a condom chemical changes may slow up the motility of the sperm and give a false impression. The specimen should be examined within an hour or two after it is obtained. The normal ejaculate will have a volume of three to five cubic centimeters. The specimen should be kept as near as possible at body or room temperature until it is examined.

Having noted all the characteristics mentioned above, the doctor may be able to correct the deficiencies and the man will no longer be sterile.

At any rate the examination of the female is so complex that in every case of infertility the male member of the partnership should be examined first. If the man is found to be normal then the woman should be examined. In some cases both parties should be examined.

For some strange reason many men have a false pride that makes them think that the fault could not possibly be theirs and so it is the woman who is usually examined first; and only after much persuasion does the man consent to an examination.

GLOSSARY

Condom   cover for penis
Ejaculation   expulsion of semen
Enzyme   chemical formed by living cells
Genitourinary   genital and urinary organs
Permeate   enter without being ruptured
Spermatozoa   male germ cells

FRIGIDITY IN THE FEMALE

Cause and Nature

The word "frigidity" to describe a woman has been used for a long time and it has come to have many meanings.

The real definition of frigidity is probably as follows. A woman who never attains an orgasm during intercourse. This is sometimes called total frigidity and is quite rare.

There are other forms of relative frigidity ranging from women who are difficult to arouse sexually to those who find displeasure or discomfort in intercourse.

The relatively frigid woman may desire intercourse only on rare occasions or she may be one who may achieve an orgasm only on rare occasions.

It has been estimated that the average female does not always achieve an orgasm during coitus. Kinsey determined that the average woman reaches an orgasm about seventy-five percent of the time during marital intercourse. Males always experience an orgasm during coitus.

For a woman, an orgasm (sometimes called a climax) means a mounting sexual excitement which gives rise to such physiologic changes in the genitalia as venous engorgement and culminates in a sensory peak which may be followed by a gradual diminution of excitement and a feeling of release.

Signs and Symptoms

There are very few physical signs or symptoms of frigidity in a female. At least ninety-nine percent of the women who suffer from varying forms of frigidity do so because of their state of mind.

The large percent of functional disorders are usually caused by the woman's attitude toward sexual intercourse. In many cases she has been taught from childhood that the sexual act is evil or dirty and she cannot rid herself of this idea. In some cases she may be trying to punish her husband by not cooperating, and in others she may be unable to enjoy the act because of her feeling of guilt.

The rare physical causes may be:

1. Alcoholism
2. Central nervous system disease
3. Irritation or disease of the genital tract
4. Malformation of the genitalia
5. A deficiency in hormones.

Treatment

The physical causes, which are so rare, may be easily detected and should be treated by a physician.

The psychological causes are a great deal more difficult. The family physician, by listening to the patient's story with an uncritical attitude, by showing a sincere desire to straighten out her thinking and to improve her well-being may bring about an improvement. If these efforts on the part of the family doctor fail on account of embarrassment on the part of the patient or the doctor, then the patient may be referred to a psychiatrist who can help her.

Usually some relative improvement can be achieved although a completely successful treatment of the condition is not always possible.

GLOSSARY

Coitus   sexual intercourse
Genitalia   reproduction organs
Hormones   internal secretions having special action on cells
Physiological   function of body organs
Venous engorgement   increased amount of blood in the veins

MENOPAUSE OR CHANGE OF LIFE

Cause and Nature

When the ovaries cease to function, the woman will stop having periods. This usually occurs after the age of forty-five, but may vary greatly as to the time of onset and the duration of symptoms.

Signs and Symptoms

Most women pass through the change of life without any trouble and this is a normal condition which comes to every woman. The periods may become shorter, the time between periods may vary greatly, or in some cases the periods may be very heavy until they cease entirely. In a very small percentage of women, about ten to fifteen percent, there may be hot flashes, nervous instability, increase in tension, pains in the breasts, or various rheumatic pains.

Treatment

For those in whom the emotional disturbances and vascular phenomena (such as hot flashes) are severe, mild sedation is useful, and in some cases estrogens such as theelin or diethylstilbestrol may be used under strict supervision of a doctor.

In most cases the fact that this is a normal process is understood, and if the physician treating the case uses sympathy and understanding, very little medication is needed. In other cases, the symptoms may be very severe, and these women definitely need help from adequate medication. There should be very little, if any, lessening of sexual desire in women who have passed through the menopause. The sexual urge does not depend upon ovarian secretions to any great extent, and may not be affected by the menopause at all. In some women it may be enhanced, for there is no longer any fear of pregnancy.

GLOSSARY

Enhance   improved or increased
Estrogens   hormones
Menopause   change of life

PREGNANCY

Of all the events in the life of a woman, there is perhaps none as important as pregnancy. A proper understanding of this condition and intelligent management during the prenatal period should be the goal of every prospective mother.

In the first place, the woman must realize that this is a normal phenomenon, and that, according to recent statistics, about four million babies are born in the United States every year. Therefore, there should be no cause for alarm. As a matter of fact, pregnancy should be a cause for great happiness, for only after a woman has brought a new life into the world does she feel that she has accomplished her purpose in life.

The early signs of pregnancy are manifold. One of the first is a missed period. This may mean that the ovum or egg has been fertilized or penetrated by a spermatozoon in the Fallopian tube, and has passed on down to the uterus, where it has become imbedded in the soft inner lining of the uterus, and has begun to grow. Hence, no period.

There are many laboratory tests which can determine whether or not the woman is pregnant. Among these are tests which consist of injecting some of the patient's urine into a female rabbit. After a few weeks, the ovaries of the rabbit are examined to see if they are inflamed or en-

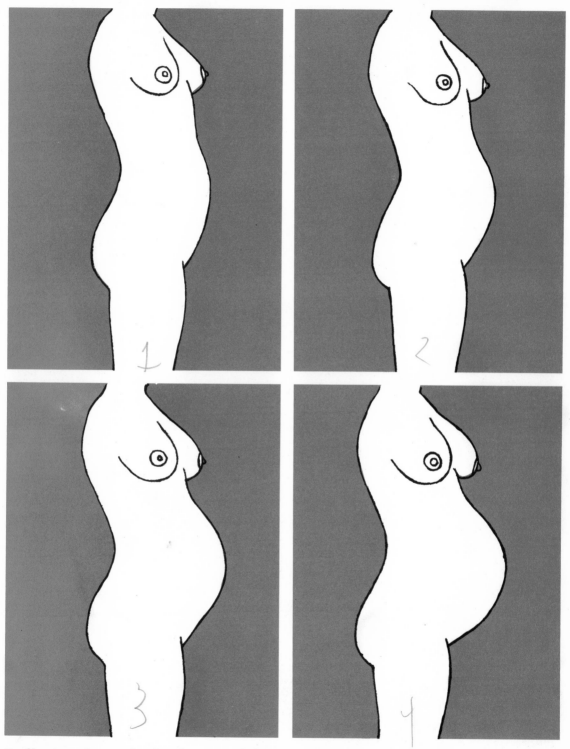

Profile views showing height of uterus and shape of abdomen at about five, seven, eight and nine months. Baby settles during last month. Breasts become larger.

larged. This will indicate that the urine came from a pregnant woman.

After about two months, a doctor can usually tell whether the uterus or womb is enlarged, and with the help of other signs, determine whether pregnancy exists. It is hardly possible for a doctor to detect this change in the size before two months.

Other signs are numerous; change in the color of the cervix, engorgement or enlargement of the veins of the breasts; change in color around the nipples; it has even been said that a mother or grandmother can tell that a girl is pregnant by looking at her eyes. This is known as "grandmother's sign," and of course cannot be relied upon.

When pregnancy is suspected, a woman should go to her doctor for an examination. He will take external and internal measurements of her pelvic region to determine if the patient is capable of having a child in the usual manner. He will also instruct her in what she is to expect during the coming months, and ask her to return for examination about once a month. At this time she should bring a urine specimen which he will examine each month. He will also take her blood pressure each month, measure the height of the womb, and weigh the patient. This is important because about twenty pounds is all any woman should gain during a pregnancy. If she is gaining too fast, the doctor will advise her about her diet. A blood test will be taken early to be sure that syphilis is not present, and to determine whether the mother is Rh positive or Rh negative. This blood test will also determine if the patient is anemic. This latter condition is present in a fair percentage of pregnancies and can be combated easily by taking liver and iron—usually in the form of a pill.

The diet will be discussed, especially with regard to calcium content. With this in mind, an adequate amount of milk should be consumed every day. The baby's bones will need calcium, and if the mother does not take enough calcium in her diet it may be withdrawn from her teeth or other parts of her body. This may be the reason that long ago a mother might be expected to have trouble with her teeth after childbirth. Some doctors give additional calcium in the form of dicalcium phosphate with viosterol, which comes in a capsule. The diet should also be well balanced, with an abundance of protein and vitamins.

During these monthly visits, the doctor will be able to discuss with the patient ways of treating minor complications which may occur. Six of these are listed and discussed below:

1. Nausea and Vomiting

About sixty percent of pregnant women may experience these symptoms in varying degrees. The cause is unknown, but they are thought to be caused by a combination of physical and psychological factors.

Whatever the cause, nausea or morning sickness usually occurs in the early part of pregnancy, and at the end of about three months it usually disappears. Various drugs may be used by the doctor to make the symptoms less severe. Eating small amounts of food at frequent intervals sometimes helps, and eating some crackers upon first awakening has been known to help morning sickness. Fluids should be taken liberally, and carbonated soft drinks not only supply fluids, but carbohydrates also.

If a woman welcomes the pregnancy and does not have any subconscious fears—in other words, if she understands the process and realizes that the chances of anything really dangerous occurring are very slight, she is not so likely to have nausea and vomiting.

The cases of maternal death have greatly decreased during the past twenty years. According to statistics, in 1920 there were 616 maternal deaths for every 10,000 births. In 1953 this had been reduced to only 4.4 maternal deaths in 10,000 births. The reasons for this wonderful improvement in such a short time have been: first, the use of antibiotics such as penicillin to combat infection; second, the better understanding and treatment of the severe toxemias of pregnancy; and third, the liberal use of transfusions to combat hemorrhage. There is no doubt that as time goes on this record will be improved.

2. Constipation

This is a common complaint during pregnancy and can usually be corrected by close attention to bowel habits,—that is, having a bowel movement every day at the same time, and taking a diet liberal in fruits and fruit juices. If these do not correct the condition, the doctor will usually order some milk cathartic such as mineral oil or milk of magnesia. Enemas should not be used during pregnancy.

3. Heartburn

This unpleasant symptom is very common in pregnant women. It is not caused by too much acid in the stomach, but by a slowing up of the motion of the stomach, and a reverse peristalsis which allows the stomach content to be regurgitated back into the lower end of the esophagus, causing a burning sensation.

Soda bicarbonate should not be used to correct the symptom, since the sodium ion causes water retention. Instead, some form of aluminum hydroxide should be taken in tablet form to stop the burning—three or four tablets a day.

4. Insomnia and Frequency of Urination

These two usually go together. Because of the pressure of the baby on the bladder, the mother has the urge to urinate frequently, and hence her sleep is interrupted. The distention of the abdomen sometimes causes a mild shortness of breath which may make it difficult to go to sleep. It is considered safe to take small doses of such hypnotics as Nembutal and Seconal now and then in order to get a good night's sleep. As a matter of fact, it is far less harmful to take occasional small doses of these sleeping pills than it is to lose too much sleep.

5. Hemorrhoids

On account of the extra abdominal pressure, hemorrhoids often occur during the latter part of pregnancy. They usually disappear after the baby is born. If they cause too much discomfort, they may be treated by local anesthetic ointment or suppositories.

6. Dependent Edema

In many pregnancies there may occur swelling of the feet and ankles especially in the last few months. This unpleasant manifestation can usually be lessened by going on a salt-poor diet, and by not being on the feet any more than is necessary.

GLOSSARY

Edema   swelling or filling up with fluid
Fallopian tubes   tubes that conduct the egg from the ovary to the uterus

Hemorrhage   bleeding
Hemorrhoids   piles
Menopause   change of life
Spermatozoa   male seeds
Syphilis   venereal disease
Uterus   womb

NORMAL TERMINATION OF PREGNANCY

The average pregnancy terminates about 280 days from the first day of the last menstrual period, as computed in the following tables. This date is not absolute, but it can be said that about fifty percent of all pregnancies come to delivery within one week of this date. The fact that the other fifty percent may be more than a week early or more than a week late and still be perfectly normal should lessen the worry of many expectant mothers who go past their estimated date of confinement.

GLOSSARY

Confinement   end of term of pregnancy
Menstrual period   monthly period

THE MAJOR COMPLICATIONS OF PREGNANCY

As stated above, dangerous complications of pregnancy are very rare, but they should be recognized and treated early and conscientiously if they are to be cured.

The cause of these complications known as pre-eclampsia and eclampsia is not known. They are characterized by high blood pressure, albuminuria, headaches, visual disturbances, generalized edema, and finally by convulsions. A doctor should treat a patient with pre-eclampsia or eclampsia, as self-treatment of these conditions is very dangerous.

Bleeding in pregnancy is another important complication. Of the serious causes of bleeding during pregnancy, abortion is the most common. Abortion and ectopic (or tubal) pregnancy cause bleeding during the first three months. Placenta previa (afterbirth over the mouth of the uterus), abnormal separation of normally placed placenta, and premature labor cause bleeding in the last three months of pregnancy.

Other minor causes of spotting or bleeding during pregnancy are erosion of the cervix, and polyps of the cervix. Any case of bleeding during pregnancy should receive a doctor's care.

GLOSSARY

Abortion   termination of pregnancy before baby is alive
Albuminuria   presence of albumin in urine
Eclampsia   attack of convulsions
Edema   swelling or filling up with fluid
Pre-eclampsia   toxemia of late pregnancy, preceding eclampsia

ABORTION

The word "abortion" is used to define the termination of a pregnancy before the baby is viable, or alive—usually before eighteen weeks.

It is well to remember that in about sixteen percent of all pregnancies abortion is threatened, and that spontaneous abortion occurs in about ten percent. Often this happens so early that the woman is not quite sure that she is pregnant.

As a general rule, spontaneous abortion occurs when the fertilized ovum is defective and a normal baby would not result. In any event, this may be considered a blessing, and it should always be remembered that the occurrence of one abortion does

HOW TO ESTIMATE DATE OF CONFINEMENT

Find the first day of your last menstrual period in the following calendar (in red). The date opposite (in black) is your estimated day on confinement.

January *		February *		March		April	
1	Oct. 7	1	Nov. 7	1	Dec. 5	1	Jan. 5
2	8	2	8	2	6	2	6
3	9	3	9	3	7	3	7
4	10	4	10	4	8	4	8
5	11	5	11	5	9	5	9
6	12	6	12	6	10	6	10
7	13	7	13	7	11	7	11
8	14	8	14	8	12	8	12
9	15	9	15	9	13	9	13
10	16	10	16	10	14	10	14
11	17	11	17	11	15	11	15
12	18	12	18	12	16	12	16
13	19	13	19	13	17	13	17
14	20	14	20	14	18	14	18
15	21	15	21	15	19	15	19
16	22	16	22	16	20	16	20
17	23	17	23	17	21	17	21
18	24	18	24	18	22	18	22
19	25	19	25	19	23	19	23
20	26	20	26	20	24	20	24
21	27	21	27	21	25	21	25
22	28	22	28	22	26	22	26
23	29	23	29	23	27	23	27
24	30	24	30	24	28	24	28
25	31	25	Dec. 1	25	29	25	29
26	Nov. 1	26	2	26	30	26	30
27	2	27	3	27	31	27	31
28	3	28	4	28	Jan. 1	28	Feb. 1
29	4	(29) †	(5)	29	2	29	2
30	5			30	3	30	3
31	6			31	4		

* Subtract 1 day if leap year.

† Use only if leap year.

How to Estimate Date of Confinement (Cont.)

(See page 59 for information on how to use this table)

May		June†		July†		August†	
1	Feb. 4	1	Mar. 7	1	Apr. 6	1	May 7
2	5	2	8	2	7	2	8
3	6	3	9	3	8	3	9
4	7	4	10	4	9	4	10
5	8	5	11	5	10	5	11
6	9	6	12	6	11	6	12
7	10	7	13	7	12	7	13
8	11	8	14	8	13	8	14
9	12	9	15	9	14	9	15
10	13	10	16	10	15	10	16
11	14	11	17	11	16	11	17
12	15	12	18	12	17	12	18
13	16	13	19	13	18	13	19
14	17	14	20	14	19	14	20
15	18	15	21	15	20	15	21
16	19	16	22	16	21	16	22
17	20	17	23	17	22	17	23
18	21	18	24	18	23	18	24
19	22	19	25	19	24	19	25
20	23	20	26	20	25	20	26
21	24	21	27	21	26	21	27
22	25	22	28	22	27	22	28
23	26	23	29	23	28	23	29
24	27	24	30	24	29	24	30
25	28	25	31	25	30	25	31
(26) *	(29)	26	Apr. 1	26	May 1	26	June 1
26†	Mar. 1	27	2	27	2	27	2
27†	2	28	3	28	3	28	3
28†	3	29	4	29	4	29	4
29†	4	30	5	30	5	30	5
30†	5			31	6	31	6
31†	6						

† Subtract one day if next year is a leap year.

* Use only if leap year.

How to Estimate Date of Confinement (Cont.)

(See page 59 for information on how to use this table)

September†		October†		November†		December†	
1	June 7	1	July 7	1	Aug. 7	1	Sept. 6
2	8	2	8	2	8	2	7
3	9	3	9	3	9	3	8
4	10	4	10	4	10	4	9
5	11	5	11	5	11	5	10
6	12	6	12	6	12	6	11
7	13	7	13	7	13	7	12
8	14	8	14	8	14	8	13
9	15	9	15	9	15	9	14
10	16	10	16	10	16	10	15
11	17	11	17	11	17	11	16
12	18	12	18	12	18	12	17
13	19	13	19	13	19	13	18
14	20	14	20	14	20	14	19
15	21	15	21	15	21	15	20
16	22	16	22	16	22	16	21
17	23	17	23	17	23	17	22
18	24	18	24	18	24	18	23
19	25	19	25	19	25	19	24
20	26	20	26	20	26	20	25
21	27	21	27	21	27	21	26
22	28	22	28	22	28	22	27
23	29	23	29	23	29	23	28
24	30	24	30	24	30	24	29
25	July 1	25	31	25	31	25	30
26	2	26	Aug. 1	26	Sept. 1	26	Oct. 1
27	3	27	2	27	2	27	2
28	4	28	3	28	3	28	3
29	5	29	4	29	4	29	4
30	6	30	5	30	5	30	5
		31	6			31	6

† Subtract 1 day if next year is a leap year.

not indicate that the woman cannot go ahead and have normal pregnancies in the future.

On the other hand, if a threatened abortion is treated and the baby lives, it will be normal as a rule. Otherwise, the threatened abortion could not have been successfully treated. During the early months of pregnancy threatened abortion is indicated by spotting or bleeding with abdominal cramps or pain. In any case of this kind, the doctor should be consulted.

Rh FACTOR

In recent years, it has become the practice to determine the Rh factor for all expectant mothers. In case the mother is Rh positive, there is no cause for further study. If the mother is Rh negative, however, she should be watched carefully, especially if this is her second, third, or fourth pregnancy.

The Rh factor is present in the red cells of about eighty-five percent of all white women, and in about ninety-two percent of all Negro women. If the Rh factor is present, the woman is said to be Rh positive. If the substance is not present, she is Rh negative.

If an Rh negative woman marries an Rh positive man, their child is likely to be Rh positive, and while it is in the uterus some of the baby's blood escapes into the mother's circulation. The Rh negative mother then builds up protection or antibodies against the Rh factor in her baby's blood. These antibodies will then flow back into the baby's body and attack its blood. This may result in the so-called erythroblastosis in the newborn baby.

Since such a small amount of the baby's blood gets into the mother's circulation carrying with it a small portion of Rh factor, the mother only builds a very small amount of protective substance against the Rh factor. Therefore, the first baby is very seldom affected, but with repeated pregnancies more and more anti-Rh substance is formed until in some of the future pregnancies the baby may have its blood damaged. Erythroblastosis in the newborn can be corrected by massive blood transfusions.

If an Rh negative woman gets a transfusion of Rh positive blood, she builds up a large amount of anti-Rh factor, and this is much more dangerous than the small amount she may get from her Rh positive babies. As a matter of fact, an ill advised transfusion—Rh positive blood into an Rh negative woman—may render her incapable of ever having a baby. For this reason, no woman in the childbearing age should receive a transfusion of any other than Rh negative blood.

GLOSSARY

Erythroblastosis disease of red blood cells; excessive red blood cells are developed
Rh blood factor
Transfusion introduction of blood into a patient's veins
Uterus womb

FALSE LABOR

In many cases, especially when having her second or third child, the mother will experience painful uterine contractions before her estimated date of confinement. These contractions are called false labor and it is important to be able to differentiate between these and real labor contractions. The following will illustrate some of the differences.

True Labor Pains

Occur at regular intervals
Pains gradually become harder
Time between pains gradually becomes shorter
Pains start chiefly in the back
Walking makes the pains stronger
Some show is usually present

False Labor Pains

Occur at regular intervals
Pains remain about the same intensity
Time between pains remains the same
Pains located in abdomen
Walking has little effect—may relieve pain

False labor may occur several times many weeks before delivery, and it is always best to notify the doctor or even go to the hospital, for there is no disgrace in going home from the hospital after a false labor. But there may be some inconvenience or even damage done by remaining home too long, believing a true labor to be false.

LUMPS OR MASSES IN THE BREAST

Cause and Nature

The two principal causes of lumps or masses in the breast are cancer and cystic disease of the breast—so-called fibrocystic disease of the breast.

These lumps may be divided into two main classes, the ones with a single, discrete mass in one breast, and those with multiple or many masses in one or both breasts.

The single mass is by far the most dangerous. In women over thirty-five years of age 15.1 percent of these lumps are malignant.

In a recent study which was conducted in a reputable medical clinic, 17,111 women were examined over a period of five years. Of these, 966 were found to have breast masses or lumps; 804 of these patients were followed for a period of four to eight years and of the 804 only 76 patients were found to have definite cancer or malignant disease of the breast. This is only about 9.5 percent. Of these 804 patients, 49.5 percent had single masses and 50.5 percent had multiple masses. These latter were all diagnosed as fibrocystic disease.

These figures would make it seem that all cases of multiple masses (many lumps in the breast) are benign; that is, not cancer. But in the follow-up of the patients with many lumps, 2.2 percent or nine patients out of 406 had cancer.

By the same token one would think that nearly all of the cases with single lumps turned out to be cancer; but from the follow-up statistics it was found that of the 398 patients with single masses only 67 had cancer and 331 had benign or non-cancerous lesions.

Signs and Symptoms

Lumps or masses in the breast usually do not cause any pain but are discovered by the patient through self-examination. Because the percentage of cures is so much higher in cancer of the breast which is discovered early, it is very important for every woman to examine her breasts at least once a month in order to see if there are any lumps. This examination should be made when the patient is lying flat on her back. It is especially important in a woman over thirty-five years of age.

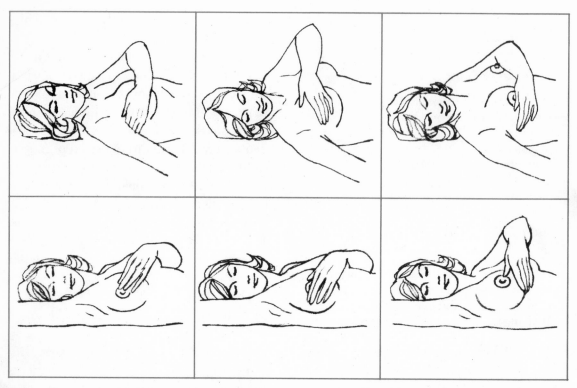

Every woman should examine her breasts once a month after her period. Flat on back, pillow between shoulders. Regular routine—four quarters, outer upper and lower inner upper and lower. Use flat of hand. See doctor if lump is found.

Some of the masses which produce pain are abscesses of the breast. These lumps are painful and hot.

Bleeding from the nipple is another sign which should be investigated by a doctor, as this is often the first sign of a certain form of malignancy of the breast.

Treatment

As seen by the above figures, most lumps in the breast are not cancer, but they are all potential cancer and all of them should be seen by a doctor, who will advise the proper treatment. When he is at all in doubt he will advise a biopsy. This is a simple operation in which the small lump is removed and is studied under a miscroscope by a pathologist. If the lump is benign that's all there is to it. If, however, the pathologist in studying the cut sections of the lump finds cancer cells, the breast must be removed. This is very often a life-saving procedure.

Sometimes a biopsy is not needed, as in the case of an abscess. Then the doctor will follow the case carefully until the mass disappears or is incised and drained.

GLOSSARY
Benign mild character
Biopsy removal of a piece of tissue for laboratory examination
Fibrocystic fibrous sac
Incised cut into
Lesion wound or sore

Chapter 4

The Male Genital System

THE MALE GENITAL system includes the testicles or testes, the prostate gland, and the penis. (See illustration on next page.) The testes are glands that have two functions:

1. Production of androgen, which gives rise to the secondary characteristics of a male —deep voice, distribution of hair, body shape, etc.
2. Production of spermatozoa, which are responsible for reproduction

The spermatozoa are gathered in a tube which runs from the testes to the prostate gland. This is called the vas deferens. The part of the tube, or vas deferens, which is connected to the testes and collects the spermatozoa is called the epididymis. The spermatozoa are stored in the prostate gland, which has a small opening into the penis, until the time of ejaculation, when they pass out into the penis and from the penis into the vagina of the female. Then the spermatozoa are very active, and swim up through the cervix of the uterus of the female and into the tubes; and if they meet an ovum, or egg, coming down the tube they penetrate it, and thus the egg becomes fertilized and a new life is begun.

ORCHITIS

(Inflammation of the Testes)

Cause and Nature

This is usually caused by infection with mumps, or injury to the testes. Vary rarely is it caused by other systemic infections.

Signs and Symptoms

The testicle is swollen and extremely tender.

Treatment

The scrotum should be elevated on a pillow or sling, and cold applications will often relieve much of the discomfort. The patient should remain in bed, and daily doses of five milligrams of diethylstilbestrol will

65

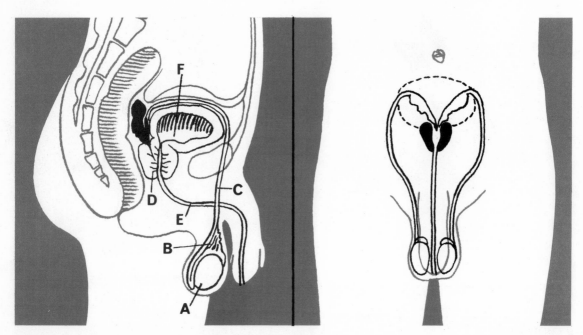

Front and side views showing: Testes (A), epididymis (B), Vas deferens (C) carrying sperm to prostate gland (D). Urethra (E), a tube leading from the urinary bladder (F) through penis, passing through prostate gland.

help to hasten the cure. Aspirin can be taken for comfort, and the patient should realize that if properly taken care of, there are seldom any after-effects.

GLOSSARY

Scrotum   the external pouch containing the testicles

Testes   male genital glands or reproductive organs

PROSTATIC HYPERTROPHY

(Enlarged Prostate)

Cause and Nature

For the prostate gland to be overgrown in men, especially past the age of sixty, is a common thing. In some cases of overgrown or hypertrophied prostate, there are symptoms that may be troublesome. The cause of the enlargement is not understood.

Signs and Symptoms

The most common symptoms are caused by urinary retention or obstruction. This may come on gradually and be characterized by frequent urination, especially at night. Difficulty in starting the stream, the diminishing of the force and size of the stream, and sometimes painful urination are also symptoms.

At times, there may be mild pain or discomfort in the region of the rectum and if this condition progresses—that is, the prostate becomes larger—there may occur complete inability to urinate. This is a painful emergency and requires catheterization by a doctor observing sterile precautions.

Prolonged inability to empty the bladder may lead to urinary tract infection, which may be accompanied by chills, fever, and pain.

Treatment

If the symptoms become severe enough, the only treatment is surgery. This will depend upon what part of the gland is enlarged. In some cases, the median bar can be removed by transurethral resection—that is, performance of the surgical procedure by going through the urethra. In other cases, the entire gland must be removed.

GLOSSARY

Aseptic   free of germs; sterile
Catheterization   withdrawing urine from the bladder by introducing a tube
Hypertrophied   overdeveloped; excessively enlarged
Median bar   middle section of the prostate gland
Prostate gland   male genital gland
Urethra   canal from bladder

ACUTE PROSTATITIS

Causes and Nature

Any invasion of pathogenic bacteria into the ducts of the prostate gland may cause acute prostatitis.

These organisms or bacteria may reach the prostate through the blood stream from other points of infection, such as infection of the tonsils, abscesses of the teeth, or infections of the sinuses.

The bacteria may come from the outside up through the urethra or may come from above when the kidneys or bladder are infected.

Signs and Symptoms

There may be fever and irritability of the urinary bladder. There is usually a sense of fullness around the rectum and this may at times result in acute pain which may be ac-

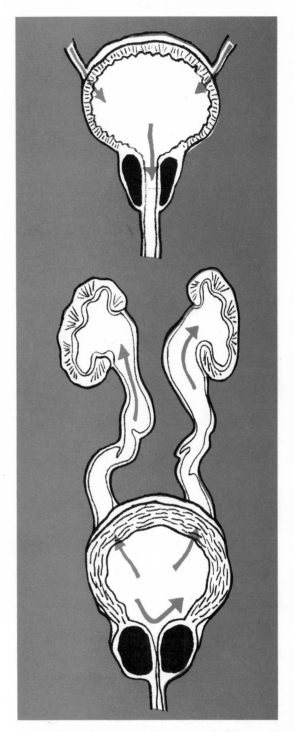

Top: Normal prostate. **Bottom:** Bladder wall thickened by enlarged prostate; and tubes to kidneys enlarged from back pressure.

companied by some difficulty in urinating. The pain may be referred (seem to occur in) to the lower part of the abdomen.

Treatment

If the gland is palpated gently with the finger and found to be extremely tender it should not be massaged.

Sometimes a culture of the urine will identify the causative organism and sensitivity tests will tell what antibiotic could be used to the most advantage. In the meantime it is well to give large doses of Procain Penicillin intramuscularly twice a day or perhaps some broad-spectrum antibiotic by mouth.

For the pain, a rectal suppository with opium in it will sometimes give local relief or it may be necessary to give narcotics by mouth.

This treatment should be only in the hands of a medical doctor.

GLOSSARY

Bacteria   germs or organisms
Culture   a growth of microorganisms
Foci   areas of infection
Intramuscularly   into a muscle
Palpated   to examine by the hand or to feel
Pathogenic   disease producing
Urethra   canal from bladder through which urine passes

CHRONIC PROSTATITIS

As stated above, benign prostatic hypertrophy is one of the most common ailments to affect men, especially those over sixty years of age.

In a large percent of cases this enlargement may be accompanied by infection of the glandular substance and this infection may be acute or chronic.

Cause and Nature

Many reasons have been given for the development of chronic prostatitis. Some of them have been proven, others are just suspected. Among the proven cases are:

1. Surgery, such as a transurethral prostatectomy. This is when a wedge of the prostate is removed by going in through the urethra.
2. Wearing of an indwelling catheter, i.e., Foley catheter. This is sometimes inserted when a person cannot urinate or is unable to control his urine.
3. Instrumentation, such as passing sounds up through the urethra or performing a cystoscopy, that is, looking at the inside of the bladder and the prostate by passing a tube or cystoscope up through the urethra.
4. Any infection of the urethra such as gonorrhea or a nonspecific urethritis.
5. Infections of the upper urinary tracts such as tuberculosis of the kidney.

Among the causes for chronic infections of the prostate which have been suspected, but not proven are:

1. Infected teeth.
2. Stones in the kidney, ureter, urinary bladder, or prostate.
3. Infections of the skin and even upper respiratory infections.

These last are suspected of causing the chronic prostatitis when the causative organism passes from the site of infection through the blood and comes to rest in the prostate.

When there is a chronic infection of the prostate it may be caused by bacteria and the most common pathogens or bacteria which cause these infections are:

1. Streptococcus faecalis and viridans
2. Aerobacter aerogenes
3. Neisseria gonorrhea or gonococcus

4. staphylococcus aureus and albus
5. Escherichia coli
6. Pseudomonas aeruginosa
7. Micrococcus pyogenes
8. Klebsiella

All cases of chronic prostatitis are not caused by bacteria. Some are caused by sexual activities or lack of activities; for instance a man who has been out of contact with civilization for some time and has not had intercourse may have his prostate engorged, enlarged, and chronically inflamed. By the same token a young man who becomes sexually excited often without having an orgasm or discharge of the prostatic fluid may have an enlarged and chronically inflamed prostate.

One other cause for chronic prostatitis is acute prostatitis. The disease may appear to be cleared up, only to have a chronic inflammation show up after many months or even years.

Signs and Symptoms

Chronic prostatitis may be manifested by many symptoms, or the person may have no symptoms at all, only to have this condition discovered during the course of a routine physical examination.

The signs may be noted by a doctor, who places his finger in the rectum and palpates the prostate. He then massages it gently expressing some of the prostatic fluid on to a glass slide.

He examines this smear for pus, red blood cells, and bacteria. The consistency of this gland will give the doctor some clues. It may be enlarged, soft and mushy, or hard. There may also be nodules in the gland which can be felt.

Among the symptoms noted by the patient are:

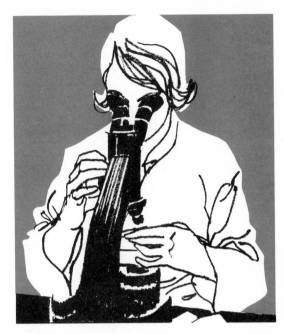

Looking through a microscope one can see pus, red blood cells and bacteria in prostatic fluid if these are present.

1. Pain. This may be back pain or a dull pressure around the rectum, or it may be just a tired feeling in the lower back. At times there is pain in the groin.
2. The urinary symptoms may be frequency of urination, painful urination, urgency, and decrease in the size and force of the urinary stream. There may also be slowness or difficulty in getting the stream started. A man may have to get up often at night to urinate—this is nocturia.
3. At times there are sexual symptoms which may range from complete impotence to premature ejaculation. However these symptoms are not always present and a man may have benign enlargement of the prostate or even inflammation of the prostate without knowing it.
4. Symptoms which affect the entire body may be:
   a. weakness of the legs and thighs
   b. anxieties
   c. tension headaches
   d. nervousness

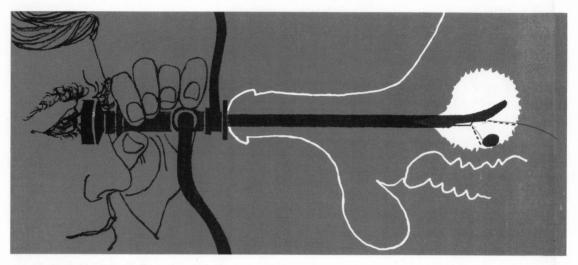

An Urologist can look through a cystoscope and detect stone, tumors in the bladder and condition of the prostate. He can through the same instrument run a catheter up each ureter and find out if there is infection in either kidney.

A more revealing form of diagnosis is made by using a cystoscope. This should be done by a genitourinary specialist. He will be able to see what the opening of the prostate into the urethra looks like and if there is inflammation or chronic prostatitis, this will have a certain color. He will also see if there are stones in the bladder or an inflammation of the urinary bladder. By a special examination through the cystoscope he can get urine from each kidney and determine whether the infection has gone up into the kidneys. Another advantage of this cystoscopic examination is that the doctor can tell whether the entire gland is enlarged and needs to be removed, or whether a more simple operation called transurethral resection can be done. This procedure is cutting a trench through the prostate at the time of the cystoscopy. This is a much simpler operation although neither operation is really simple. A cystoscopy should always be performed in a hospital by a specialist.

Finally it must be remembered that chronic prostatitis is not a simple condition. It can range all the way from engorgement of the gland to widespread chronic infection, from formation of multiple small abscesses in the gland, to stone formation, and sometimes to cancer of the prostate.

Treatment

The great majority of cases of prostatic enlargement and chronic prostatitis can be treated in a doctor's office. Their treatment may consist of simple things such as understanding and explanation on the part of the doctor. If one of the causes is sexual maladjustment this can be explained and sometimes corrected. If the size of the prostate needs to be decreased by massage, which the doctor performs with his finger, this should be done about once a week at first and then once a month until the symptoms are gone and the gland is smaller.

If bacteria are found to be coming from the gland then these should be cultured and sensitivity tests performed which will determine which chemotherapeutic agent or antibiotic would be most effective in doing away with the infection. Such pills as mandelomine and pyridium will often help. Among the numerous antibiotics are tetrocycline and chloromycetin.

Finally chronic prostatitis is a very common condition and every man over fifty should have his prostate examined and massaged by a doctor to see if pathogenic bacteria are present. In most cases the condition can be greatly improved by simple methods such as prostatic massage or taking medicine. The patient should allow a specialist to perform a cystoscopy examination if his family doctor has advised it. Neglecting these things may lead to serious complications as mentioned above.

There is one other thing to know about chronic prostatitis or prostatic hypertrophy. In about one third of these cases there is no infection or bacteria, in another third there may be only harmless bacteria, (nonpathogenic) and in one third there may be pathogenic bacteria (bacteria capable of causing disease).

GLOSSARY

Benign   mild in character
Cystoscopy   examination of the urinary bladder
Engorged   swollen with fluid
Genitourinary   pertaining to the sex and urinary organs
Glandular substance   material of which glands are made up
Groin   area between lower part of abdomen and thigh
Hypertrophy   overdeveloped; excessively enlarged
Indwelling catheter   a tube that must remain in the bladder
Instrumentation   use of instruments
Nodule   little knot
Retention   inability to urinate
Spermatozoa   male seeds

Urethra   canal from bladder through which urine passes
Urethritis   inflammation of the urethra

MALE SEXUAL DISORDERS

In considering sexual behavior, normal and abnormal, in either the male or female, it should be emphasized at the beginning that the psychological attitude of a person plays a tremendous part in his or her sexual behavior.

In the first place, many of us have been taught or have some way come by the idea that sex is something evil. Thinking this, some people are handicapped by a sense of guilt which prevents them from engaging in the sexual act in a satisfactory manner. It is, therefore, very important to realize that the act of sexual intercourse is a true expression of love, and should be considered as one of the most sacred and important urges to which human beings are subject. If it were not for this act, the human race would not survive. A sound understanding of sex and sexual disorders in both the male and the female is of utmost importance.

The laws of our society make it obligatory that this act of love is only consummated after marriage. These laws do a great deal toward protecting the children, all of whom should be born with a father and mother to love and care for them. The laws also protect the health of individuals, for venereal disease is usually spread by the promiscuous disregard of our social code.

In discussing sex, two terms are used frequently, and the meaning of these terms should be understood. The word "libido" means interest in or thinking of sex; potency or potentia means the ability to perform the sexual act. When a person no longer is interested in or thinks of sex, there is said to of be a loss of libido. When a person is unable to perform the sexual act, he is said to be impotent. Of course, there are many stages of the above conditions. The sexual urge, or libido, is usually at its height during puberty and for a time thereafter. Sometimes people who in later life do not have proper physical, emotional, and intellectual outlets, may become emotionally unstable, highly excitable, and sexually overactive.

When a male begins to have a decrease in potentia, this is usually manifested through premature ejaculation or inability to obtain a satisfactory erection. This is nearly always caused by some psychological maladjustment. There may be nervous tension, anxiety, fatigue, worry, preoccupation, or excess of masturbation. The important thing to know is that once the above causes are corrected, the man will resume his previous ability to perform the sexual act. It is very rare, indeed, for these symptoms to have a real physical cause.

Often a feeling of inadequacy will cause a man to be unable to have an erection, and as his failures are repeated, he will feel more and more inadequate, and the condition will become worse. If he realizes the cause and is able to get rid of this feeling of inadequacy, he will soon return to normal. For once the male has shown himself able to have an erection and to go through with the sexual act, this ability will never be lost until he has reached a very old age. Of course, it will decrease as he becomes more advanced in years, but it will very rarely leave him due to physical reasons. Therefore, realizing that the causes are psychological he should be able to correct them.

Other sexual symptoms which the male may experience are:

1. Painful ejaculations, which may be caused by some obstruction to the ejaculatory ducts such as stricture or benign prostatic hypertrophy
2. Bloody ejaculations, which usually have no significance, and will clear up without any treatment

Another symptom, sterility, may be caused by impaired ability to form spermatozoa. Also, the ducts may be stopped up, or the sperm may be sluggish and lack the proper motility. To correct these, assistance from a doctor will be necessary.

GLOSSARY

Benign   mild character
Ejaculation   sudden act of expulsion, as of the semen
Promiscuous   indiscriminate
Puberty   age when sexual maturity is reached
Sperm   seed
Spermatozoa   male seeds

IMPOTENCE

Cause and Nature

In about ninety percent of the cases there is a psychogenic cause for impotence, and in the other ten percent there may be some physical cause such as a severe case of mumps during puberty.

Impotence is usually the inability to obtain an erection. This failure to gain, or early loss of, an erection occurs in most cases of psychogenic impotence. Other complaints are premature ejaculation or retarded ejaculation, and in some cases there is a complete lack of sexual desire or pleasure. Impotence is not a disease but is a symptom of some underlying condition which in nearly all of the cases is psychogenic or "in the head."

The stimulus for sexual arousal, and

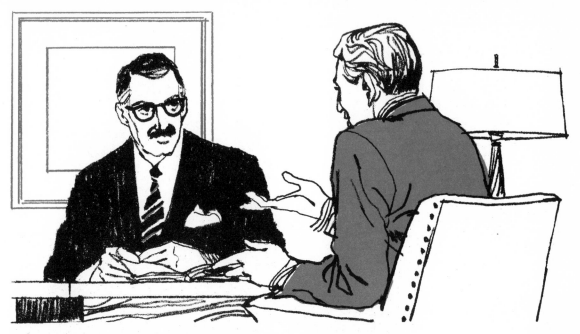

Frank discussions with a doctor will often do more good than medicine.

hence for an erection, is very delicate and it can be easily interfered with by such emotions as anxiety, anger and depression. The cause for these emotions, when psychogenic, can usually be discovered and in most cases these causes can be done away with and the person will be returned to normal sexual behavior. There is no reason why anyone who has had satisfactory sexual intercourse when a young man, should not continue to do so up into his late sixties or early seventies.

Signs and Symptoms

There may be an inability to obtain an erection, or once having obtained one the person may not be able to maintain it for a satisfactory length of time.

Premature ejaculation is another sign which is often complained of and in some cases there may be retarded or delayed ejaculation.

One other symptom of impotence may be an absolute lack of desire for the sexual act or a lack of pleasure in it. Since the cause of this impotence is usually "in the head" or psychogenic, there are different stages of it and it is important to find the cause early and do away with it.

Anxiety is one of the main causes and this may be deep rooted or relatively mild. The man may have been unable to obtain an erection on one occasion and the next time he wishes to have intercourse, he may be anxious and tense, fearing that this will happen again. It may start on the honeymoon when a temporary situation may arise, such as staying in the house with the wife's mother and father, or being too tired and excited after the wedding. Sometimes too much alcohol is taken at the wedding reception and this may interfere with a normal erection. All of these things are temporary and should not be worried about. There should never be any fear or anxiety that things will not be all right later.

If these small situations are not corrected and the failure to obtain an erection persists for over a month the man's attitude may change from concern and anxiety to one of deep humiliation. Again, if he knows that this is just a temporary condition and does not worry about it, chances are that nature will take its course and things will be all right.

Sometimes there is hostility toward the wife which may cause impotence. In nearly all cases of retarded ejaculation there is hostility toward the wife. This may be so deeply hidden that the man is not aware of it, but if he is carefully questioned by a doctor, the cause for this hostility may be brought out and done away with.

Often, guilt will prevent a man from having an erection. He may have some entirely unjustified guilty feeling because he masturbated when younger or because he had sexual relations before he was married. If these things are talked over frankly with a doctor they are usually shown in their true light and the feeling of guilt disappears and so does the impotence.

After having failed in sexual intercourse over a period of many months the man may have a great feeling of depression and may suffer from insomnia, loss of appetite, or constipation. These problems can be cured if the man will go to a doctor and discuss things with him. If the doctor thinks it necessary, he will refer the patient to a psychiatrist who can help a great deal if the patient cooperates with him.

Treatment

A thorough history should be taken and a physical examination should be performed by a doctor to rule out any physical cause for impotence. Then by frank discussion the hidden cause of the condition can be brought out and usually corrected. If this fails, the man should be referred to a psychiatrist who can nearly always help in correcting a psychogenic condition. There is no disgrace in going to see a psychiatrist. His treatment will usually be successful.

GLOSSARY

Ejaculation   sudden expulsion, as of the semen
Insomina   inability to sleep
Masturbation   self-induced sexual excitement
Psychogenic   originating in the mind
Psychiatrist   a doctor specializing in mental or nervous disorders

EUNUCHOIDISM OR EUNUCHS

Cause and Nature

A eunuch is a man or boy who has been deprived of testes; eunuchoidism denotes a defective state of testicular function with impaired sexual power and eunuch-like symptoms. The testes have two main functions, one being to form sperm or spermatozoa and the other to secrete a substance called androgen, which is responsible for the secondary male characteristics in a man—the deep voice, male distribution of pubic hair, libido and potentia (the ability to perform the male part in sexual intercourse).

When the second part of the testicular function is impaired or absent, eunuchoidism occurs.

The cause may be castration, that is, surgical removal of testes, or partial castration caused by diseases such as mumps, or by accidents such as crushing the testes, or the testes may be small or absent.

When this loss of testicular function occurs before puberty, a eunuch is the result, but when the loss occurs after manhood has been achieved, any degree of eunuchoidism may result depending upon the amount of loss.

Signs and Symptoms

Loss of testicular function before puberty results, usually, in very tall stature but this is not always the case. Some eunuchs are medium size. The shoulders are narrow, and there are excessive fat deposits around the hips, abdomen, and thighs. The breasts also may have an abnormal amount of fat resulting in large breasts. Muscular development is usually poor and strength is reduced. There may be a very slight growth of pubic hair and the voice remains high pitched. The skin shows characteristic wrinkles about the face and the color of the skin is usually pale. There is no acne and baldness does not occur. There is usually an absence of sex drive and of ability to perform. There may be marked anemia. These signs all vary with the amount of testicular function. If castration occurs after manhood, then there may be a regression of the secondary sex characteristics. That is, there will be less growth of the beard and body hair and fine wrinkles will appear around the mouth and eyes. A reduction of sexual activity will occur but it is not always entirely absent.

Treatment

The treatment of loss or reduction of testicular function consists of the administration of testosterone. There are different forms of this androgen and these forms may be administered in different ways.

Testosterone propionate may be given by intramuscular injection. This substance

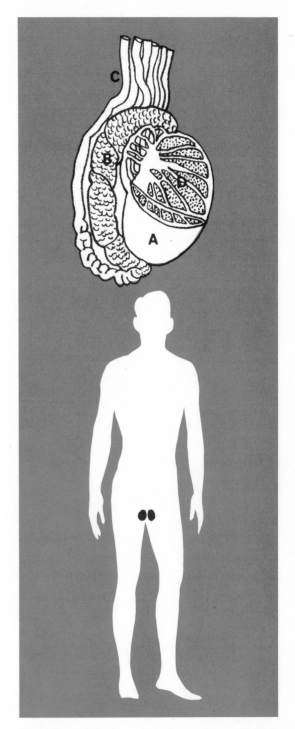

Testicle: A. The sperm are formed here. B. Epididymis collects the sperm. C. Vas deferens tube carrying sperm to prostate. D. Androgen or male hormone formed here.

is in oil and is liberated slowly so that it is effective when injected every three or four weeks. This is the method that most patients prefer.

Methyl testosterone can be taken in tablet form or can be held under the tongue until it is absorbed into the blood stream. When swallowed, the dose should be about twice as much as it would be if held under the tongue.

Another effective way of administering testosterone is to implant pellets under the skin. This a simple operation and the implantation of a pellet containing about one thousand milligrams will usually last about four to six months.

All such treatment should be under the strict supervision of a doctor.

GLOSSARY

Acne   disease of glands in the skin
Anemia   deficient blood
Sperm   germ cell of the male
Testes   male sex glands

MALE CLIMACTERIC OR CHANGE OF LIFE IN MEN

Cause and Nature

Although the change of life in women is an occurrence expected when the ovaries cease to function, this same phenomenon has never been proven to occur in men when the testes decrease in function. There has been a great deal of controversy over this subject, but the general opinion is that the change of life does not occur in men.

Signs and Symptoms

If men suffer hot flashes and changes in temperament when they are in their sixties or seventies, then by taking a biopsy of their testes, and testing their urine for an increased secretion of gonadotropin the diagnosis of change of life may be made. These symptoms are usually caused by psychoneurotic changes in middle-aged and elderly men, and not by loss of testicular function.

Treatment

If the symptoms are relieved by the administration of testosterone propionate or methyl testosterone and not by the injection of a placebo, then it may be assumed that these symptoms are not of psychoneurotic origin.

GLOSSARY

Biopsy   examination of a piece of tissue
Gonadotropin   a stimulating substance
Ovary   a female sex gland
Placebo   medicine given to please the patient (sugar pills having no medicinal qualities)
Psychoneurotic   resulting from a disorder of the mind
Testes   male sex glands

Chapter 5

Sex Life

NORMAL SEXUAL INTERCOURSE

Sexual life should be thought of as something normal and very important. The normal love between a man and a woman should contain a feeling of real tenderness for each other and sexual intercourse should be an expression of this tenderness and love.

When the act is regularly practiced between man and wife, the man should be able to control his ejaculation so that he gives his partner three to five minutes in which to reach a climax or orgasm. Some women take longer to reach this climax than others and some men are not able to refrain from ejaculation for that long. An effort should be made by the man to do this.

The woman will usually be able to reach the orgasm in about the same time as her partner.

The highest peak of pleasure for adults should be the orgasm, and the aim of the sexual act should be to build up as much pleasure as possible in order to obtain a complete "letting go," such as occurs in an orgasm. In a man, the orgasm occurs at the same time as the ejaculation. The woman experiences the orgasm, but not the ejaculation.

In order for two people to reach this climax in the proper manner their minds should be free from any other thought. If a man cannot refrain from ejaculation, or suffers so-called premature ejaculation, this is a sign of neurosis and has not a physical but a mental origin.

The so-called "petting" or preparatory acts or manipulations which take place before intercourse are all considered normal only if they are preparatory to regular intercourse.

The average young adults, after having been married for some years, have intercourse about twice a week. Too much emphasis cannot be placed upon the fact that a great deal of the success of this act depends upon the mental attitude toward it, and it is well for young people who are about to be married to understand these facts.

The sexual act as practiced between husband and wife should result from a spontaneous desire on the part of both of them. In order for the act to be satisfactory to

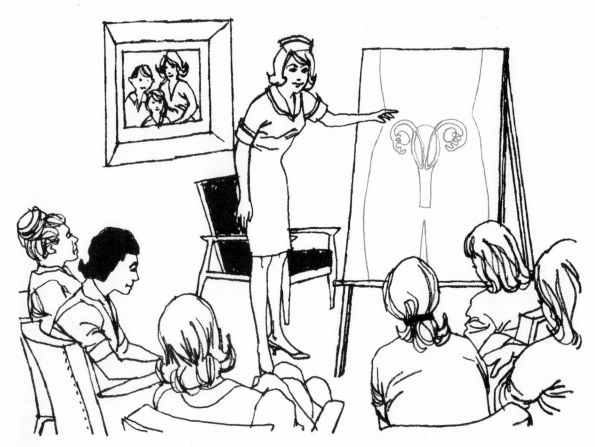

Health education classes: prospective mother should know about her reproductive organs.

both of them a great deal of understanding and cooperation on the part of the husband and wife is very important. For instance, this act may be painful to the wife at first, or the husband may not be able to prevent a premature ejaculation. They must realize that this is not a permanent state of affairs and know that by mutual understanding and a sincere effort to help each other the act will, as time goes on, become as successful as it should be.

One of the things the woman should know is that every woman does not arrive at the climax on each occasion in which the sexual act is consummated. Knowing this she should not be disappointed because she does not reach this successful conclusion every time.

This act, which is important to married life, takes a great deal of understanding and it takes time in some cases to arrive at a level of performance which is satisfactory to both partners. Always remember that this is an expression of love. It can be worked out properly if both the man and the wife try to cooperate and understand what is to be expected.

GLOSSARY

Climax the sexual orgasm
Ejaculation ejection of semen by the male
Orgasm the crisis of the sexual act for either man or wife

FAMILY PLANNING

Much has been written about a population explosion and a great deal of research has gone into so-called family planning—that is, having as many children as the couple desires and at the time when they can best afford to have them.

It is a popular pattern now in large cities to have Family Planning Clinics in county hospitals. But these are only for people who are on the county welfare rolls and the person who is not eligible for county welfare must go to the family doctor or to a specialist for instruction.

All of these activities or precautions should be guided by the religious and moral belief of the couples involved.

The Family Planning Clinics as a rule do not accept unmarried persons unless two doctors advise that these persons be instructed.

The time-honored methods of contraception as outlined below are still taught in these clinics and the women involved can usually get help from the Public Health Nurse in following up on the instructions. A great number of women throughout the United States and in some foreign countries have taken advantage of these clinics and the number is growing all the time.

In all cases of contraceptive counseling a thorough physical and pelvic examination should be performed first. This should include a "Pap" smear.

METHODS OF CONTRACEPTION

One of the oldest methods of contraception is the so-called "rhythm method." This means abstaining from intercourse during the period when the woman ovulates, or produces an egg that goes down the Fallopian tube to the uterus. This egg usually comes from the ovary about halfway between two periods. So to be safe, intercourse is practiced only during the days just before or just after a period. One fault with this system is that a woman cannot be sure just when she does ovulate. To correct this fault and be doubly sure, if you are going to use the rhythm system, a basic temperature chart should be kept by the woman for several months (*See* chart on page 51). The mouth temperature should be taken every morning before arising and it should be charted. This chart will show a change, as shown in the diagram, when the egg comes forth. If this occurs several months on the same day, say the sixteenth day of her cycle, then she can be reasonably sure that she ovulates on the sixteenth day, and by avoiding intercourse for a day or two before and after the sixteenth day she may avoid pregnancy. By the same token, when a baby is wanted, the best time to have successful intercourse is the sixteenth day or a day before or after this presumed day of ovulation. Sometimes a woman can check her basic temperature chart and find that during ovulation there is a little mid-period pain or discomfort; she can use this in the future to determine just when the egg comes out of the ovary.

The various mechanical means of contraception have many degrees of effectiveness. Intra uterine devices such as plastic coils are easily inserted by a doctor and are quite effective. If the person wishes to have a baby the device may be removed by a doctor to allow pregnancy to occur. The use of an intra uterine device is considered by some women to be easier than taking the "Pill". The diaphragm pessary, properly used by the woman, is considered a safe device. Next is the condom, used by the man. Either one of these should be used with contraceptive jelly that can be purchased in tubes. This jelly usually contains lactic acid, which may kill the spermatozoa or seal off the cervix (or the entrance to the womb) in case the other mechanical appliance fails.

For a newly married couple it may be better for the husband to use a condom, for it may be difficult for a woman to properly insert a diaphragm. After a short while, the diaphragm can be used instead of the condom. The woman should have this diaphragm fitted by a doctor, who will give her instructions as to the proper insertion and care of this appliance.

A diaphragm should be left in place after intercourse and not disturbed for at least eight hours. Then a douche should be taken in the reclining position before the diaphragm is removed. A good douche to use is one teaspoon of lactic acid U. S. P., to two quarts of warm water. After the douche, the diaphragm may be removed, washed, dried thoroughly, and put away.

Medicinal suppositories are used but they are far less effective as a contraceptive agent. For one reason, they do not melt quickly and may not cover the entire vagina.

Withdrawal just before orgasm should never be practiced. First, because it is not safe, and second, because it is not good for the husband or wife.

There is one type of contraceptive that is mentioned only to be condemned—the so-called stem pessary. This is a metal pessary that is inserted into the cervix and left there indefinitely. It is not only inefficient as a contraceptive method, but is most dangerous because of the constant irritating effect upon the cervix and may tend toward producing cancer of the cervix. The stem pessary should never be used.

THE PILL

There Are Better Things Coming

The American College of Obstetricians and Gynecologists has recently made a favorable report on the success of oral contraceptives—that is, pills taken by mouth to prevent pregnancy. During the last few years a great number of oral contraceptives have been placed on the market by the various drug companies and most of them have been successful. It is estimated that there are over a hundred types of these pills now being sold.

With the most popular type used now, the woman takes a pill the fifth day of her period and one each morning thereafter for twenty days. She then stops to allow her period to occur.

These pills are made of various combinations of estrogen and progesterone and were originally used to regulate periods. When it was discovered that they would stop ovulation or the production of the egg, they really became popular.

There have been few cases of complications arising from the use of the pill. In some cases there has been spotting which stopped after a month or so. Some women have complained of nausea which subsided after changing to a different pill. There have been reports of weight gain which is thought to result from the woman's relief of anxiety about becoming pregnant rather from than the pill itself.

Many articles have been written about

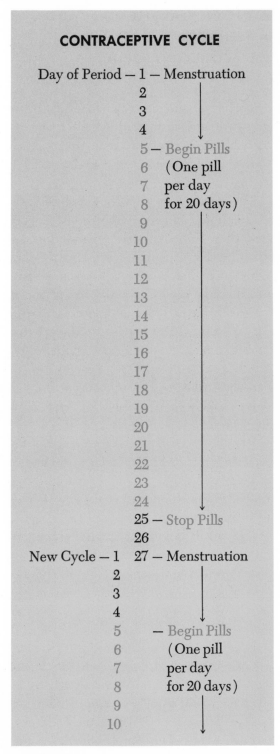

CONTRACEPTIVE CYCLE

Day of Period — 1 — Menstruation
2
3
4
5 — Begin Pills
6 (One pill
7 per day
8 for 20 days)
9
10
11
12
13
14
15
16
17
18
19
20
21
22
23
24
25 — Stop Pills
26
New Cycle — 1 27 — Menstruation
2
3
4
5 — Begin Pills
6 (One pill
7 per day
8 for 20 days)
9
10

Birth Control: The above diagram explains the correct method of taking birth control pills.

the occurrence of phlebitis or thrombophlebitis while taking the pill, but there is no reliable evidence that this was connected with the medicine and in nearly all cases the occurrence of this condition was thought to be a coincidence. That is, the woman would have had phlebitis even if she had not been taking the pill.

Women admit that they are forgetful and fail to take the pill on some mornings with a pregnancy resulting. Many husbands complain that their wives do not know how to count or to use a calendar properly. Some wives agree that this is so.

With this in mind doctors who are doing research have tried to develop a pill which can be taken once a month and prevent ovulation from taking place during that month. In some of the clinics this has been remarkably successful and it is hoped that in the future the counting of twenty days will not be necessary. These pills are composed of various combinations of the hormones produced by the ovaries, which are released slowly into the system.

In addition to "The Pill," or instead of the pill, many women who are forgetful or do not want to take a pill every morning prefer a device that is placed in the uterus to prevent conception. These intra-uterine devices are usually small plastic curly objects that look like a small apple skin that has been recently peeled or like a small spring. They are made of plastic and have a small thread on one end which is left hanging out of the cervix or mouth of the womb; thus the patient can have a doctor remove the device when she wishes to become pregnant.

These coil-like devices may be easily inserted in a doctor's office and the insertion should take place within seven weeks after having a baby or on the fifth to seventh day after the beginning of a period.

There have been few complications. In a small number of cases the device has been expelled and had to be reinserted. In a few cases the thread was absent from the cervical mouth and a new coil with a thread on it had to be inserted after the defective one was removed. In only one case a healthy baby was delivered along with the coil.

Other doctors have used injections, or implantation under the skin, which will prevent ovulation for a month.

It is to be hoped that these will prove to be efficient and free of side effects.

Always remember that the use of contraceptive methods should be under the supervision of a doctor and should be compatible with the moral and religious beliefs of the couple involved.

GLOSSARY

Condom   a cover for the penis to prevent impregnation

Contraception   prevention of pregnancy

Contraceptive jelly   a non-greasy jelly to be used in the vagina for contraception

Diaphragm pessary   an instrument used for contraception

Douche   a stream of water directed into a cavity

Ovulate   produce an egg

Ovary   the female organ in which eggs are produced

Pap smear   (Papanicolaou's smear) a staining method by which secretions are obtained from various parts of the organs for examination of exfoliated cells.

Phlebitis   inflamation of a vein

Spermatozoa   male germ cells

Suppository   medicated mass to be introduced into the vagina

Thrombophlebitis   a condition in which inflammation of the vein wall has preceded the formation of the thrombus

Thrombus   a plug or clot in a blood vessel

Uterus   womb

Vagina   the canal in the female genital organs

A PARENT'S ADVICE TO A TEENAGER OR ADOLESCENT CHILD

To begin with, in order for a parent to give good advice and aid to a son or daughter who has arrived at the age of puberty, the parent must believe the advice which is given.

This advice is an explanation of the sexual functions, and the parent must believe that these functions are pure and clean, and that there is nothing bad about them.

When one stops to think about it, how can there be anything really bad about an act that brings a little baby into the world? The newborn baby is pure, so the act that caused him to be born must be pure.

Advice about sex should come to a son or daughter from the parent, and not from an older child who probably does not know the true facts.

It is far better if this advice is given before the child actually reaches the age of puberty so that he may be prepared in advance for the wonderful changes which his body is to undergo.

The explanation of sexual functions should be made in a "matter of fact" way, just as you would explain any other function of the body or, for that matter, the function of an inanimate object, such as an automobile.

Some children are very inquisitive and ask such questions as "Where do babies come from?" These questions should be answered in full, using exact terms, and not beating around the bush. If the child does not ask questions, he or she should be told anyway and, as stated above, before the age of puberty is reached.

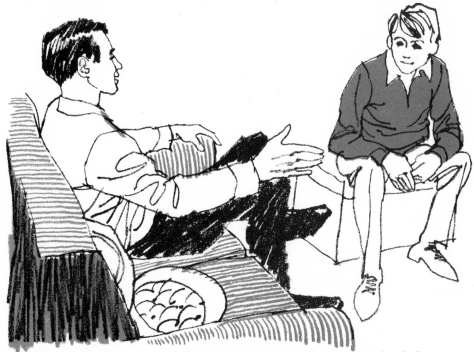

One of the most important phases of a boy's education. Frank talks with his father.

In discussing the real facts about the body with a young child who has reached the age of puberty or one who is almost at that stage perhaps the most important single subject that should be explained is masturbation. This requires tact and understanding on the part of the parent and unfortunately many parents were misinformed when they were growing up and do not really understand the significance of this act. Before discussing it with the child they should be sure that they have in their own minds a good idea of what masturbation means.

In the first place the act should not be emphasized and the approach to an explanation should be casual. The child should be told that all of us have curiosity about the different parts of our body and when a boy or girl attempts to find out what his or her sexual organs are there is nothing sinful or bad about this. The only harmful part about this act is to overdo it or perform it too often. By explaining that nearly all boys and girls when they are growing up may experiment in this way, the parent may do away with the great feeling of guilt or shame which some children feel after attempting or performing this perfectly normal act.

Because of lack of proper information about masturbation I am sure that many children have had their lives seriously affected. This can be prevented by explaining what the sexual organs are for and how they will be used after a person is married to bring other little boys and girls into the world.

A girl should be prepared for her first menstrual period and one good way to prepare her is to have her look forward to it. I once heard a doctor say that one of the proudest moments of his life occurred when a young girl, who had been his patient since childhood, made an appointment and came to his office alone. She proudly showed him a new addition to her charm bracelet. This new charm had a date on it, and she said, "That is the date when I became a woman." She meant, of course, that she had experienced her first period. Her mother had prepared her for it properly, so that instead of being shocked and frightened she was very happy about it.

Adolescence is a very trying period to both boys and girls, but it can be made much easier if the mother and father make it a point to explain sexual affairs fully. This may require some study and some changing of ideas on the part of the parents, but the results will certainly compensate them for their efforts.

During this strange and disturbing period in which the sexual urges of the boys and girls come to life, it will be wise to warn both girls and boys that they are too young to assume the responsibility of having a family and that any act of this kind may result in a baby. This is especially true when children are still in high school. Some girls feel that to be popular they should be promiscuous, which is not true. As a matter of fact, most boys will admire them more, and they will be more popular if they do not participate in sexual intercourse. There seems to be a general letdown in this re-gard and probably it is because the parents have not impressed it upon both boys and girls that this sexual act is a sacred thing which is to be saved until they are married. If they indulge in it too soon their future life may be affected in a way that will prevent them from being as happy and healthy as they would have been had they used self-control and restraint. It should be explained that when they are going through this period of change they have not become mature enough to use good judgment in selecting a mate for the remainder of their lives.

Another reason for not entering into matrimony too early is that they have not been fully educated and are not yet ready to assume the roles of breadwinner or housewife. In addition to the religious aspect of these affairs, it should be pointed out that our society is governed by a set of rules and standards, unwritten laws so to speak; and the good citizen does not break these laws.

In case the parents are uncertain about how to give the proper advice to their adolescent children, they may call upon the family doctor.

GLOSSARY

Adolescence   growth from childhood to maturity
Masturbation   self-manipulation of the genitals
Menstruation   monthly flow of blood from the genital tract of women
Puberty   the physical beginning of manhood and womanhood

The Human Anatomy

ON THE following pages are illustrations showing various parts of the human anatomy which are intended to familiarize the reader with terms often used by doctors in describing a disease.

These diagrams are made as simple as possible in order to promote a ready understanding. They do not include all the parts of the anatomy in the various segments shown.

It would be wise for every person to have some knowledge of the location and approximate shape of some of the important anatomical structures in order that he may better understand terms used in describing injury and disease.

CONTENTS

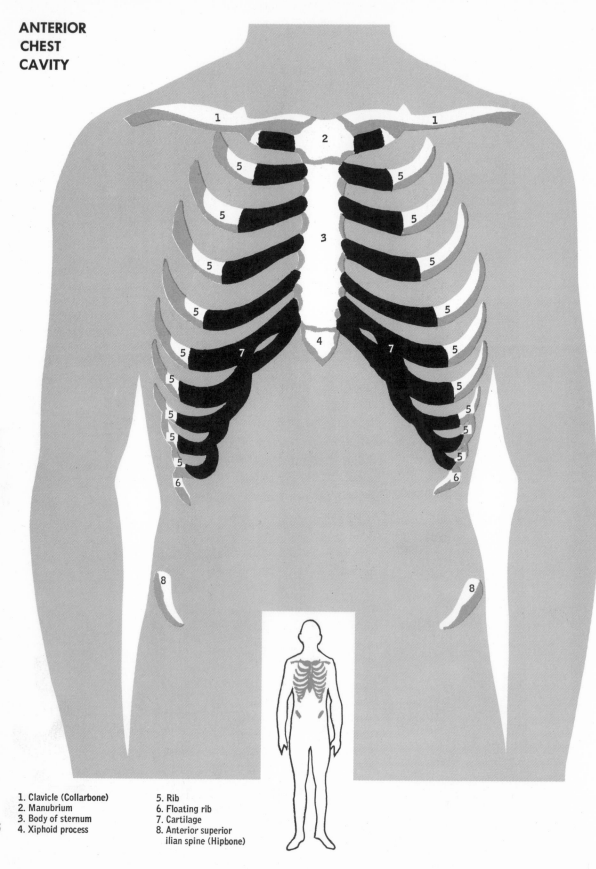

ANTERIOR CHEST CAVITY

1. Clavicle (Collarbone)
2. Manubrium
3. Body of sternum
4. Xiphoid process
5. Rib
6. Floating rib
7. Cartilage
8. Anterior superior ilian spine (Hipbone)

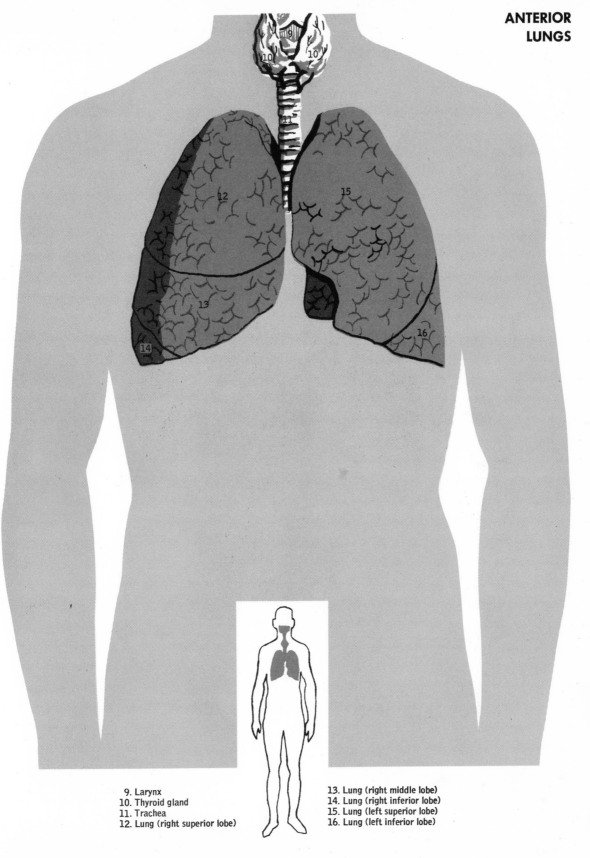

9. Larynx
10. Thyroid gland
11. Trachea
12. Lung (right superior lobe)

13. Lung (right middle lobe)
14. Lung (right inferior lobe)
15. Lung (left superior lobe)
16. Lung (left inferior lobe)

87

ANTERIOR LIVER AND SMALL INTESTINE

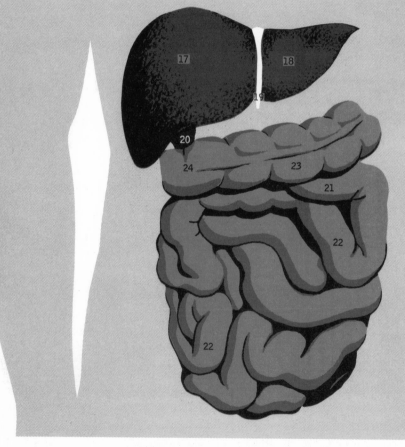

17. Liver (right lobe)
18. Liver (left lobe)
19. Falciform ligament
20. Gall bladder

21. Jejunum
22. Small intestine
23. Transverse colon
24. Taenia

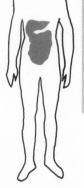

88

ANTERIOR STOMACH AND COLON

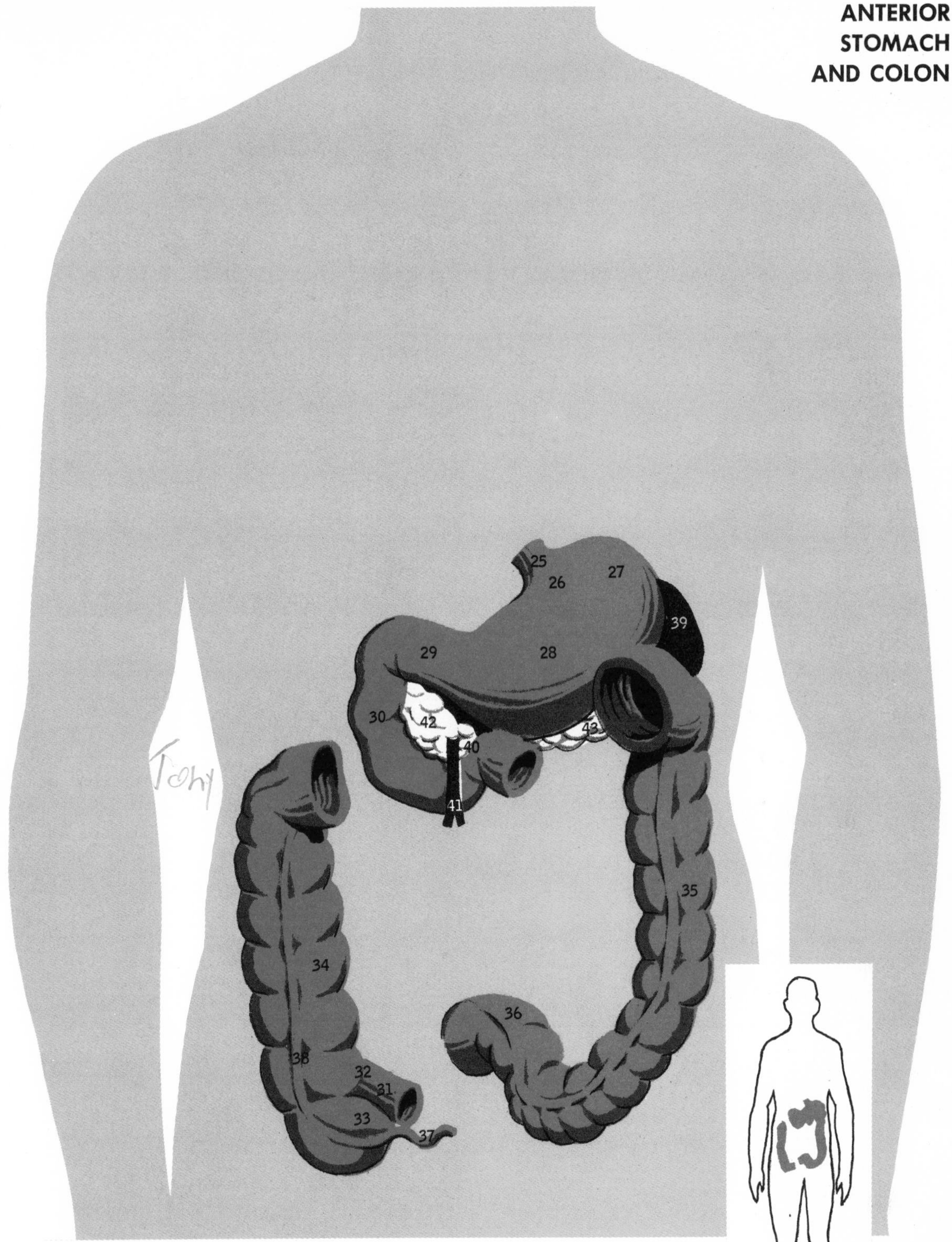

25. Esophagus
26. Stomach (cardia)
27. Stomach (fundus)
28. Stomach (body)
29. Stomach (pylorus)
30. Duodenum
31. Ileum
32. Ileocolic junction
33. Caecum
34. Ascending colon
35. Descending colon
36. Sigmoid colon
37. Vermiform appendix
38. Taenia coil
39. Spleen
40. Superior mesenteric artery
41. Superior mesenteric vein
42. Pancreas (head)
43. Pancreas (tail)

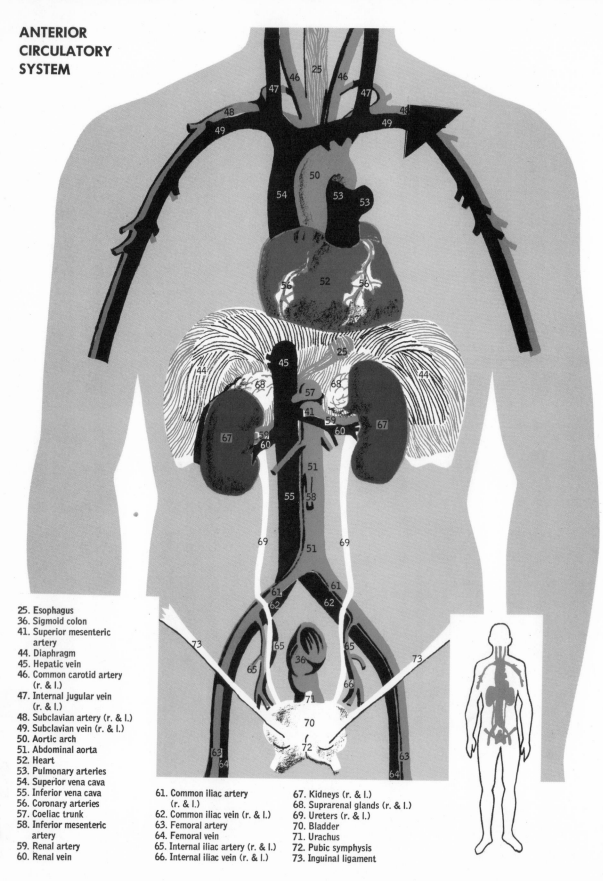

ANTERIOR CIRCULATORY SYSTEM

25. Esophagus
36. Sigmoid colon
41. Superior mesenteric artery
44. Diaphragm
45. Hepatic vein
46. Common carotid artery (r. & l.)
47. Internal jugular vein (r. & l.)
48. Subclavian artery (r. & l.)
49. Subclavian vein (r. & l.)
50. Aortic arch
51. Abdominal aorta
52. Heart
53. Pulmonary arteries
54. Superior vena cava
55. Inferior vena cava
56. Coronary arteries
57. Coeliac trunk
58. Inferior mesenteric artery
59. Renal artery
60. Renal vein

61. Common iliac artery (r. & l.)
62. Common iliac vein (r. & l.)
63. Femoral artery
64. Femoral vein
65. Internal iliac artery (r. & l.)
66. Internal iliac vein (r. & l.)

67. Kidneys (r. & l.)
68. Suprarenal glands (r. & l.)
69. Ureters (r. & l.)
70. Bladder
71. Urachus
72. Pubic symphysis
73. Inguinal ligament

90

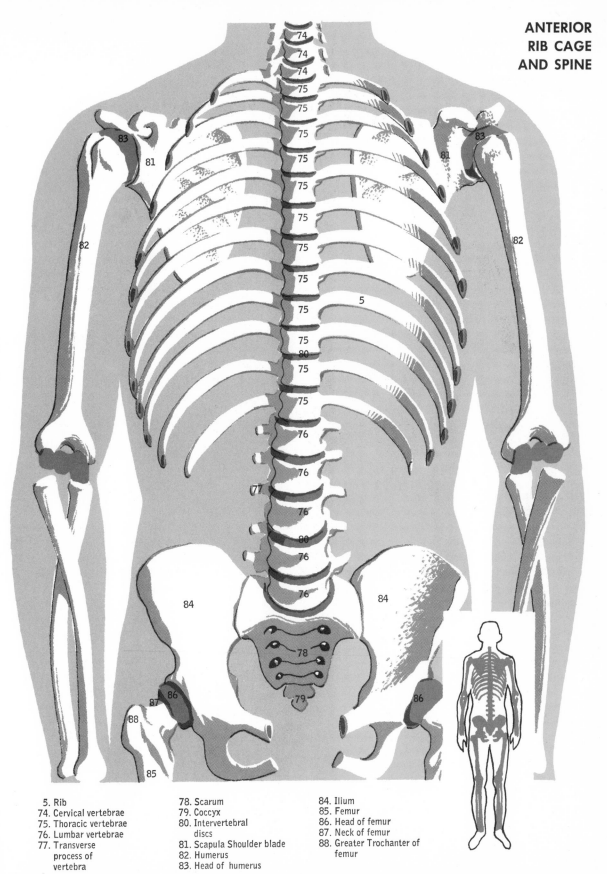

ANTERIOR
RIB CAGE
AND SPINE

5. Rib
74. Cervical vertebrae
75. Thoracic vertebrae
76. Lumbar vertebrae
77. Transverse
    process of
    vertebra

78. Scarum
79. Coccyx
80. Intervertebral
    discs
81. Scapula Shoulder blade
82. Humerus
83. Head of humerus

84. Ilium
85. Femur
86. Head of femur
87. Neck of femur
88. Greater Trochanter of
    femur

91

Index to
The Human Anatomy Section
Pages 86 to 91

PART 2

Diseases of Mankind

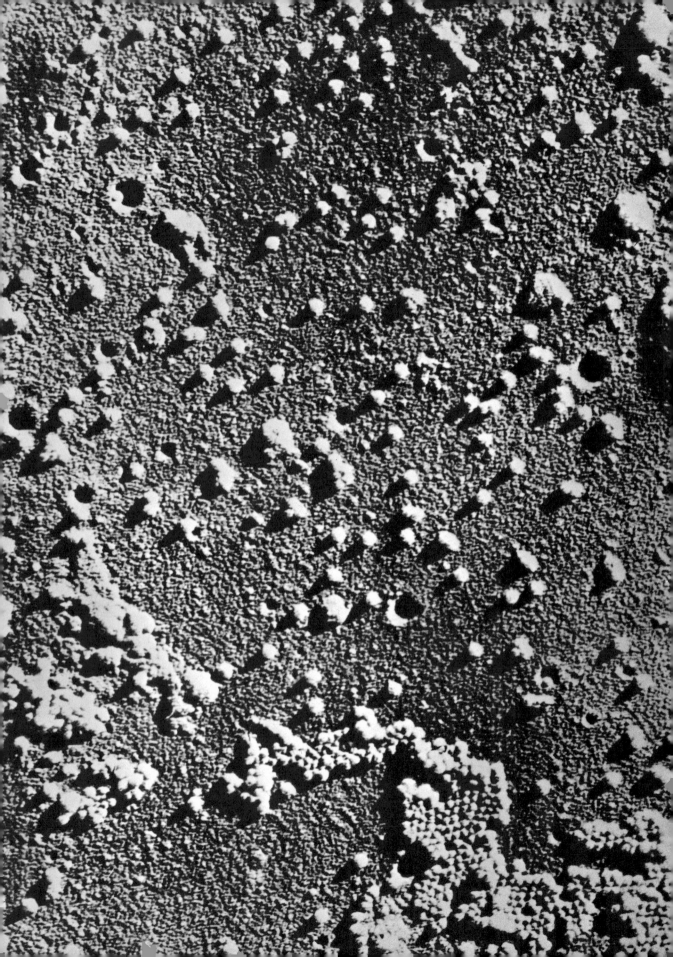

Chapter 6

Venereal Disease

THE MOST COMMON venereal diseases seen today are gonorrhea and syphilis. Other rare venereal conditions are chancroid—granuloma inquinale and lymphogranuloma venereum.

The fact that both gonorrhea and syphilis can be cured by treatment with penicillin has made the public more complacent, and these diseases are not dreaded as they were in the past. As a matter of fact, in spite of the availability of penicillin, there are still a great number of cases of gonorrhea and syphilis reported every year. The public should know that these diseases are still dangerous and should take precautions against contracting either of them. A knowledge of what causes these diseases may help in the all-out fight which is being made to eliminate them.

GONORRHEA IN THE MALE

Cause and Nature

This disease is caused by a diplococcus which is passed from person to person by direct contact. Despite the fact that cases of this disease have been blamed on dirty toilet seats, dirty towels, etc., it is usually passed on through sexual intercourse. The gonococcus is not very hardy and does not survive for any great length of time in an unfavorable environment—that is, outside the warmth and moisture of the human body.

Since gonorrhea is manifested differently in the male and female, the signs and symptoms will be discussed separately.

Signs and Symptoms

In the male, gonorrhea usually appears as a urethritis—that is, an infection of the canal inside the penis which runs from the urinary bladder to the end of the penis. It may appear from three to five days after exposure—that is, sexual intercourse with someone who has gonorrhea—and almost always appears within nine days, if it has been contracted.

Complications of gonorrhea may be gonorrheal arthritis or, in rare cases, gonorrheal myocarditis, which may be fatal if untreated.

The first sign is an itching at the end of

95

Strains of poliomyelitis virus magnified 77,000 times

the penis followed by a burning during urination and then by a discharge which rapidly becomes almost pure pus. A doctor can take a smear of this pus on a glass slide, stain it, and identify the gonococci under a microscope, thereby making the diagnosis. There are rare cases in which a non-specific or non-gonorrheal infection of the urethra causes a pus-like discharge. This type of discharge can be caused by injury, by chemical irritation, or by an infection due to some other bacteria. But it must be remembered that non-specific urethritis is extremely rare.

The gonorrheal urethritis may extend down into the prostate gland, into the vas deferens (the tubes that lead from the prostate to the testicles), and into the epididymis that is in the scrotum, causing swelling and pain there. In severe, untreated cases the vas deferens, or tubes which carry the spermatozoa from the testicle to the prostate, may become fibrotic or closed, thereby rendering the individual incapable of having children.

Treatment

Treatment since the advent of penicillin is comparatively simple. One injection of 300,000 units of penicillin will usually effect a cure. To be sure, four or five injections may be given. When the discharge ceases and there are negative smears on three successive days, the cure is considered complete. All of the patient's contacts should be watched closely and the patient should wash his hands after he handles his penis; for if the pus in transferred to his eyes he may develop a gonorrheal conjunctivitis which, if untreated, may lead to blindness. It is very poor treatment to plug the end of the urethra with cotton, as this prevents the pus from coming out. The patient should be put on a bland diet and should not use alcohol in any form, as this tends to irritate the urethra.

GLOSSARY

Arthritis   disease of the joints
Bland   not stimulating
Chancroid   veneral sore
Granuloma   growth containing granular tissue
Gonococcus   pus-producing bacteria
Gonorrhea   contagious disease; "clap"
Myocarditis   inflammation of the muscular part of the heart wall
Penis   the male organ
Syphilis   contagious disease

GONORRHEA IN THE FEMALE

Cause and Nature

The cause is the gonococcus, just as in the male, and the disease is usually contracted by sexual contact. The urinary symptoms are not as marked in the female, as there may be no burning during urination, and the smear taken from a female is not nearly so likely to be conclusive as that from the male. Therefore, the disease in a female may go undetected until one of many complications occurs. It is also possible for a female to pass the disease on to many persons without being aware of the fact that she has it.

The complications in the female may be many, ranging from an infected cyst on the vulva, to infection of the tubes—resulting in a pelvic abscess.

If a mother has gonorrhea when she is delivered of a child, the gonococci get into the eyes of the baby and may cause blindness. This has been the cause of a great many cases of blindness and has caused most states to pass a law making it obligatory for the doctor to have some drops of medicine (silver nitrate or penicillin) placed in the baby's eyes immediately after birth.

Little girls are quite susceptible to gonorrhea; when they sleep with their parents they may become infected if some of the pus comes in contact with their vagina.

Signs and Symptoms

In the female, symptoms of gonorrhea may be mild at first, but become very severe if untreated and undetected. The first sign may be an endocervicitis—that is, inflammation of the glands of the cervix. Salpingitis, or inflammation of the tubes, is quite common in untreated cases, and this may occur after a period. There is pain and fever with inflammation of the tubes, and this inflammation may progress into a pelvic abscess.

Treatment

This may be difficult, as in addition to penicillin injections there may have to be drainage of abscesses, such as Bartholin cysts and pelvic abscesses, before a cure is obtained.

GLOSSARY

Cyst   pouch or sac
Smear   a sample of mucus used for analysis under the microscope
Vulva   outer parts of female genital organs

CHANCROID

Cause and Nature

This venereal disease is characterized by a small ulcer on the penis which is caused by a bacteria known as Ducrey's bacillus. The ulcers may be multiple, and they are painful. They must be carefully differentiated from a chancre, as seen in syphilis.

This is done by examining smears under a microscope with what is known as a darkfield illumination. In addition to this, blood tests for syphilis should be taken every two weeks for four months.

Signs and Symptoms

The lesion usually begins as a pustule which ruptures, leaving a round ulcer with sharp, red undermined edges. There is no hardness around the ulcer as there is around a chancre. This hardness is called induration. These ulcers are painful, and there is usually a large, swollen lymph gland in the inguinal region which may contain pus.

Treatment

The treatment for this disease should consist of large doses of aureomycin. The suppurating lymph gland, or bubo, should never be incised, but should be aspirated with a sterile needle.

GLOSSARY

Aspirated   withdraw by suction
Chancre   sore with hard edges
Incised   cut into
Inguinal region   region of the groin
Penis   male organ
Suppurating   producing pus
Syphilis   contagious disease

LYMPHOGRANULOMA VENEREUM

Cause and Nature

This is a systemic disease caused by a virus, and is usually acquired by sexual intercourse.

Signs and Symptoms

The first sign is a small blister or pimple on the penis, which is not painful and will disappear. But within thirty days the lymph glands in the groin or inguinal region swell up and may become abscesses which drain from many openings.

Treatment

Aureomycin or terramycin given in large doses for about three weeks usually will clear up the condition. The bubo, or lymph gland containing pus, should not be incised.

GRANULOMA INGUINALE

Cause and Nature

This condition is caused by an organism known as a Donovan body. It spreads slowly and usually involves the groin.

Signs and Symptoms

The first lesion is in the groin. It gradually becomes an ulcer with a red granular base. This ulcer bleeds easily. Scarrings may eventually occur.

Treatment

Streptomycin by injection and aureomycin by mouth, given in adequate doses should clear up most cases.

SYPHILIS

Cause and Nature

Syphilis is one of the most dreaded of all diseases. It is caused by a spirochete and is acquired nearly always by direct contact with an open sore, as the spirochete which causes the disease dies almost immediately when it becomes dry. Hence it does not survive long after leaving the body. These open sores which harbor the spirochete are usually on the genitals, the penis of a man or the vagina of a woman. The primary sore, or chancre, as it is called, can be on any part of the body. The lips are often involved, and sometimes the sores are seen on the fingers. This disease has been called "the great imitator," because it can imitate almost any disease. If it is not diagnosed and treated properly it can lead to many severe complications.

Syphilis can be passed from the mother who has it to her unborn baby. Hence, a child may acquire congenital syphilis.

The fact that penicillin is almost a specific cure for syphilis has caused a great decrease in the number of cases in recent years; but the disease is still present and should be watched for carefully.

Signs and Symptoms

The manifestations of syphilis should be divided into various stages of the disease in order to understand them more clearly. These stages may be called:

1. Early syphilis
2. Latent syphilis
3. Late syphilis

Early syphilis. The first sign is the development of a small sore that is usually painless and is usually in the form of an open sore that is firm around its borders. This is called a chancre and may be seen on any part of the body where contact has been made with an open sore containing spirochetes—usually on the penis, vagina, lips, or fingers. There may be, and usually is, an enlarged lymph gland in the region of the chancre.

The chancre, or sore, usually appears three weeks to a month after the infection has taken place. In the meantime, the spirochete has entered the body almost on the moment of contact and has spread throughout the body.

The chancre should be examined and fluid from it looked at under a special microscope to see if spirochetes are present. The blood should also be tested, as a positive blood test usually develops about thirty-five days after infection. If untreated, the primary sore or chancre usually disappears in two to six weeks.

About six weeks after the appearance of the chancre, a rash usually appears over the entire body. The chief characteristic of this rash is that it never itches and may be so light as to escape notice. There may be a general feeling of malaise, headache, sore throat, etc. All of these symptoms and signs disappear, then another rash may appear which is darker and more generalized than the first. It may be seen on the palms of the hands and soles of the feet. Again, there is no itching. Another sign which may appear now is the so-called mucous patch which appears on the throat or in the mouth.

All of these early lesions have a great number of spirochetes in them and may be highly contagious. This disease should be detected early by the signs and symptoms, by searching for the spirochete, and by blood tests. After the diagnosis is made, the disease should be treated thoroughly, and great care taken to prevent its being spread to other people.

Latent syphilis. After the early signs and symptoms disappear, which they will do even without treatment, the disease may go into a quiescent stage which may last from one year up to twenty-five years. During this period there is no visible sign of the disease and it is not contagious, but the blood remains highly positive for syphilis. This is the stage that is usually detected by routine blood tests.

Late syphilis. after a period the organisms finally settle in some organ of the body, and if the patient has had no treatment or insufficient treatment, the terrible results of syphilis become evident. Some patients may become blind, others may have tabes dorsalis (inability to control their legs); others may have paresis (it has been called softening of the brain), in which the patient becomes mentally ill. There are many other manifestations—the heart may be affected or the aorta, causing an aneurysm of the aorta. Any of these may be fatal. As stated above, syphilis may imitate almost any other disease.

Treatment

Vigorous and adequate treatment with penicillin will usually cure syphilis. The stage in which the diagnosis is made will determine the amount of penicillin necessary and the length of time needed to accomplish a cure.

Repeated blood tests and spinal fluid tests should be performed, and when these tests continue to be negative for one year, the patient may be said to be cured.

GLOSSARY

Aneurysm   abnormal enlargement of blood vessel
Aorta   main artery of body
Chancre   sore
Congenital   born with
Genitals   organs of reproduction
Latent   lying hidden or concealed
Penis   the male organ
Primary   first in development
Quiescent   not active
Spirochete   a bacteria or cause of disease
Systemic   involving the whole body
Vagina   a female organ
Virus   submicroscopic infectious agent

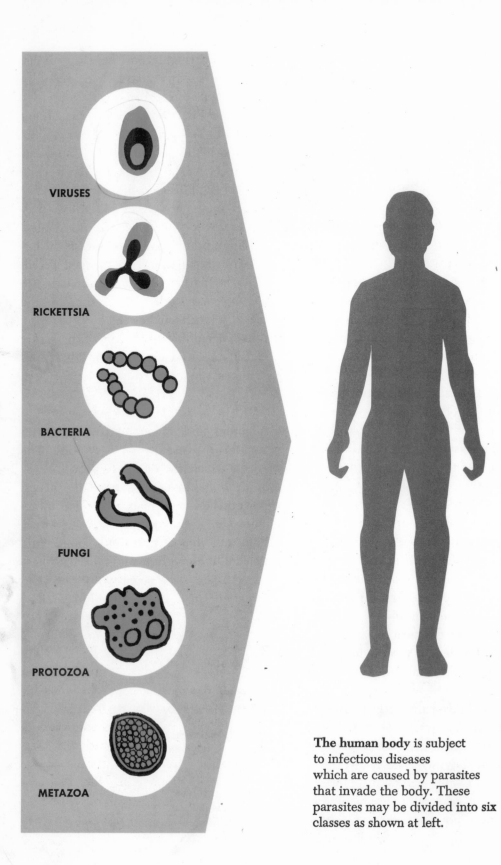

VIRUSES

RICKETTSIA

BACTERIA

FUNGI

PROTOZOA

METAZOA

The human body is subject
to infectious diseases
which are caused by parasites
that invade the body. These
parasites may be divided into six
classes as shown at left.

Chapter 7

Infectious Diseases

One of the things a young doctor learns in medical school is that as far as the human body and disease are concerned, there is no such thing as always or never. In other words, each disease described here will be outlined as it is usually seen, and the treatment recommended will be that which most generally produces favorable results. It cannot be emphasized too strongly that a doctor should be called if there is any doubt about the diagnosis of the disease, or if early treatment does not produce the desired results.

In many cases, self-treatment is not to be relied upon and, indeed, may be dangerous. If, therefore, recovery is not prompt, always call a doctor.

In considering the common acute infectious diseases, an effort has been made to follow an outline, which is about the same in most cases. A sincere attempt has been made to present material briefly, in order that in cases of emergency or stress the desired information can be obtained promptly.

Remember that the symptoms of infectious diseases will vary from person to person. It is therefore safer to consult your family doctor.

HEALTH AND DISEASE

Health may be defined as a normal condition of body and mind. This state of health is achieved by the ability a person may have to live in harmony with his surroundings. Health of mind depends upon a person's normal adaptation to the members of his family, his friends, and other people with whom he comes in contact, and the way in which he meets the stresses and strains to which he is exposed.

Health of body may depend upon the type of body a person inherits from his parents, the way in which he takes care of that body, and his ability to live in harmony with the forces of nature with which he comes in contact.

Disease is defined as any departure from the state of health and one of the most important classes of disease are infectious diseases. An infectious disease is one which is caused by parasites which invade the body and cause a disturbance of the normal body functions. A contagious disease is one that may be passed from one person to another, but all infectious diseases are not

101

contagious, for some of them may be contracted from animals or insects. It may be stated that all contagious diseases are infectious diseases, but all infectious diseases are not contagious.

The parasites which cause infectious diseases may be divided into six different classes, according to their size and other structural differences, and the diseases which they cause differ widely in their characteristics. These classes are called viruses, rickettsia, bacteria, fungi, protozoa and metazoa.

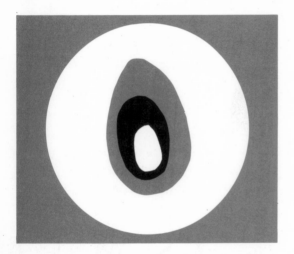

The smallest infectious agent is called a virus, and this microorganism is so small that it can be seen only with the very highest powered microscope, i.e., the electron microscope. There are about fifty different diseases that are known to be caused by viruses, and viruses are presumed to be the causative agent of many other diseases although absolute proof is lacking. Among the more common diseases caused by viruses are the common cold, influenza, herpes simplex or cold sores, herpes zoster, infectious hepatitis, infectious mononeucleosis, measles, mumps, rabies, warts, chickenpox, smallpox, and poliomyelitis.

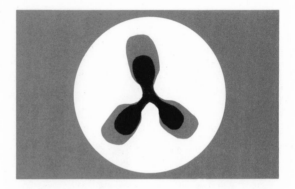

The next infectious agent in size to the virus is called rickettsia, after the man who discovered them, Dr. Ricketts. These rickettsia cause serious diseases and the common ones are typhus fever and Rocky Mountain spotted fever.

Next in size and perhaps the most important group are the bacteria. There are three main types of bacteria which may cause disease.

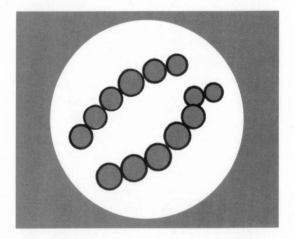

I. The cocci are small round bodies. They may occur in strings, streptococci; in groups, staphylococci; and in pairs, as pneumococci and gonococci. These small bacteria cause hundreds of different diseases, such as boils, pneumonia, scarlet fever, gonorrhea and meningococcal meningitis.

II. Many bacteria are shaped like rods. Among these the common ones are the tubercle bacillus which causes tuberculosis, typhoid bacillus, leprosy, bacillary dysentery, plague, tularemia, glanders, anthrax, gas gangrene, cholera, and other diseases almost too numerous to name.

III. The third type of bacteria is the spirochete. These are spiral shaped, like a cork screw. The most common disease caused by a spirochete is syphilis. Another disease caused by a combination of spirochetes and bacteria is known as trench mouth.

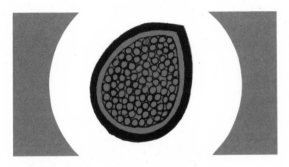

The next class of infectious agents are called fungi. Some of the well-known diseases caused by a fungus are athlete's foot, monilia infections, actinomycosis, blastomycosis, histoplasmosis, and many others. These diseases caused by fungi are classified as the mycoses.

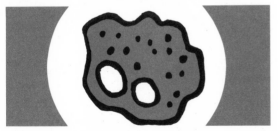

The next group of infectious agents are called the protozoa. These are one-celled organisms which cause such diseases as amebiasis and malaria.

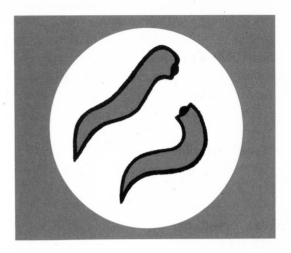

The metazoa are invertebrate animals made up of many cells and they are responsible for many infectious diseases. These metazoa can be divided into about four main groups:

1. The Platyhelminthes or flat worms
   a. tapeworms (Trematoda)
   b. flukes (Cestoda)
2. Nemathelminthes or roundworms
3. Hirudinea or leeches
4. Arthropoda or insects

The infections caused by the worms are too numerous to name, but some of them are very common, such as trichinosis (sometimes called porkworm disease), hookworms, pinworms, and tapeworms. Some of the insects causing diseases are scabies or itchmite, lice or pediculosis, fleas, chiggers, maggots, scorpions, centipedes, wasps, ticks, and ants.

All of the agents which may cause infectious disease—the viruses, rickettsia, bacteria, fungi, protozoa and metazoa—have one thing in common. They are living organisms and require food and the proper environment in which to live. Sometimes when they find conditions just right in the human body, they may multiply very rapidly causing serious illness or death.

On the other hand, we must realize that we are living in a world with these organisms. They surround us and live in our bodies without doing any harm until conditions become just right. Our bodies are covered with bacteria, our throats always have in them a few staphylococci and streptococci which ordinarily do no harm.

Some of these organisms do not live in animal or human flesh at all; they can exist only on dead matter.

The organisms that are capable of causing disease in mankind are called pathogens, while those which are found only on dead matter are called saprogens.

Some pathogens may cause disease by passing from person to person as in the case of contagious diseases—measles, for instance.

When an organism is living in an animal, this animal is called a host. Other types of organisms do not pass directly from man to man, but must go through an intermediary host, as in the case of malaria. This organism goes from a man with malaria to a mosquito that bites him, and after being in the mosquito for some time, the organisms are passed on to another man and he comes down with malaria. This information is useful, for in order to stop the spread of malaria, all that needs to be done is to do away with the intermediary host or mosquito.

As a matter of fact, bacteria help to digest our food and they work in many ways to make it possible for us to live. The reason why the pathogens become dangerous to us is that they may suddenly develop great strength and invasive powers and they invade our bodies when our resistance is low or not up to par.

Resistance to this invasion of organisms is sometimes called immunity. It may be that we inherit immunity to certain diseases. For example, measles is not considered a dangerous disease in the United States because for generations nearly everyone has had measles and our bodies have built up a resistance or immunity to it. But, if measles were introduced on one of the South Sea Islands, where it had never been seen, half the people on the island might die of the disease.

Another example of the increase in virulence or strength in infectious organisms may be seen in our epidemics of influenza. One form of influenza may occur in occasional mild cases for about three successive years and then we can expect an epidemic in which thousands of cases will occur. This same influenza will then quiet down and almost disappear for another three years, only to flare up again. No one knows just why this increase in virulence or invasive strength occurs.

Knowing these things about the causes of infectious diseases, we should do all within our power to escape them. We should keep our bodies strong and healthy by getting enough rest and a good diet. We should take advantage of all forms of prevention, such as vaccination against smallpox and immunization against poliomyelitis.

Last of all, we should avoid contact with known cases of contagious disease, and if we do contract a disease a doctor should be consulted early so he can start the proper treatment.

Man is subject to many diseases in addition to the ones caused by the parasites described above. He may suffer from forces in his environment such as changes in the weather, or from chemical injuries, or from deficiencies in his diet.

Then, there is that large group of diseases called the degenerative diseases that are caused by a breaking down of some part of the body. An example of this is the disease called arteriosclerosis.

THE COMMON COLD

Cause and Nature

Definite cause of the common cold has not been determined. There is much evidence to prove that it may be caused by a virus or several viruses.

New vaccines made from various live attenuated or weakened viruses have been used on human subjects with some success and we may be nearing a point where all of us who want to may be vaccinated against the common cold.

This disease is more common than all other diseases of man combined. In mild, uncomplicated cases, the course is from four to seven days. There may be all degrees of severity, and children are more susceptible than grown people. Uncomplicated cases usually affect the upper respiratory tract only. Predisposing factors include fatigue, long exposure to damp and cold, poor ventilation, and malnutrition.

The incubation period is from twelve hours to four days following exposure.

Signs and Symptoms

The earliest symptom is usually a scratchy or burning sensation in the throat or behind the nose. A watery nasal discharge appears. The nose becomes stuffy and there may be sneezing. The throat may be sore and red. A cough may appear and there is a general feeling of not being up to par. There may be a mild aching in the back and extremities. Headache is often present. The sense of smell is impaired and there is sometimes a loss of appetite.

As the disease progresses the nasal discharge becomes thick and yellow. Cold sores sometimes appear. There may be a slight rise in the temperature—100 to 102.

Complications

The most frequent complications are caused by the invasion of bacteria—so-called secondary infections. This may be noted in the form of bronchitis, sinus infections, and middle ear infections.

Treatment

There is no specific medication. Penicillin and antibiotics do not help and should not be used unless complications occur. Rest is the single most important factor in treatment. In order to rest, the patient should be comfortable. Aspirin, ten grains three times a day, will help relieve the pain.

A light diet. Keep the bowels open. Force fluids and fruit juices.

It is thought that the watery discharge from the nose is an allergic reaction to the invading organism. Therefore, at the first sign of a cold it is wise to take one of the antihistaminic drugs such as Co-Pyronil, one capsule, three times a day, for three days.

Bed rest is imperative when fever is present. The room should be kept warm, especially at night, and the air should be moist. A steam kettle on the stove or a vaporizer in the room will keep the air moist.

If the cough is troublesome, a cough syrup, such as syrup of Hycodan for adults and Cheracol for children, is good.

The prolonged use of nose drops is not advisable and thought to do more harm than good.

In giving children aspirin, it is very important never to give over one grain for each year of age. For example, at two and a half years, the child can have one-half of a five-grain aspirin tablet or two, one-grain baby aspirin tablets.

An attempt should be made to protect others, particularly children and sick people, from exposure to nasal discharge or cough spray, as in some cases a cold can be transmitted from one person to another.

GLOSSARY

Allergic reaction   itching or swelling; breaking out in hives or rash
Bacteria   germs
Bronchitis   inflammation of bronchial tubes
Incubation   time between exposure to disease and the illness
Respiratory tract   organs for breathing
Transmitted   passed from one person to another
Vaporizer   steam kettle

SINUS TROUBLE

Cause and Nature

There is probably no other complaint which is heard more often by doctors than "sinus trouble," and by far the majority of people who say and actually believe that they have sinus trouble do not have that at all. This is because there are so many symptoms which may be experienced around the upper respiratory system, the mouth, nose, and throat, which are caused by many different conditions which are not related to the sinuses at all. It is easy to blame all of these symptoms on "sinus trouble," and unfortunately many doctors have heard patients make this statement so often that they finally despair of being able to make the patient understand that his symptoms are not caused by sinus trouble.

The sinuses are cavities or caves in the bone which are found on each side of the nose, in the cheek bone, in the forehead or frontal bones of the skull, and in the bones behind the nose.

These are called paranasal sinuses because they are all lined by mucous membranes which extend directly from the nose and form a lining for these cavities. This is the same tissue that lines the nose or an extension of it, and any unusual condition that affects the upper air passages may or may not cause infection of the sinuses.

It is not particularly important whether or not these symptoms are caused by "sinus trouble" as long as they are understood. The air passages through the nose perform very important functions. For instance, the sense of smell and the sense of taste (which is closely related to the sense of smell) can be damaged if the nasal or nose passages aren't healthy. The mucous membrane of the nose is lined with very fine hair called cilia. These hairs wave all the time and they wave in the direction of the outlet of the nose. Thus the nose acts as a filter of the air and picks up small particles of dust, which are carried to the outside by the waving

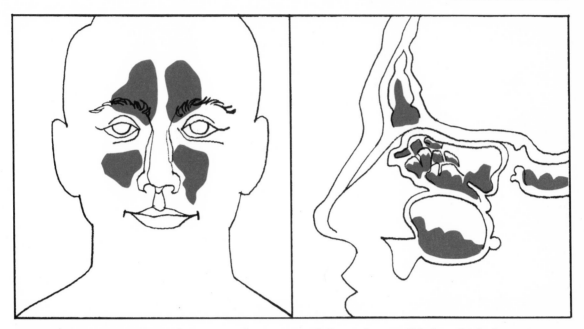

Infection may spread from the nose to the sinuses. If the outlet, small holes which drain sinus are swollen closed, fluid and pus gathers in sinus causing pain.

hair or cilia. The nose also air conditions the air which is breathed in and warms it up before it reaches the lungs. The mucous membranes lining the nose always secrete a fluid which is sticky and helps trap bacteria and dust particles which are in the air. This fluid is capable of killing bacteria; hence, the nose is a protector of the body. Last but not least, the nose or nasal passages form an airway through which we breathe most of the air which is used by the body. Any of us who has a stopped-up nose and must breathe through the mouth knows how important this function is.

Anything which interferes with the above functions of the nasal passages has been referred to as sinus trouble when, as often as not, the sinuses are not irritated at all.

Signs and Symptoms

Pain is one of the most important of all symptoms, and in acute sinusitis the pain is usually severe. This results from the lining of the maxillary sinus (the one in the cheek at the side of the nose) becoming infected, swollen, and inflamed. Pus is formed and cannot drain out through the small opening from the sinus to the nose, and pressure builds up, causing pain. It is not easy to confuse this pain with any other type of pain and it may be accompanied by fever.

The mucous membranes of the nose may swell up because of allergy, as in the case of "hay fever," which causes the nose to run. This very seldom causes sinus trouble.

Any infection in the nasal cavities, such as a cold or any irritation by smoke from cigarettes or fire, may cause inflammation of the nasal passages which may be acute or chronic.

The nose may be easily stopped up because of a crooked nasal septum—that is, the partition which runs down through the middle of the nose. If it is pushed over to one side, that side will be difficult to breathe through. Nasal polyps also cause obstruction to breathing.

The posterior nasal drip or some phlegm which may drip down the back of the throat from the nose is often spoken of as sinus trouble, when actually the sinuses may not be involved at all. The condition may be caused simply by an infection, acute or chronic, of the nasal mucous membrane.

Treatment

In real sinus trouble with acute pain, the object of treatment is to secure drainage of the sinuses. This is done by using antibiotics or drugs to kill the infection, and decongestant tablets (taken by mouth) that shrink the mucous membranes, which may be swollen. An operation may be performed to drain the sinuses. Sometimes this operation is simply the insertion of a needle into the sinus to wash it out, but in very bad cases, the floor or wall of the sinus must be operated on to form a window. Since the advent of antibiotics to kill infections, very few sinuses have to be operated on, and this has become a rare operation.

Too frequent use of nose drops is definitely to be frowned upon because the repeated use of nose drops, especially in young children, may hinder the natural defenses of the mucous membranes of the nose and stop the cilia from waving. Indeed after the initial shrinking effect that nose drops are supposed to have, they may actually cause the mucous membrane to swell more if used over a long period. So do not be fooled by advertisements for nose drops because the too frequent use of this method may damage the nasal passages. If you think you have sinus trouble it is best to see a good doctor.

GLOSSARY

Cilia   hair
Maxillary sinus   sinus in cheek on side of nose
Mucous membrane   soft, moist lining of nasal passages and throat
Nasal polyps   tumors or growth from mucous membrane
Septum   division between the two nasal passages
Sinusitis   inflammation of a sinus

CHICKENPOX

(Varicella)

Cause and Nature

Chickenpox is caused by a virus found in the blisters or lesions on the skin. It is transmitted by direct contact with the sick person or with objects which have the live organisms on them. One attack confers permanent immunity. The incubation period (between time of exposure and the first appearance of symptoms) is 15 to 21 days.

Signs and Symptoms

The onset is usually abrupt, with appearance of red spots or pimples. The rash develops over trunk, scalp, face, and extremities, in this sequence, and there may be a slight fever.

Large, dimpled blisters may appear in some, but not all, of the red spots. One of the features of the rash which helps to identify the disease is that the lesions seem to be all different sizes appearing at one time—everything from a small red spot to a pimple, to a blister containing pus. The lesions may be in the mouth, on the palms of the hands, and on the soles of the feet.

The blisters dry up and form crusts. These may itch, and if scratched will become secondarily infected and cause small scars.

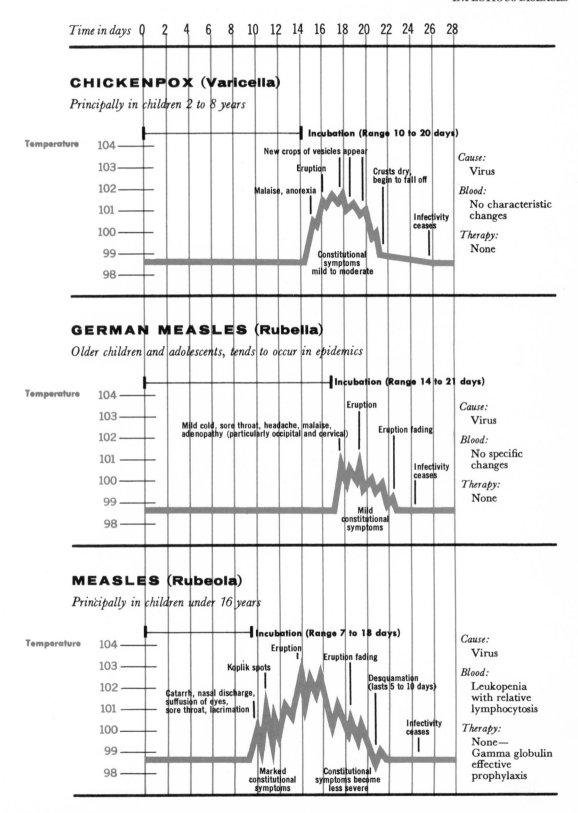

CHICKENPOX (Varicella)

Principally in children 2 to 8 years

Temperature

Incubation (Range 10 to 20 days)

New crops of vesicles appear

Eruption

Crusts dry, begin to fall off

Malaise, anorexia

Infectivity ceases

Constitutional symptoms mild to moderate

Cause: Virus

Blood: No characteristic changes

Therapy: None

GERMAN MEASLES (Rubella)

Older children and adolescents, tends to occur in epidemics

Temperature

Incubation (Range 14 to 21 days)

Eruption

Mild cold, sore throat, headache, malaise, adenopathy (particularly occipital and cervical)

Eruption fading

Infectivity ceases

Mild constitutional symptoms

Cause: Virus

Blood: No specific changes

Therapy: None

MEASLES (Rubeola)

Principally in children under 16 years

Temperature

Incubation (Range 7 to 18 days)

Eruption

Koplik spots

Eruption fading

Desquamation (lasts 5 to 10 days)

Catarrh, nasal discharge, suffusion of eyes, sore throat, lacrimation

Infectivity ceases

Marked constitutional symptoms

Constitutional symptoms become less severe

Cause: Virus

Blood: Leukopenia with relative lymphocytosis

Therapy: None— Gamma globulin effective prophylaxis

Time in days 0 2 4 6 8 10 12 14 16 18 20 22 24 26 28

Treatment

All articles in contact with patient should be sterilized.

Isolation is maintained for ten days, or until all crusts have disappeared.

Bed rest and restraint from scratching.

Warm soda baths sometimes help itching, as does chlortrimeton (four milligrams, twice a day).

Aspirin will make patient more comfortable.

There is no specific medicine.

Cut fingernails short and keep patient's hands clean to lessen chance of secondary infection from scratching lesions.

Calamine lotion may be used on lesions which become troublesome.

Diet

Milk and bland diet.

GLOSSARY

Isolation   to place a person apart from others to prevent spreading a disease
Lesions   sores or abnormal spots
Sequence   the order in which the disease progresses

GERMAN MEASLES

(Rubella)

Cause and Nature

The cause is a virus found in secretions of the nose and mouth. It is transmitted by direct contact, and the incubation period is 14 to 21 days. Babies up to six months have a good immunity. It is most contagious a day or two before the rash appears.

There is a short period of illness before the rash appears—usually an upper respiratory catarrh—and the lymph glands on the back of the neck become swollen.

One attack usually confers immunity for life.

Signs and Symptoms

The onset is sudden, with a fine red rash, slightly raised, varying in size from a pin head to a small pea. The lesions may be discrete (by themselves), or confluent (running together).

The rash first appears on face or neck, or behind the ears. Within a day, the rash usually extends over the entire body.

Treatment

Patient is kept in isolation and in bed.
Aspirin.
Force fluids and orange juice or other fruit juices.
Quarantine should be observed for seven days.

Pregnancy

German measles contracted by a mother in her first three months of pregnancy quite often will cause abnormalities in the baby. It is very important for an expectant mother who is exposed to measles to see her doctor for injections of gamma globulin, which will offer passive protection against measles.

To prevent this situation from arising, it is thought wise today to allow young girls to contract measles in order to acquire immunity. A vaccine against German measles has been developed and used in New York City with great success. This vaccine, made from a live attenuated or weakened virus, when it becomes available to the public will greatly diminish the number of babies who are born with deformities caused by the mother contracting German measles during pregnancy.

MEASLES

(Rubeola)

Cause and Nature

This is a serious disease and is highly contagious. It is one of the most common infectious diseases. The cause is a virus found in the nasal secretions. The greatest period of infectivity is during the catarrhal period before the rash reaches its height. It is passed from person to person by direct contact. One attack gives lifelong immunity.

Infants usually have fairly good immunity during the first six months of life, but should not be exposed to the disease. All babies should be vaccinated against measles beginning when they are nine months old.

A live attenuated or weakened vaccine should be used.

Children exposed to the disease may sometimes have the attack modified or made less severe by an injection of gamma globulin.

The incubation period, that is the time between exposure and the first appearance of the symptoms, may be nine to sixteen days.

Signs and Symptoms

The early symptoms resemble those of a common cold. These may include a mild fever, headache, vomiting, loss of appetite, and sometimes diarrhea. The eyes become red. There is sneezing, nasal discharge, and a dry hard cough. The eyes are sensitive to light, and lacrimation (tears) is present. The swollen face and watering eyes give a characteristic picture. On the second or third day, red spots with white centers may appear on the inside of the cheeks (Koplik's spots).

The invasion period lasts three or four days. By the third or fourth day the rash appears. It appears first on the scalp, temple, or behind the ears and also on the neck, then covers the entire body except the extremities. Later, the extremities are covered even to the soles of the feet. This occurs about thirty-six hours after the first appearance of the rash. The fever is now higher.

The rash begins to fade after about two days and the improvement in general condition is rapid. The rash usually begins to disappear after five days. The lesions are small pink, raised spots which afterwards darken in color. The individual spots may be discrete (separate), or confluent (running together), and the spots feel nodular.

Sometimes a warm bath will hasten the appearance of the rash.

A brownish pigmentation may remain after the rash disappears, and then a scaling will begin on the neck, face, and thighs.

Treatment

Rest in bed during fever.

Room should be shaded, but does not have to be dark.

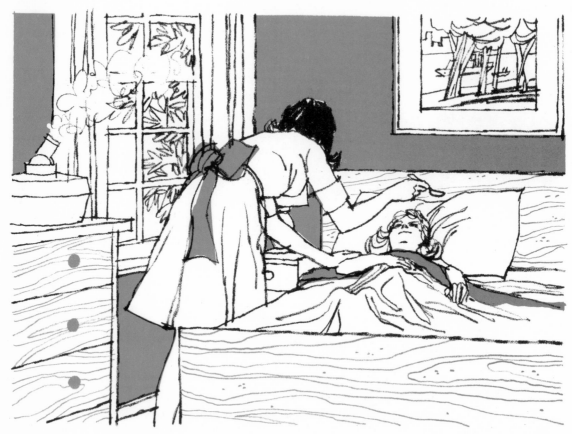

Mother's care, tender and loving. The medicine and the atomizer for moisture will work wonders.

Fluid and soft diet while fever lasts.

Wash eyes with warm water.

Cough. The room atmosphere should be kept moist by steam kettle or vaporizer. A cough syrup containing codeine should be given—one teaspoon every four hours.

A daily sponge bath is soothing.

Aspirin—one grain for each year of age up to five grains can be given three or four times a day for general comfort.

Complications

Middle ear disease, or otitis media, characterized by pain in ear and persistent fever.

Bronchopneumonia.

These should be treated by a physician.

GLOSSARY

Diarrhea   liquid discharge from bowels

Koplik's spots   red spots found in mouth of patient with measles

Nasal secretion   discharge from nose

Nodular   bumpy

Otitis media   middle ear infection

Pigmentation   brown spots found on skin

Scaling   peeling

Vaporizer   a device to produce steam for easier breathing

WHOOPING COUGH

(Pertussis)

Cause and Nature

The cause is the pertussis bacillus. The disease is characterized by spasmodic attacks of coughing which may end in a typical whoop.

This disease is especially hard on babies less than one year old. It can be prevented, or at least modified, by having early immunization starting at age three months, with injections of diphtheria-pertussis-tetanus vaccine.

One attack protects for a lifetime.

The incubation period is seven to fourteen days.

Signs and Symptoms

A typical case has three stages: catarrhal, paroxysmal, and convalescent.

1. The catarrhal stage, with running nose, sneezing, and a cough that is hard and dry, and especially bad at night. This stage may last about two weeks.

2. The paroxysmal stage. Characterized by spells of explosive coughing followed by long-drawn inspiration, and crowing sound or whoop. This spell of coughing is usually terminated by raising a thick, ropy plug of mucus. Vomiting may occur. This stage usually lasts about four weeks.

3. The convalescent stage is more like a regular bronchitis and may last about three weeks, gradually disappearing.

Complications

Bronchopneumonia in younger children. Ear infections.

Vomiting after a paroxysm. If child loses a meal, it should be fed again. Thick foods are retained better than fluids.

Treatment

See a doctor, if possible.

Antibiotics such as penicillin will help control secondary invaders and help prevent complications.

Fresh air and room temperature 70 to 75 degrees.

Codeine and phenobarbital sometimes will help control paroxysms.

Frequent small feedings.

A boosting dose of vaccine will sometimes help a person who has been vaccinated previously.

GLOSSARY

Bacillus organism or germ
Catarrhal pertaining to discharge from inflamed mucous membrane
Convalescence period of recovery
Immunization protection from disease produced by use of serum or vaccine
Inspiration breathing in
Modify change
Paroxysm coughing seizure
Pertussis whooping cough

MUMPS

Cause and Nature

This is an infection of the salivary glands. The cause is a virus found in the saliva of infected persons. Incubation period is twelve to twenty-one days.

Transmitted by contact with secretions of infected persons, or soiled articles.

May be communicated until swelling disappears from glands.

One attack gives immunity for life. A person may, however, have mumps on one side only and subsequently have them on the other side. This is very rare.

A new vaccine against mumps is being worked on but it has not yet been perfected.

Signs and Symptoms

Pain and stiffness in angle of jaw in front of ears.

Swelling in region of parotid glands in front of ears, on side of face. The lobe of the ear is usually about the center of the swelling after it is fully developed.

Fever and general malaise.

Swelling goes down in about ten to fourteen days.

Treatment

Patient should be isolated.

Keep in bed in a warm room with fresh air.

Aspirin may be given for comfort.

To prevent orchitis, or involvement of testes, male patients over twelve years should have five milligrams stilbestrol daily for about three weeks.

Mouth hygiene is important.

Adults usually kept in bed for two weeks to prevent complications.

Complications

In women, rarely, the ovaries are involved. In males, the testes are sometimes involved. This rarely occurs under the age of ten. The testicular involvement rarely results in impotence or sterility. Scrotum and testes should be supported on a pillow. Aspirin given for comfort and stilbestrol given to modify the attack and make it lighter. Sometimes an ice bag or heat to testes will make patient more comfortable.

GLOSSARY

Hygiene   cleanliness; sanitary habits
Impotence   inability to obtain an erection
Incubation   time between exposure to disease and the illness
Malaise   lack of energy; feeling bad all over
Ovaries   female reproducing organs
Parotid glands   glands just in front of ears
Saliva   secretion in mouth
Scrotum   the male pouch containing the testes
Testes   male reproductive organs

POLIOMYELITIS

(Infantile Paralysis)

Cause and Nature

An acute infection caused by a virus. The principal mode of dissemination is not known, but human carriers are probably an important source of infection. This disease is most prevalent during the late spring, summer, and early fall.

One attack may offer lifetime immunity to the type of virus causing the attack. The attacks vary from a very mild form with no aftereffects to a more severe form, with paralysis of muscles.

The introduction of Salk vaccine has made it possible to protect children by the injection of the vaccine on four different occasions. The vaccine is harmless and has proven to have a high percentage of protection. After the first injection, 60 percent protection has been noted; after two injections, 75 percent; and after three injections, as high as 90 percent. There have been no known deaths among children who have had four injections.

Recently, the Sabin oral vaccine has come into general use. This vaccine is so effective and so easily administered that the Salk injections are very seldom used now. (See *Newer Vaccines*.)

Since this disease attacks people up to forty years of age, and even on rare occasions after that, it is to be devoutly hoped that every person up to forty years of age will be immunized against polio, and in that way the disease, which has caused so much disability and suffering, will be almost completely wiped out—just as diphtheria has been—by vaccination.

Everyone up to forty years of age should be immunized against poliomyelitis.

Chilling, overexertion, crowds, and contact with ill persons should be avoided during epidemics.

Signs and Symptoms

A mild attack may show headache, fever, generalized aches and pains, vomiting, and irritability; and all symptoms may subside in four to six days.

A severe attack with sudden onset may present similar symptoms with higher fever and neurological signs showing up early—pain and muscle tenderness, stiffness of the neck and back, pain on bending the neck. The fever may be as high as 105 and may persist for as long as ten days.

The residual paralysis may vary from a mild weakness which will finally diasppear, to a crippling paralysis of large muscle groups.

Treatment

Treatment should be in the hands of a physician, and since there is no specific drug which can be used, the doctor should treat the patient symptomatically, trying to:

1. Prevent and treat complications
2. Prevent deformities
3. Reeducate the muscles, and rehabilitate the patient
4. Make the patient as comfortable as possible

Patients should be isolated for three weeks, with concurrent disinfection.

GLOSSARY

Concurrent at the same time; from hour to hour
Disability damage to body from disease or accident
Disinfection killing organisms by boiling all articles in contact with patient
Dissemination scattering
Epidemic large numbers of cases in a given area
Neurological pertaining to the nervous system
Paralysis inability to move muscles
Prevalent widely existing
Rehabilitate to teach a patient to become as independent and useful as possible in spite of handicaps
Residual remaining or left behind

SCARLET FEVER

Cause and Nature

This is an acute infectious disease characterized by sudden onset with sore throat, high fever, and vomiting. The cause is Group A Beta hemolytic streptococci. Transmitted by direct contact with sick persons or their discharge, by contaminated food or milk, or by contact with carriers.

Signs and Symptoms

Abrupt onset. Vomiting, high fever, sore throat, red flush over soft palate and throat, strawberry tongue after third day. A red rash or uniform blush appears within thirty-six hours over neck and chest, spreading over entire body. There is a pale circle around the mouth (so-called circumoral pallor) since the rest of the face is flushed. Rash fades about the eighth day, and desquamation (peeling off of skin) begins. The neck and chest shed fine flakes. Shedding may continue for a long time.

Treatment

Penicillin is specific, and given early in sufficient doses should hold the disease and prevent complications such as nephritis and middle ear disease. Sore throat may be relieved by an ice collar for children, or in adults by irrigation with hot salt water solution.

Aspirin, ten grains for adults, for headache or pain. Aspirin for children, one grain for every year of age. May be given every four hours.

Itchy skin may be relieved by antihistaminic ointments or soda baths.

Liquid diet and bed rest; force fluids. The patient should drink lots of water or fruit juices to help protect the kidneys by diluting the poison.

GLOSSARY

Hemolytic   destructive to red blood cells
Irrigate   to wash out place of infection
Streptococci   germs causing disease

SMALLPOX

Cause and Nature

This disease is rarely seen any more because most children are vaccinated against it, and this affords absolute protection. It is caused by a virus and is characterized by a sudden onset with fever, vomiting, diarrhea, generalized pain, and headache. It is transmitted by direct contact.

One attack confers lifelong immunity.

Signs and Symptoms

After three days of fever, headache, generalized aches, and vomiting, there appears a rash on the face and forearms, then on upper arms and trunk, then on the lower extremities. The lesions are separate, but may be so thick as to become confluent. They are first red, then raised, then blisters, then filled with pus, and afterwards become a crust. If the lesions are discrete, pitting of the skin very seldom follows. If the lesions run together scars are often left.

Treatment

Every person should be vaccinated, and then the disease will not occur. Babies from six months on should be vaccinated, and if there are cases of smallpox around, the people who have been vaccinated before should be revaccinated. If they still have protection, there will be a very mild reaction at the site of the vaccination. If not, the vaccination will take.

Isolation of the patient is imperative for from four to six weeks.

All utensils and linen should be disinfected by boiling.

Light diet; force fluids.

Aspirin for comfort.

Penicillin or some other antibiotic to prevent secondary infection of lesions.

Itching may be alleviated by applying nupercain ointment.

GLOSSARY

Alleviate   relieve
Imperative   necessary
Pitting   scarring
Vaccinated   immunized

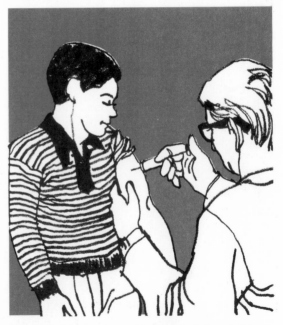

Immunizations are well tolerated by children. The injections cause very little pain.

TETANUS

(Lockjaw)

Cause and Nature

Tetanus is an acute infectious disease caused by the poison from Clostridium tetani. This organism has spores which allow it to survive for long periods of time, and these spores may be found in any soil— most often where there is manure. The fact that a nail is rusty does not mean it has tetanus spores on it. A bright, new nail with soil on it could be more dangerous.

The disease occurs after implantation of spores in any wound. It is more likely to occur following a deep puncture wound, or following a severe, dirty wound where there is a lot of dead tissue. The organism likes to grow where there is no oxygen— hence the importance of preventing the disease by immunization. Rather than trying to treat it, all children should have vaccination against tetanus by giving them tetanus toxoid along with diphtheria and pertussis vaccine. Then this immunity should be kept up through life by having booster injections about every four years.

Signs and Symptoms

There are two kinds of tetanus.

I. Localized, where the muscle group in the region of the wound becomes unyieldingly rigid three days to three weeks after the wound. This may persist for weeks and disappear. This is the less fatal of the two.

II. Generalized tetanus usually appears first as stiffness of the jaws (lockjaw) followed by restlessness, immobility, stiffness of the neck, and difficulty in swallowing. There may be a fever of 101 to 104 if the initial symptoms are not successfully treated. Convulsions may appear.

Treatment

This disease must be treated by a physician and should be prevented by active immunization as outlined above.

In case of a wound or burn in a previously immunized person, a booster injection of toxoid should be given at once, for it takes several days for this to become effective.

GLOSSARY

Convulsions   spasms of voluntary muscles
Fatal   deadly
Initial   first
Localized   in one spot
Oxygen   one element of the air
Spores   reproducing element of organism causing tetanus
Tetanus   lockjaw
Tetanus toxoid   a serum used for protection against tetanus

TYPHOID FEVER

Cause and Nature

Typhoid fever is an acute, generalized infection caused by the bacillus typhosus, which usually enters the body through the intestinal tract from contaminated water, infected food, or milk.

The onset is not acute. Prodromal symptoms may be chilly sensations alternating with hot flashes, headache, backache, loss of appetite, diarrhea or constipation, nosebleed, and generalized aching.

The fever usually rises slowly to a height of 103 or 104. In the beginning there may be pink or rose spots on the abdomen. The pulse is slow in comparison to the fever. The abdomen is usually tender and the spleen is enlarged.

There are all degrees of typhoid. Some people may have light cases and not go to bed—the so-called walking typhoid.

Treatment

Good nursing care is all-important and a doctor should always be in attendance. A high carbohydrate, high caloric, soft diet is essential. Fluids should be given freely, as sometimes the patient hemorrhages from the intestinal tract. In this case, feeding by mouth should cease. Chloromycetin, one of the antibiotic drugs, may be of great value in treating this disease.

Strict isolation should be observed and all linens and bed cloths thoroughly disinfected. All discharges should also be carefully disinfected.

GLOSSARY

Abdomen   belly
Caloric   pertaining to amount of food value
Carbohydrates   starches and sugars in foods
Constipation   lack of regular bowel movement
Hemorrhage   excessive amount of bleeding
Intestinal tract   organs in body to digest food
Prodromal   occurring before disease
Spleen   internal organ of the body

TUBERCULOSIS

Cause and Nature

Tuberculosis is an infectious disease caused by the tubercle bacillus. The bacteria may gain entrance into the body by being breathed in from the air or by being swallowed. The organism may be in the air or in droplets from a cough by a person with a positive sputum, or on articles which may have been soiled by a person with tuberculosis.

There are two main types. One is the so-called childhood type which may involve the lungs or the lymph nodes, and is usually healed in a caseous-like node or tubercle which contains a few live bacteria. This may remain in the person, alive but harmless, for many years; or these nodes may break down and allow the disease to spread.

The second type, the adult type, may involve any tissue, but it is usually found in the lungs. It may be acute or chronic, and it may be possible for a person to have it for a long time, until the disease is far advanced, without knowing that he has it. This is the reason why everyone should have an X ray of the chest every year.

Tuberculosis can be cured, and when found early it can be cured in a shorter period of time, with the use of new drugs and rest in bed. If not found, it may be the cause of death.

A person who is tired and undernourished is more apt to be susceptible to tuberculosis.

Signs and Symptoms

These may include easy fatigability, loss of weight, loss of appetite, feeling below par, fever, coughing up blood, a cough which may vary from a slight hack to the severe, persistent, productive type, and night sweats.

The important thing to remember is that a person may have it for years and spread it to others without knowing that he has it. Hence, the extreme importance of having chest X rays every year.

Treatment

This must be supervised by a doctor.

Rest in bed is the most important single treatment, and this may take from six months to a year or longer. The new drugs, such as streptomycin, para-aminosalicylic acid, isoniazid, and others have been proven to be effective.

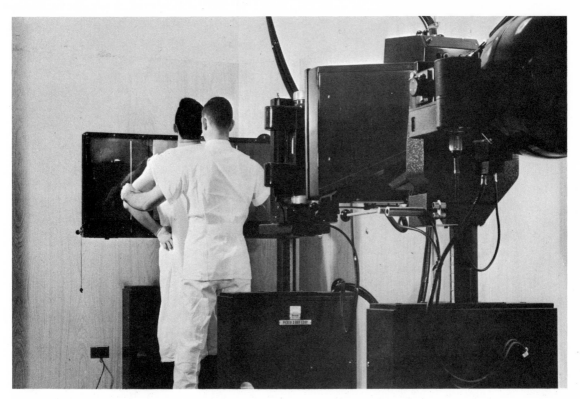

Yearly chest x-rays after 35 are important for early detection of tuberculosis and cancer.

Although rest is the most important single item, surgery, such as collapse of the lung or removal of the diseased area, may be deemed advisable.

It is important to know that now tuberculosis may be cured, and a person may live a perfectly normal life after having it. The important thing is to detect it early and treat it adequately.

An X ray of the chest every year will help detect early cases and help in preventing the disease from being spread to others by a person who does not even know that he has it.

The disease may be fatal to one person, although the man who gave it to him by coughing, or some other means, may not know that he has tuberculosis.

A person does not inherit tuberculosis—he catches it from another person. Since the new forms of cure have been used, tuberculosis is no longer among the first ten causes of death. With early detection and treatment, it may be possible to make this disease become one of the rare ones, like diphtheria and typhoid.

GLOSSARY

Adequately   enough
Caseous   composed of cheese-like material
Chronic   long standing
Collapse   immobilize by removing air
Fatigability   tendency to tire
Inherit   to derive from parents
Node   lump
Productive   having ability to produce sputum
Supervised   under watch
Susceptible   lacking resistance to disease
Tubercle   tube-shaped lesion
Undernourished   inadequately fed

MENINGITIS

Cause and Nature

The word "meningitis" means an inflammation or infection of the central nervous system or its coverings. These coverings are membranes called the meninges.

The picture presented by the condition will depend upon the extent of the invasion by the causative organism.

The most commonly seen causes for meningitis are the microorganisms such as the meningococcus, the influenza bacillus, staphylococcus and hemolytic streptococcus and the tubercle bacillus. Almost any of the pathogenic organisms which cause disease in man may cause meningitis.

The bacteria may attack the meninges or central nervous system through the blood, through direct invasion as in the case of infected sinus or middle ear disease, by skull fracture, or by spinal taps.

Signs and Symptoms

The signs and symptoms of meningitis may present many different clinical pictures. A history of previous disease or infection, contact with a person who has meningococcus meningitis, head injuries, or spinal taps, are all important things to consider when meningitis is suspected.

When meningitis is suspected an examination of the spinal fluid will usually show the presence of pus or bacteria or both. There are certain conditions known as aseptic meningitis or non-purulent meningitis which can be caused by a large number of organisms, such as certain viruses as in mumps or herpes simplex. No bacteria are seen in the spinal fluid.

Meningitis should be suspected when there is an acute onset of headache, vomiting, fever, and a stiff neck.

Most cases of influenzal meningitis are seen in children under two years of age and incidence decreases with age.

Since the introduction of so many antibiotics which kill the causative organisms in meningitis the outlook is usually good if diagnosed and treated with the proper drug.

These cases must always be treated by a doctor.

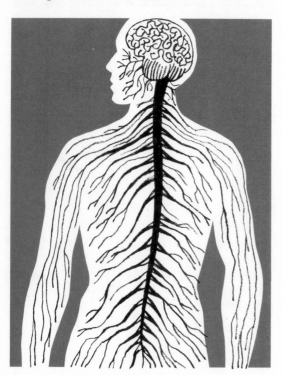

A **pinched nerve** in the neck may radiate pain down an arm through the nervous system.

GLOSSARY

Acute onset sudden appearance of symptoms
Antibiotics drugs given to kill germ caused disease
Clinical course of disease—symptoms found in examination
Diagnoses determination of cause and nature of disease
Hemolytic streptococcus found in blood streams, destroying blood cells
Influenza baccillus "flu" causing germ

Micro-organism   minute germs
Non-purulent   no pus present
Pathogenic organism   capable of causing disease
Spinal tap   drawing off spinal fluid to determine disease or relieve pressure
Staphyloccus   a class of tiny organisms found in clusters, like grapes
Tubercle bacillus   germ causing tuberculosis

DYSENTERY

Cause and Nature

This is an inflammatory disease of the colon, characterized by griping pains in the abdomen, and many watery stools or diarrhea. It may be caused by many different things:

1. By bacteria
2. By amebae
3. By irritating foods
4. By small ulcers in the colon
5. By food poisoning

It may be chronic or acute.

Signs and Symptoms

The onset is usually sudden with cramp-like pains in the abdomen and loose stools. There may be a fever and prostration. The stools may contain mucus and blood.

In infants, if not checked, it may result in dehydration or starvation.

Treatment

Rest. Liquid or smooth diet. Take fluids to prevent dehydration.

There are antibiotics, such as erythromycin, which may be used to kill the infective organism. Peptobismol will reduce the irritation.

GLOSSARY

Amebae   one celled organisms
Colon   lower bowel

Dehydration   lack of fluid
Prostration   extreme exhaustion
Ulcers   sores

INFLUENZA

Cause and Nature

This is an acute, highly contagious disease, which is self-limiting (that is, the patient will recover even if no treatment is used). It is caused by a virus and transferred by droplet infection or by direct contact. Two types of virus have been identified—Influenza A and B.

Vaccines for immunization against influenza caused by certain strains of virus are available. They do not take effect for five to seven days and the protection lasts only six to nine months. In the face of a severe epidemic, it may be wise to obtain the protection afforded by these vaccines—even though it is a temporary protection.

Signs and Symptoms

The onset is sudden, with chills or chilly feeling. Generalized malaise, backache, headache, leg aches. Nausea and vomiting are present on occasion. There is fever from 100 to 105. Sore throat and a dry, irritating cough often occur. Gastrointestinal symptoms may occur, especially in children, as evidenced by diarrhea and abdominal pain.

The disease itself is not very dangerous but the complications may be exceedingly dangerous. They are:

1. Pneumonia
2. Middle ear disease
3. Sinus infection
4. Bronchitis

There are many other rare complications. These are brought on by secondary infections caused by other organisms such as streptococci, staphylococci, or pneumococci. The pneumonia may occur as a relapse after the patient is apparently recovering.

After the disease there may be a period of weakness, which may seem out of proportion to the severity of the attack.

Treatment

There is no specific treatment. The patient should be kept in a warm, well-ventilated room. Visitors should be carefully screened to prevent the patient from contracting a secondary infection from them.

The diet should be light or liquid, and the patient should have a liberal supply of fluids—up to 3,000 cc. or three quarts a day.

Aspirin or aspirin and codeine should be used to obtain comfort. Cough syrup may be helpful, such as syrup of Hycodan.

Influenza itself does not respond to penicillin or other antibiotics, but the complications, if they occur, should be treated vigorously with these products.

GLOSSARY

Epidemic   large number of cases in certain locations
Liberal   free
Nausea   sick to the stomach
Staphylococci   kind of germs
Streptococci   kind of germs
Ventilated   aired

MALARIA

Cause and Nature

Malaria is caused by protozoa of the genus Plasmodium, and is transferred from man to man by certain types of mosquitoes of the anopheles species.

It may be an acute or chronic infection. It occurs wherever conditions favor the development of parasites in the transmitting mosquito.

There are four main types of malaria. The first two may be seen in the United States, but the last two are very rare in this country.

The first and most common, called benign tertian malaria, is caused by Plasmodium vivax. The second, and more serious, is caused by Plasmodium falciparum. The other two forms, not found often in the United States, are caused by Plasmodium malariae and Plasmodium ovale.

Signs and Symptoms

As has been stated above, malaria is an acute and chronic disease characterized by acute paroxysms, then periods of remission in which the patient feels perfectly well, only to have the disease recur time and time again. In untreated cases of vivax-caused tertian malaria these attacks may occur for two or three years. In falciparum infections they may occur for one year or more.

In tertian malaria the patient may have a remittent fever (one that comes and goes) for three to five days followed by a typical paroxysm—a feeling of chilliness spreading from the back to the extremities, and progressing into a severe, shocking chill. The pulse is rapid, and there may be nausea. The chill lasts from twenty minutes to one hour. The temperature then rises, the patient becomes flushed, the eyes sparkle. There may be headache, nausea, vomiting, and sometimes slight delirium. The fever may go as high as 106, will last from one to four hours, and then the sweating stage begins. The temperature drops and the patient may go to sleep. The total paroxysm may last from eight to twelve hours, and the patient may feel well when he awakens.

These attacks may occur at intervals if the case is untreated.

The symptoms of falciparum malaria are more varied than with tertian malaria, and may be more dangerous. The severe chill may be absent and the paroxysm may be more sudden and prostrating. The temperature may rise during the first two hours to 104°, and then it may drop slightly in what is known as a false crisis, only to rise again to as high or higher than it was before. This irregularity of the fever may help to diagnose the falciparum type.

The most common symptoms and signs of malaria are chills, fever, anemia, and an enlarged spleen.

Modern drugs have been developed that are more effective in the treatment and prevention of malaria than quinine; but the most important measures are those aimed at prevention of malaria in a community. These measures are:

1. Protection of persons from the bite of the anopheles mosquito
2. Destruction of anopheles mosquito by destroying its breeding places
3. Use of protective drugs where exposure is likely

Treatment

This is aimed at cure of the clinical attack, management of the patient during the paroxysm, and prevention of relapses.

As soon as the diagnosis is made, the patient should be given Arolen (the trade name for chloroquine) in a dose of 6 grams, followed by .3 gram in six hours. Then a single dose of .3 grams daily for the following two days.

If this drug is not available, quinine may be used in appropriate doses of 2 grams a day for seven days in acute cases.

For suppression, Arolen (chloroquin) may be used in small doses—.5 gram every seven days, or once a week.

During an acute attack, a patient should be placed in bed. Liquid diet—frequent drinks of water or lemonade are good.

Chipped ice often helps the nausea.

During the chill, patient should be kept warm with blankets or by hot water bottles.

The anemia should be treated with Trinsicon, one capsule twice a day.

If convulsive seizures occur, special measures should be taken to protect the patient. One of the more important of these is to place an object such as a spoon handle, wrapped in soft cloth, between the teeth to prevent biting of the tongue.

GLOSSARY

Genus a group of animals or plants of one kind
Parasites plants or animals living on another
Protozoa microscopic one-celled animals
Species kinds
Tertian occurring every third day

RHEUMATIC FEVER

Cause and Nature

This is a general systemic disease, inflammatory in nature, and is caused by Group A, hemolytic streptococci.

Rheumatic fever is the leading infectious disease cause of death between the ages of five and eighteen years, and is a common cause of heart disease.

The attack may be acute and severe, or mild. Any degree of severity may be noted from slight soreness (so-called growing pains may be in reality a manifestation of rheumatic fever) to redness, swelling, and

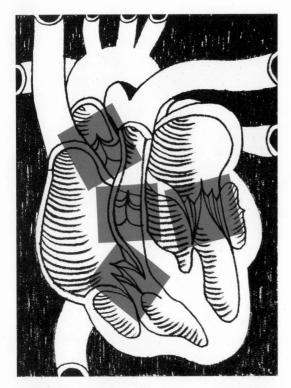

Areas of heart affected by rheumatic fever.

excruciating tenderness of the joints. One joint may recover and another become involved quickly. There is nearly always fever present.

Involvement of the heart is common, leading to damage of the mitral valve. The aortic valve is involved about half as often.

In the beginning, nosebleed may be common and, as mentioned above, in children the onset may be so insidious that it is not recognized. Easy fatigability and failure to gain weight should call for investigation by a doctor.

Signs and Symptoms

1. Fever
2. Inflammation of the joints, several joints at a time, and shifting from one to the other
3. Abdominal pain or chest pain
4. Repeated nosebleeds without injury
5. Rapid pulse
6. There may be purpura, or a red rash
7. Subcutaneous nodules are sometimes present, especially around the elbows

This disease has a tendency to recur, and special care should be taken to prevent recurrences, as the second or third attacks may cause more damage than the first. Bicillin tablets should be taken every day after an attack to prevent recurrence. This precaution should be observed for years after the attack.

Treatment

Complete bed rest, relief of pain, attention to diet, which should be high caloric, high vitamin; fluids should be pushed.

Good nursing care is important, as the treatment generally extends over a period of months.

Drugs most commonly used for relief of pain are aspirin or sodium salicylate. In most cases, one grain of aspirin per pound of body weight should be given in divided doses (every four hours) so that a child weighing 100 pounds would get 80 to 100 grains over a period of twenty-four hours in divided doses, at four hour intervals.

Penicillin should be given in large doses—1,000,000 units daily—to control the hemolytic streptococcus which is the causative organism.

Opinions vary as to the use of steroid therapy, that is, ACTH or cortisone, in the treatment of rheumatic fever. This should be left to the judgment of the doctor in each case.

The most important phase of treatment is to see that the patient has *rest*, emotional as well as physical, over a sufficient period of time until all activity of the disease has ceased.

After complete recovery, there should be a constant watch to prevent colds or sore throats. The patient should not become over-fatigued or exposed too often to drastic changes in temperature.

Prophylactic doses of penicillin should be given routinely to prevent recurrence. The dosage and frequency, if given penicillin, will be determined by your doctor. At least once a month, 1,000,000 to 1,500,000 units of penicillin should be taken to prevent another attack.

GLOSSARY

Aortic valve   valve of the heart
Bicillin   a penicillin tablet to be taken by mouth
Drastic   severe or strongest measures
Excruciating   very severe
Hemolytic   destruction of red blood cells
Insidious   coming on without warning
Manifestation   signs of
Mitral valve   valve of the heart
Nodule   hard lump
Recur   to happen again
Systemic   throughout entire body
Subcutaneous   under the skin

SAINT VITUS'S DANCE

Cause and Nature

The cause of St. Vitus's dance, also called acute chorea and Sydenham's chorea, is not known. It is sometimes a forerunner of rheumatic fever and infection by streptococcus has been suspected. It has never been proven that this is the cause. At any rate, when a diagnosis of chorea or St. Vitus's dance is made, rheumatic fever must be looked for: it may have preceded or it may follow the attack. A fairly large percentage of patients with chorea have rheumatic fever, but sometimes this amounts to only mild pains in the joints while on other occasions, murmurs are heard over the heart valves.

Acute chorea is seen more often in girls than in boys and it usually comes on between the ages of five and fifteen years. High strung, nervous, ambitious, and highly intelligent young girls are quite frequently victims of this disease. Often it is precipitated by working too hard in school, trying to get high grades or win prizes; in other cases it seems to be influenced by nervous strain which would be present when there is discord between the father and the mother or other members of the family.

This condition is rarely seen among Indians and Negroes and most often seen among young girls. It may last from eight to ten weeks or in some cases the movements may persist for months.

Signs and Symptoms

The onset or beginning of St. Vitus's dance may be very gradual and not noticed at first. A normally placid child may change in temperament and become very irritable and restless. The first signs noted may be a lack of coordination which will result in dropping things at the table or frequently knocking over a glass of milk or water. There may be pains in the limbs or headaches, and usually at some time during the disease there is a low grade fever.

After the mild symptoms have persisted for about two weeks the involuntary movements begin. These movements are usually jerky and are sometimes widespread. They vary greatly in speed and duration. At times these movements are noted only on one side of the body. The face may become screwed up as though the child were trying to make faces. The speech may be affected during an attack of jerky rapid movements.

The word "chorea" is derived from the Greek word meaning "choral dance" and these irregular, jerky, rapid movements may resemble a person going through the motions of an unusual dance.

In some cases nodules are noted under the skin.

Treatment

This disease should be treated with great care for although recovery nearly always results, there may be injury or irritation to the heart valves which will cause them to stiffen and harden. The resulting incompetence of the heart valves may handicap the person in later life.

After the diagnosis is made the child should be kept quiet, away from all sources of excitement. She should be kept in bed and often a mild sedative is needed. A good diet and warm fresh air in the sick room are important.

A doctor should be in charge of the case and he will use aspirin or salicylates to ease the pain if there is any. Due to the fact that a streptococcus may be the cause, large doses of penicillin or other antibiotics may be used over a long period.

As stated above, the outlook for recovery in this disease is good. In a few cases there are recurrences or return of the condition at a later date. This does not happen very often but the parents should try and protect the child from the things which may have brought on the attack in the first place. That is, the patient should not have to work too hard in school to get high grades or to win prizes. Excitement in any form should be avoided as much as possi-

ble and for some time after the attack the child should lead a quiet, protected life.

GLOSSARY

Coordination   ability to make brain and muscles work together
Involuntary   not controllable by person
Precipitated   set off or started by
Sedative   something to produce calm or quietness

INFECTIOUS MONONUCLEOSIS

Cause and Nature

Although the cause of infectious mononucleosis has not been definitely determined, it is thought to be caused by a virus.

This exceedingly common disease was known as "glandular fever" many years ago. It may occur at any age from seven months to seventy years but is most often seen in people who are between ten and thirty-five years of age. Because of its frequent occurrence in girls and boys of college age, it has been called the "kissing disease" although it has never been determined that the disease is spread in this manner.

There are different types of mononucleosis which range from the very mild to the quite severe and even fatal cases. As a rule, the disease is moderately severe and nearly always the outlook for a complete recovery is good. The disease may last from three to six weeks and sometimes even longer.

Signs and Symptoms

The most common sign by which infectious mononucleosis is recognized is the enlargement of the lymph glands, and the change in the white blood count which shows an increase in the number of lymphocytes. Another laboratory test that is called the heterophile agglutination test, when positive, makes the diagnosis certain.

There may be fever and a sore throat which goes along with the enlargement of the lymph glands in the neck. There is generally a certain period of weakness and loss of appetite which in some cases seems to last for an unusually long period. There may be a slight red rash in some cases but this is not always present.

Treatment

Since the cause of this disease has not been definitely determined there is no specific treatment for it. The sulfonamides and antibiotics have not been proven to help.

Rest in bed, with a diet high in carbohydrates, aspirin or aspirin and codeine for the comfort of the patient, have proven to be about the only effective forms of treatment. A doctor should be in charge because in some of the severe cases the use of the cortisone drugs has resulted in a mild improvement although these drugs have not been proven to constitute a real cure for the condition.

It is also important for the doctor to make a definite diagnosis since this disease may resemble a great many other conditions which could be cured by the use of some known drugs.

GLOSSARY

Agglutination   gathering in clumps
Lymphocytes   variety of white blood cells

CAT SCRATCH FEVER

Cause and Nature

This disease is caused by the scratch or bite of a house cat. The organism that pro-

duces the disease has not been isolated. This is usually a mild disease that is not fatal and is self limiting—that is, it will clear up even if not treated. The course of the disease is extremely variable and may last anywhere from two weeks to a year. This is a fairly common disease.

Signs and Symptoms

A few days after being scratched or bitten by a cat there will appear an ulcer or sore at the site of the lesion. This will usually scab over and may be surrounded by small blisters. The lymph glands on the side affected will be enlarged. That is, if the scratch is on the right hand there will be lumps or kernels in the right armpit and at the right elbow. These may occur about one or two weeks after the scratch and the patient will have a fever and show the signs of a generalized infection. These enlarged lymph glands may disappear in a few weeks or they may, if not treated, become filled with pus and drain when lanced. They may last anywhere from weeks to months.

Treatment

The patient is made comfortable by lowering the fever with aspirin. Some of the antibiotics like terramycin or chloromycetin will shorten the course of the disease and prevent the glands from forming pus. As stated above, this condition will disappear in time even if it is not treated.

GAS GANGRENE

Cause and Nature

Gas gangrene is a serious complication of infected wounds caused by an invasion of the wound by a spore-forming clostridia or bacteria. There are a few different kinds of bacteria which, because they form spores, are capable of remaining alive in dirt or manure for many years.

There are two main types, so designated because they put out different types of toxin or poison. One type is called the neurotoxic type because its poison attacks the nervous system. Examples of this type are tetanus and botulus. The other type is called histotoxic because its poison attacks the tissues of the body such as muscle, skin, and subcutaneous tissue. An example of the histotoxic type is gas gangrene, which as the name implies, results in the formation of gas bubbles in the tissue and eventually, in death of the tissue or gangrene.

In order for the various clostridia to multiply and cause the body to be hurt by their toxins they must have certain definite conditions. First of all, they will not multiply in the presence of oxygen. That is why they may follow puncture wounds deep into the tissue or may be caused by crushing injury to the bones resulting in a compound fracture; that is, the bone sticks out through the skin and gets some dirt on it. When the bone is placed back into the body, there may be a lack of oxygen; if there are spore-bearing clostridia on it, they may develop rapidly, causing formation of gas in the tissues and gangrene.

Signs and Symptoms

When the anaerobic bacteria multiply in the deep tissues of the wound they form gas and this can be felt. It has a peculiar cushioning feeling on pressure. The gas can be seen on X ray.

The patient appears quite ill, but the illness may come on gradually, from three to six days after the injury. The skin around the injury will be pale and shiny at first. In the later stages, after gangrene sets in, the skin becomes black. The patient has a high fever and prostration is extreme. Delirium and coma may be seen in some patients.

This is a very serious condition and should be recognized early and treated promptly by a doctor.

Treatment

All untreated cases of gas gangrene will surely die. However, if they are treated adequately and early, they can nearly all be saved. Treatment is surgical, incising or cutting into the tissues to let oxygen in and thereby stopping the growth of the bacteria. Amputation may be necessary.

The antibiotics have saved the lives of many people who had gas gangrene. Penicillin is the medicine of choice and large doses should be given, as much as 1,000,-000 units every three or four hours. This should be given by injection. One of the other antibiotics should be given with the penicillin to kill other bacteria which may be present.

Supportive treatment and constant supervision by a doctor are important.

GLOSSARY

Amputation   removal of a part
Anaerobic   grows in the absence of oxygen
Coma   complete unconsciousness
Delirium   a mental disturbance; confusion
Prostration   extreme exhaustion
Spore   a cyst or round nodule found in some organisms such as tetanus
Subcutaneous   beneath the skin

Chapter 8

Diseases of The Respiratory Tract

SORE THROAT

Cause and Nature

Streptococcic sore throat. The so-called strep throat is characterized by a sudden onset, with soreness on swallowing, fever and general malaise. It is caused by a hemolytic streptococcus, which is one of a number of species of bacteria capable of causing various acute diseases by attacking when the resistance of the patient has been reduced by a cold or some other minor ailment.

Other forms of sore throat caused by other organisms such as staphylococci are similar, but not so severe, and do not have fever and constitutional symptoms, as a rule.

Signs and Symptoms

Swelling and redness of soft palate, tonsils, and posterior pharynx (back of the throat). Sometimes there is a whitish exudate on the tonsils or around the tonsillar fossae. The lymph nodes in the neck may be swollen and tender.

There may be fever and generalized aches and pains.

Treatment

Bed rest until fever is gone.

Warm salt gargles will help, three or four times a day. One teaspoon of salt to a glass of hot water used as a gargle.

Aspirin or aspirin and codeine to keep the patient comfortable.

Penicillin, either orally or by injection.

Erythromycin, aureomycin, terramycin and other antibiotics are useful, and should be used if there is a fever.

GLOSSARY

Exudate any discharged matter
Malaise general discomfort
Nodes swollen lymph glands
Tonsillar fossa a small depression or pit on each side of the throat in which a tonsil is located

INFECTIONS OF THE LARYNX, TRACHEA, AND BRONCHI

Cause and Nature

These infections usually follow a cold in adults. Laryngitis produces hoarseness or loss of voice.

If the infection extends on down into

129

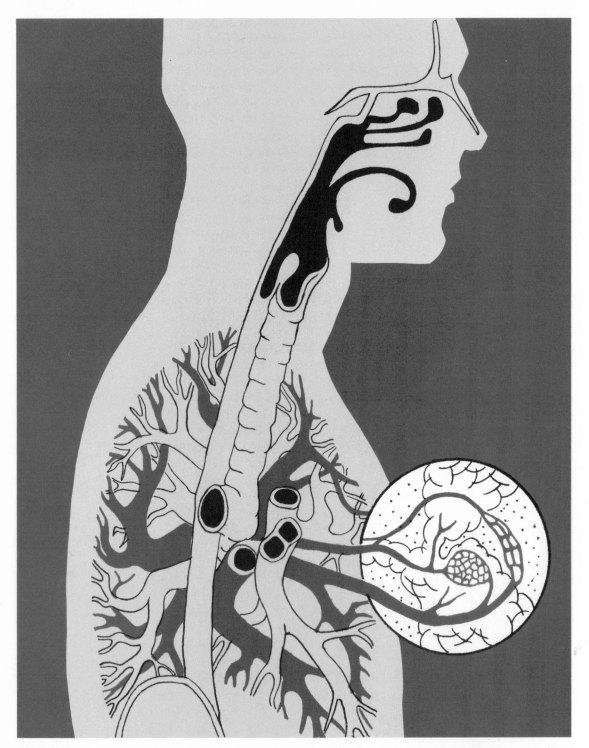

The respiratory system: This diagram shows the large bronchial tubes and the tube running from the mouth and nose to the bronchial tubes. Insert shows the air sacs where the exchanges of gases take place.

the trachea, it is usually accompanied by a harsh, dry cough and substernal pain.

The bronchial tubes may become involved, and bronchitis usually is characterized by a productive cough, substernal discomfort and tightness, and maybe a slight fever with general malaise.

Signs and Symptoms

Hoarseness, cough, pain in the chest, fever, and mild malaise.

Treatment

Bed rest in warm room. Air kept moist by steam from a kettle or vaporizer with tincture of benzoin compound (one teaspoon to one gallon of water) added. Menthol or eucalyptol may be mixed with the water instead of benzoin.

The patient should not talk any more than necessary, in order to rest the larynx.

Aspirin should be given for comfort.

Cough syrup should be used to control a dry, non-productive cough. Codeine may be used in the cough syrup for this purpose. Syrup of Hycodan is a good cough syrup.

Cold or hot compresses around the neck will often ease the discomfort in the throat.

Irritating substances such as smoke should be avoided.

GLOSSARY

Bronchi   tubes conveying air to the lungs
Larynx   organ of voice
Malaise   general discomfort
Substernal   below the breast bone
Trachea   the windpipe

PLEURISY

Cause and Nature

When an infection extends from the lung tissue to the lining of the lungs, i.e., the pleura, this inflammation of the pleura causes severe pain.

There are in general two main kinds of pleurisy:

1. Dry pleurisy
2. Pleurisy with effusion—that is, inflammation of the pleura accompanied by an accumulation of fluid

Dry pleurisy usually follows some upper respiratory infection or pneumonia, while wet pleurisy or pleurisy with effusion may follow dry pleurisy. If pleurisy with effusion comes out of a clear sky, without any known preceding infection, tuberculosis should be strongly suspected, for this is the most frequent cause. After the patient recovers from the pleurisy he should be watched carefully for the advent of pulmonary tuberculosis, and if this is detected, it should be treated promptly. This precaution may often be a life-saving measure.

Signs and Symptoms

Severe pain in the area of the chest involved, aggravated by breathing or laughing, is the most outstanding symptom. There may be fever and dry cough, and the doctor can hear a to and fro friction rub that sounds like a creaky saddle, when he listens with a stethoscope.

X ray will reveal effusion or fluid.

If the onset is insidious, without any previous infection, the fever low, not much pain, slight cough, and shortness of breath, this is called primary pleurisy with effusion, and pulmonary tuberculosis should be suspected.

Treatment

Treatment is usually aimed at controlling the pain. This can be helped by strapping around the lower part of the chest with adhesive tape.

Aspirin or aspirin and codeine can be used also to control the pain.

If the causative organism is known, then antibiotic treatment should be employed against the cause of the previous infection.

A dry pleurisy usually goes away in three or four weeks. Pleurisy with effusion lasts much longer.

GLOSSARY

Effusion escape of fluid
Insidious sly; treacherous
Pleura lining of lungs

PSITTACOSIS, PARROT FEVER, OR ORNITHOSIS

Cause and Nature

This is an infectious disease that is found in the bird family. It is often transferred to man and causes a pneumonia.

Psittacosis is most often passed on to man by infected parrots and parakeets, but it has been known to be present in pigeons, canaries, and even chickens.

The disease is caused by a virus and often is seen in groups of people who have been exposed to the same infected bird. The virus is present on the feathers of the bird, in its droppings, and in the dirt on the bottom of the cage. It is a difficult virus to kill and can live in the dust of a cage for some time. The virus is breathed into the lungs of man, causing pneumonia.

Signs and Symptoms

The incubation period or the length of time between exposure to the birds and the time when the symptoms appear is from seven to fifteen days. The disease may be mild or it may be quite severe. It starts in with a loss of appetite, fever, headache, and backache—sometimes these are accompanied by chills. There is a cough which is dry, severe, and comes in paroxysms or spells.

The fever may be quite high and can last from two to three weeks. Sometimes it takes several months to recover from a case of parrot fever. The cases contracted from parrots are usually more severe than cases from other kinds of birds.

Treatment

Care should be taken in the treatment of patients with this condition as it can be passed on from one person to another through the sputum, and the virus may be coughed out into the air.

The patient should be kept comfortable by the use of aspirin. He should be fed a light diet. Sometimes cough syrup will ease the coughing spells.

This is one of the few diseases caused by a virus in which the antibiotics are specific. Therefore a doctor should be called and he will prescribe terramycin or some similar antibiotic.

The best way to prevent psittacosis is to avoid contact with sick parrots, parakeets, or pigeons.

GLOSSARY

Paroxysm a sharp, convulsive attack
Virus a living minute organism

DISEASES OF THE LUNGS

1. Pulmonary emphysema
2. Pneumonia
3. The Pneumoconiosis
   (*miner's disease*)
4. Pulmonary embolism and infarction

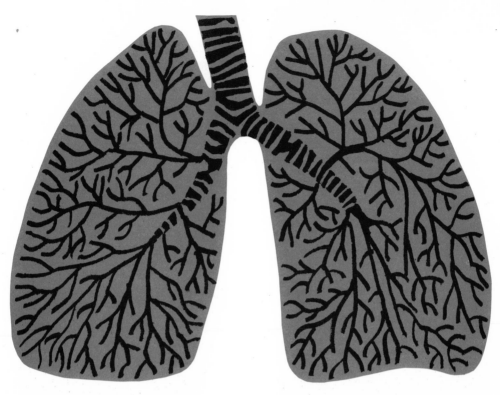

Broncial tree: The main broncial tubes branch off into smaller tubes like the roots of a tree.

5. Mycotic diseases of the lungs
   a. Histoplasmosis
   b. Coccidiodomycosis
   c. Blastomycosis
   d. Other pulmonary diseases caused by a fungus are nocardiosis, actinomycosis, aspergillosis, and mucormycosis; but because these are so seldom seen, they will not be described in this book.
6. Pulmonary tuberculosis
7. Cancer of the lung

PULMONARY EMPHYSEMA

Cause and Nature

This serious disease of the lungs is becoming more common all the time; doctors are seeing more people for the symptoms caused by pulmonary emphysema than ever before in history and the number of people with this condition is increasing every day.

The cause is usually some kind of obstruction in the bronchioles or small bronchial tubes and this is the way it works. Imagine the bronchial tree as looking like the roots of a tree. The larger branches and trunk of the tree are the bronchial tubes and these taper off into millions of small roots which are the bronchioles. At the end of the bronchioles are small air spaces, or cells, that fill with air when we breathe in. Now these air spaces have thin walls. When the new air is breathed in, the oxygen goes through these walls and into the blood stream which carries it throughout the body where it is used by muscles and all other cells of the body. When the oxygen goes into the blood stream the air in the air spaces receives in return the waste products—carbon dioxide—from the body cells. The act of breathing in oxygen and breathing out carbon dioxide is called the exchange of gases in the lung cells. The presence of sufficient oxygen in the body is absolutely essential to our well being; the lack of enough oxygen is called anoxia.

Practically every person over fifty has pulmonary emphysema to a certain extent and in some people it is a real crippling condition. Men have this condition about ten times more often than women.

When the bronchial tubes and the bronchioles are constantly irritated by inhaling polluted air, by smoking cigarettes, or by repeated infections or chest colds this causes them to be obstructed and the small air spaces become dilated. Finally the walls lose their efficiency and cease to function properly in the exchange of gases.

This condition does not come on suddenly but is very gradual in its onset and where a great number of these cells have been destroyed or impaired the exchange of gases is seriously hampered. Once the cells have been damaged they cannot be replaced by new ones and when the lungs are thus damaged the heart is affected also because it has to work harder.

Signs and Symptoms

The first symptom is shortness of breath. This usually occurs early in the morning or late in the afternoon to begin with but as the disease progresses the slightest effort may cause a struggle to get enough air.

Soon a person may notice weakness, loss of appetite and weight; just walking a short distance will make him feel out of breath.

Treatment

The best treatment of course is prevention and this is accomplished by avoiding anything that will cause irritation of the bronchial tree and thereby produce obstruction.

The doctor will tell you at first to stop smoking—this is a must. Avoid polluted air (smog) such as is found in large cities. Try to avoid any infection of the lungs or bronchial tree. A doctor will be able to give medicine to help this. There are many medicines which will help dilate the bronchial tree. Then the doctor may prescribe breathing in a special kind of air with medicine in it. This is done with breathing machines. The Bird respirator and the Bennett are two examples. Exudate in the bronchial tree should be thinned out if possible. Breathing moist air or drinking hot drinks may help this. Some doctors think that certain medicines such as potassium iodide drops will help thin the secretions.

A diet which is easy to digest and regular bowel habits will help.

By avoiding strenous exercise the patient can often help relieve his symptoms.

X rays of the chest will show the presence of emphysema if it is far enough advanced.

So remember that this condition can be prevented, it can be helped if treated early, and it is very important to prevent it because pulmonary emphysema puts an extreme load on the heart and causes certain forms of heart disease.

GLOSSARY

Bronchioles fine subdivisions of the branched bronchial tree

Exudate any substance deposited in or upon a tissue by a vital process or disease

PNEUMONIA

Cause and Nature

Pneumonia is an infection of the lungs that may be caused by a great number of organisms. The pneumococcus, streptococcus, tubercle bacillus and many other bacteria may cause pneumonia. There is the atypical pneumonia caused by a virus. The infection goes from the bronchial tubes into the lung cells causing an exudate to form in one or more lobes of the lung.

There are two main types:

1. Lobar pneumonia, in which one lobe or the entire lung is affected and becomes congested.
2. Bronchial pneumonia, which is a scattered infection with congestion around the small bronchial tubes.

Lobar pneumonia is the more serious, and bronchial pneumonia, while less serious, is more frequently seen. The various types of causative organisms show different types of clinical pictures in pneumonia.

One attack does not give immunity, and pneumonia is not contagious—that is, it is not passed directly from one person to another.

Signs and Symptoms

Pneumonia should be suspected when fever persists more than four or five days in a bronchitis. A sudden onset of cough, prostration, and elevation of temperature in the course of another disease should make one suspect pneumonia.

X rays will usually reveal congestion, and a doctor can detect the signs of pneumonia by listening to a patient's chest with a stethoscope. "Rales" (fine crackling sounds) are heard in bronchial pneumonia. Breath sounds are absent in lobar pneumonia.

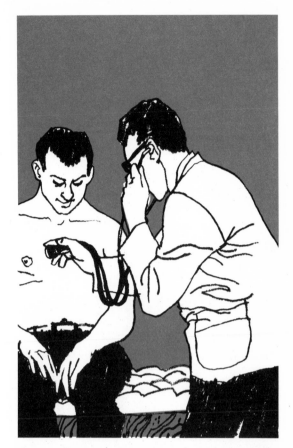

Doctor listening to a patient's chest using a stethoscope.

Treatment

The antibiotics are usually specific in the more common forms of pneumonia. Penicillin is still considered the best in most cases, and should be given in adequate doses.

Bed rest is very important, and a cough syrup to control the cough helps. The patient is able to throw off the condition more readily if he is comfortable, so aspirin should be given for discomfort.

If possible, the patient should be hospitalized, and if he does not respond quickly to treatment the causative organism should be found by taking sputum cultures. Sensitivity tests should be done to determine which one of the antibiotics will be more effective in killing the particular organism that is causing the disease.

GLOSSARY

Congestion   accumulation of fluid
Culture   growth of organisms or culture media
Exudate   any substance deposited in or upon a tissue by a vital process or disease
Organism   any living thing (i.e., bacteria, virus, etc.)
Sputum   saliva mixed with mucus
Stethoscope   instrument for hearing body sounds
Virus   a living minute organism

PNEUMOCONIOSIS

Cause and Nature

Pneumoconiosis is caused by deposits in the lung tissue of particles of dust.

It has sometimes been called miner's disease because hard rock miners breathing in particles of silica are very often affected by this disease. However there are many other types of dust which will settle in the lungs and cause pneumoconiosis.

There are two types of pneumoconiosis. One is the inert or harmless, inactive type in which the patient does not feel any effects of the dust and does not even know that it is present until an X ray of the chest is taken. The second type is the harmful or active type which causes symptoms.

Workers or people in contact with the following mineral dusts may have pneumoconiosis:

a. silica
b. beryllium
c. bauxite
d. asbestos
e. coal dust

These cause active disease from which

symptoms may be noted. The time of exposure varies. Sometimes, as in pneumoconiosis caused by silica dust, one must be exposed for years. On the other hand, sometimes just a short exposure to dust such as beryllium may produce dust disease.

Various occupations may be considered hazardous because of exposure to mineral dust particles in the air. Silica may be inhaled in hard rock or silica bearing rock mining (which causes silicosis), glass manufacturing, dressing of granite, sandstone and flint work, sand blasting, metal grinding, and ceramic manufacturing.

Coal dust is a hazard to people engaged in bituminous coal mining.

Asbestos may be inhaled in the installation of insulating material, asbestos products manufacturing, and the spinning or weaving of asbestos with other materials.

Beryllium is encountered in the extraction of that metal from the ore, in the manufacturing of neon lights or tubes, in the salvaging of fluorescent lamps, or in neighborhood contamination. It must be added that beryllium is no longer used in the manufacture of fluorescent lamps.

Bauxite is used in the manufacture of synthetic abrasives.

Signs and Symptoms

The diagnosis of pneumoconiosis is usually made by taking an X ray of the chest which will show the deposits of these various minerals.

The symptoms vary a great deal depending upon the length of time exposed and, to some extent, upon the complications which may follow the deposit of dusts in the lungs. There may be shortness of breath or pulmonary heart disease. In many cases, pulmonary tuberculosis may be superimposed upon pneumoconiosis, the so-called miner's consumption.

In some acute cases there may be cough, pneumonia with little or no fever, and blood streaked sputum. These symptoms appear in acute beryllium poisoning.

During the early stages of the inactive form of dust inhalation there may be no symptoms and the disease may be discovered only when an X ray of the chest is taken.

It is thought that cancer of the lung may be influenced by these irritating dusts, causing pain in the chest, spitting of blood, and coughing.

Treatment

It must be remembered that some types of pneumoconiosis produce no symptoms and require no treatment. In other types, where complications such as tuberculosis occur, specific treatment for that disease is indicated.

The real treatment is prevention. Manufacturers and mining concerns are using many safety factors today which prevent the inhalation of these mineral dusts.

GLOSSARY

Complications a disease existing with another disease
Sputum spittle; saliva
Superimposed a thing over another

PULMONARY EMBOLISM

Cause and Nature

A pulmonary embolus or embolism is caused by the passage of any abnormal material through the blood vessels to the lungs, where this material may plug up branches of the pulmonary artery. This ma-

terial is usually a blood clot which may break off from a clot in other parts of the body, such as the veins in the leg, and circulate through the blood until it becomes stuck in an artery in the lungs, thereby stopping the flow of blood through that artery. Other materials which may circulate in the blood stream and cause a pulmonary embolus are air, fat, or pieces of bone.

Signs and Symptoms

The signs and symptoms of pulmonary embolism vary greatly. There may be a very small embolus that will cause no symptoms, or there may be a large clot which obstructs one of the major lung arteries causing sudden and unexpected death. Many of the sudden deaths following surgery or severe fractures, which may occur when the patient is apparently doing well and ready to go home, are caused by pulmonary embolism.

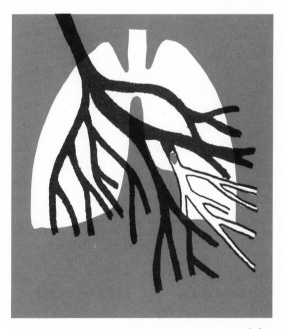

Pulmonary embolism: A clot in an artery of the lung which cuts off the blood flow.

Symptoms that may be brought on by pulmonary or lung embolism are sudden acute shortness of breath, a sudden onset of extreme weakness, and chest pain. The patient usually sweats excessively and appears pale.

Treatment

The best treatment for pulmonary embolism is prevention. Absolute prevention is not always possible, but people with clots in the leg veins, (thrombophlebitis) should be treated with care to prevent a piece of the clot from breaking off. Early ambulation after operations—that is, getting the patient out of bed the next day after surgery, prevents pooling of blood and the formation of clots.

The use of medicines such as heparin or dicumorol will prevent the clots from becoming larger.

After the embolism has occurred, early and intensive treatment is indicated. The use of oxygen and morphine to ease the pain are immediate steps to be taken. In order to prevent further embolism the anti-clotting drugs such as heparin or dicumorol or both should be used.

Sometimes when repeated clots are breaking off from a thrombus or clot in the leg veins in spite of all medicines, the femoral vein should be tied off in order to prevent further emboli from going to the lungs.

All of these treatments require the immediate and careful attention of a physician.

GLOSSARY

Arteries   vessels that carry blood from the heart
Blood vessels   tubes for carrying blood
Embolus   a clot or plug
Femoral   pertaining to the thigh
Pulmonary   pertaining to lungs

MYCOTIC DISEASES OF THE LUNGS

Histoplasmosis

Cause and Nature

The cause of histoplasmosis is a tiny yeast that grows in the cells of the body. It may cause lesions of granulomatou and exudative nature that will lead to caseation (cavity formation), fibrosis or scar formation, and calcification or formation of calcium deposits in various parts of the body such as the lungs, liver, adrenal glands, central nervous system, heart valves, and spleen. The disease as it is seen in the lungs will be described here.

In the United States, the Mississippi River Valley, portions of Virginia and North Carolina have so many cases that these areas are said to have a high endemic prevalence of this disease. It is also found in other parts of North America as well as Latin America, Africa, and Southeast Asia.

The disease is usually found in people who work in dusty places which are alternately damp and dry, as in spelunking, and cleaning out chicken coops or old silos.

Histoplasmosis is seen more often in white people than in Negroes. It is found equally in boys and girls before puberty but in grown people it is seen much more often in men than in women.

The disease that affects all different parts of the body is seen most often in the very young and the old, that is, after sixty. This condition or disease is not passed on from one person to the other.

Signs and Symptoms

Histoplasmosis of the lungs produces a varied group of symptoms and signs. The disease may occur without any symptoms and be healed without treatment only to be discovered when a skin test is positive to histoplasmin and X rays of the chest show old scars of deposits of calcium.

The acute disease may resemble pneumonia with marked fever, fatigue, dry cough, and sweats. The condition may occur seven to twenty-one days after exposure to the yeast cells in dust, and usually the acute symptoms last only a short time from a few days to two weeks. The signs are noted in X rays of the chest which may show soft, widespread, mottled densities throughout both lungs. After two or three years some of these spots leave scars or deposits of calcium.

The chronic form of pulmonary histoplasmosis occurs most often in farmers. The onset may be slow, with a slight sore throat, and the cough may last a long time with prevalent sputum which may show streaks of blood. There may be a loss of weight, weakness, fatigue, and chest pain.

X rays of the chest will show scarring and sometimes many cavities of different sizes. Rare cases may show a single coin lesion which may be thought to be cancer but after operation and removal of the coin lesion from the lung it will be seen to contain these little yeast cells known as "histoplasma capsulatum."

In diagnosing histoplasmosis, the yeast cells can be recovered from the dust or soil to which the patient has been exposed. Skin tests are positive and the X rays show lesions. The sputum may contain the yeast cells. Patients with lung lesions should always have skin tests for histoplasmosis.

This disease must be differentiated from pulmonary tuberculosis as they have much in common, and in chronic cases both diseases may occur at the same time.

Treatment

Acute pulmonary histoplasmosis requires only symptomatic treatment, rest in bed, aspirin for discomfort, cough syrup for cough, and the course is usually mild.

In the chronic form bed rest for periods of from six months to a year may be needed. Smoking is absolutely forbidden and the prompt treatment of complications such as pneumonia or tuberculosis is indicated.

There are a few drugs such as the steroids and antibiotics which may be helpful in stabilizing this chronic lung disease.

GLOSSARY

Calcium   the basic element of lime
Caseation   degeneration of tissue into a cheese-like substance
Endemic   prevalent in a particular area
Lesion   any wound or destruction of tissue
Mycotic   caused by a fungus or yeast

Coccidiodomycosis

Cause and Nature

Coccidiodomycosis is caused by a fungus known as "Coccidioides immitis." This disease is found most often throughout the southwestern United States and the causative organism grows more readily in hot, dry climates with low altitude and alkalin soil. The fungus enters the body by being breathed in on dust particles in the air. It is not passed on from person to person, but it is seen more often than the other pulmonary diseases caused by a fungus. The diagnosis is made by skin tests, sputum tests, and blood tests.

Signs and Symptoms

The pulmonary form of the disease may be without symptoms, and the site of infection in the lungs is often self-limited—that is, it heals by itself—and may be localized to one spot in the lungs. The diagnosis often depends upon a positive skin test called coccidiodin skin test.

If the disease spreads from the lungs throughout the body the disease may be very serious. In some pulmonary cases there are symptoms such as chest pain, fever, cough, loss of appetite, and sometimes spitting of blood.

Only in rare cases does this disease spread through the body, and may be discovered only when an X ray of the chest and a skin test are positive.

Treatment

As the disease is usually mild and self-limiting, symptomatic treatment is all that is needed. When the disease spreads there is no drug that has been found which will effect it, although the antibiotics and anti-fungal drugs are being tried and it is to be hoped that a cure will be found.

Blastomycosis

Cause and Nature

Blastomycosis is a chronic infectious disease caused by a yeast-like fungus known as "Blastomyces dermatitidis."

The lesions produced are granulating and pus-forming tumors in the lungs, on the skin, and in other tissues of the body.

The causative organism has not been found in soil or any other external environment but has been demonstrated in animals and man. Dogs are the animals most frequently affected.

North American cases have been found in the Mississippi River Valley and in North Carolina. It is seen at all ages.

Signs and Symptoms

There are two main types—the pulmonary type which may have serious results, and the type affecting the skin, which may be cured if treated over a long period.

In the pulmonary form there is a cough with purulent sputum, a moderate fever, loss of weight, and easy fatigability. Skin lesions may break out while the pulmonary disease is in progress.

X rays may show spots on the lungs with cavitation—especially in the apex or top portion of the lungs—which resemble pulmonary tuberculosis and make the diagnosis difficult.

The causative organism can be isolated and identified from the pus of the sputum or from the lesions themselves if seen on the skin. This fungus must then be cultured and grown in a laboratory to confirm the diagnosis.

Treatment

The treatment of this disease may be somewhat more successful than in pulmonary disease caused by other yeasts or fungi. Potassium iodide and certain anti-fungal antibiotics have been used successfully. The cases should be treated by a physician.

GLOSSARY

Cavitation formation of cavities
Granulating division into small particles (in a healing lesion, granulations are red, bumpy areas of tissue sometimes called proud flesh)
Purulent containing pus

CANCER OF THE LUNG

Cause and Nature

As in the case of other cancers we do not know the cause of cancer of the lung. In the last ten years cancer of the lung has become a very serious problem and apparently its incidence is increasing rapidly. The condition is now considered the most common form of cancer causing death among men in some cities. Cancer of the lung is seen more often in men than in women. The ratio is about six in men to one in women.

The cancer usually starts in one of the bronchial tubes and the most common form, which arises from the lining of the tubes, is known as bronchiogenic carcinoma. The less frequently seen type arises from the mucous glands of the bronchial tubes and is known as adenocarcinoma of the bronchus or of the lung.

Since the bronchial tree spreads throughout the lung, the cancer, which is a wild growth of cells, may occur close to the main bronchial tube or may begin out near the edge or outer portion of the lung.

Other conditions which may be confused with cancer of the lung are pulmonary embolism, chronic abscess of the lung, a healed tuberculosis lesion of the lung, a small localized pneumonia, or at times a lipid or fat pneumonia of the lung which may be caused by using oily nose drops too often and inhaling or breathing them into the lungs, or by breathing in some mineral oil which is being swallowed.

Cancer of the lung is seen more often in men who live in cities than in people who live in the country. A great number of men who have cancer of the lung are heavy cigarette smokers, hence any form of irritation to the bronchial tree is thought to have some influence in starting cancer of the lung. Pollution of the atmosphere as seen in the smoke or "smog" in large cities needs to be studied further to find out if this plays a role in causing cancer of the lung.

Men who work in certain occupations

CIGARETTES AND DEATHS FROM ALL CAUSES*

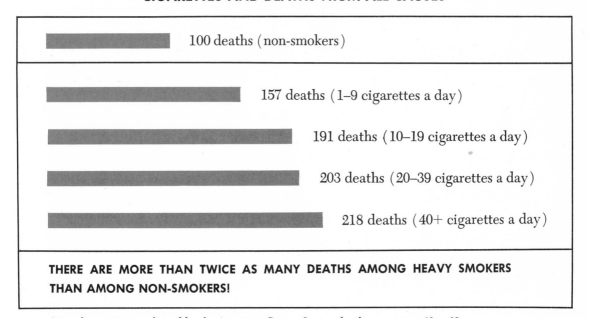

100 deaths (non-smokers)

157 deaths (1–9 cigarettes a day)

191 deaths (10–19 cigarettes a day)

203 deaths (20–39 cigarettes a day)

218 deaths (40+ cigarettes a day)

THERE ARE MORE THAN TWICE AS MANY DEATHS AMONG HEAVY SMOKERS THAN AMONG NON-SMOKERS!

*Based on statistics released by the American Cancer Society for the age group 40 to 69.

are found to have cancer of the lung more often than other men. These occupations cause the workers to breathe in irritating substances such as radioactive dust or certain chemicals such as the chromate compounds.

Cancer of the lung is usually fast growing, and if not detected early and operated upon may be fatal within a year of the time it is first detected.

Since the lungs are body organs to which cancer from other parts of the body can metastasize or spread, it is very important when a lesion is found in the lungs to examine the other parts of the body for a cancer. It would not do any good to operate on the lungs to remove cancer which had spread through the blood to the lungs from a cancer which arose in some other part of the body. When a cancer starts first in the bronchial tubes of the lungs it is called a

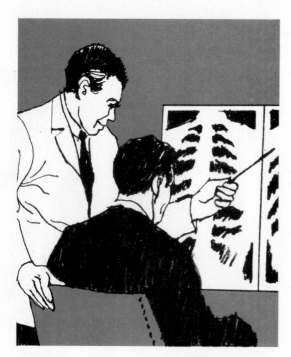

A **doctor** explaining an X ray of the chest to a patient.

primary cancer of the lungs, and if found early enough this may be operated upon and perhaps cured. If it has spread to the lungs from some other part of the body it is called metastatic carcinoma, and an operation on the lungs will not cure it.

Signs and Symptoms

The signs of cancer in the lung are not numerous and may be absent until the cancer is far advanced. This depends upon where the cancer first starts. If one of the main bronchial tubes is partially obstructed there may be a wheezing which will lead to an X ray of the lungs. If there is a congestion of the lining caused by blocking of a bronchial tube out near the periphery, dullness may be noted on percussion or tapping the chest with the finger. Sometimes there will be a collection of fluid or effusion if the cancer involves the pleura or lining on the outside of the lung. On rare occasions rales may be heard when listening to the chest with a stethescope.

X ray of the chest is the most reliable way to detect cancer of the lung and should be used about twice a year if the person if over forty-five and cancer is suspected.

Chronic cough is the most common symptom, but because cancer is seen most often in heavy cigarette smokers who nearly always have a cough, this symptom is often ignored or called a "cigarette cough" and the diagnosis is missed.

Sometimes there is sputum with the cough which may be bloodstreaked, or the cough may be dry and nonproductive at first. Coughing up blood and pain in the chest may be present. Progressive loss of weight and increasing weakness may be the only symptoms. Hoarseness may be

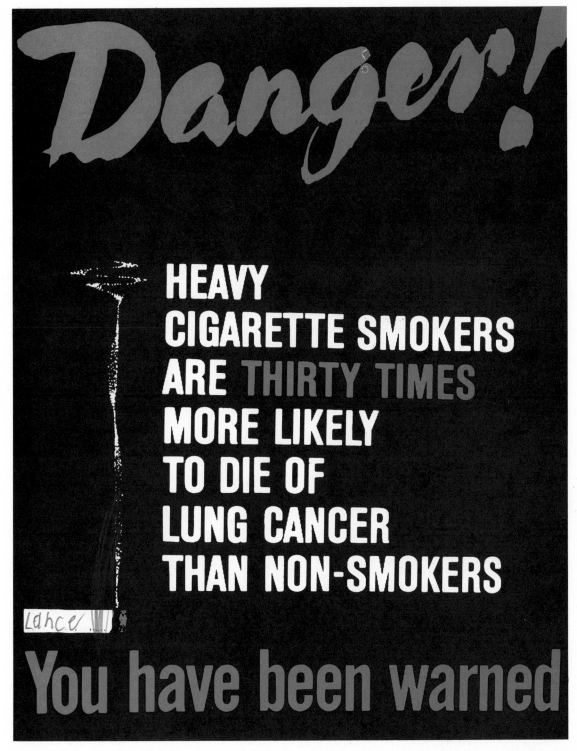

Poster used in England to inform people of the harmful effects caused by cigarette smoking. This danger has been proven.

noted, as well as shortness of breath. If the cancer is near the top of the lung, there may be pain in the shoulder on that side.

X ray of the chest should be performed early if symptoms are present. Looking into the bronchial tubes with a bronchoscope may permit detection of a tumor. Study of the cells in the sputum (called cytology) will often reveal cancer cells.

All of these methods of diagnosis may be used, but X ray is the most important one. One term used by doctors in describing a spot on the lung which may be cancer is "coin lesion." This means that there is a white spot on the X ray of the lung about the size of a nickel or a dime and perfectly round. In some cases this is the only abnormality; but it should be investigated because it may be early cancer, although in many cases it may be harmless.

Treatment

When cancer of the lung is found to be primary cancer (one arising in the lung), it should be removed by surgery. The methods for doing this have been improved greatly, but it is still a major procedure. The cancer is removed by excising or cutting out one lobe of the lung, or in some cases by removing the whole lung. It is possible for a person to live without one lung.

Emphysema, which is present in some older people, will often be a complication which prevents removal of a lung. Since cancer of the lung and emphysema are both seen in older people, this condition should be investigated before surgery is attempted.

When there is a single small "coin lesion" near the outer edge of the lung it is considered wise to remove only the lesion, to determine whether or not it is cancer.

Deep X ray therapy or treatment is often used to slow up the growth of the cancer, but it will not cure it. When the lobe of the lung or the whole lung is removed, the lymph gland nearby should be removed also to prevent an early spread of the cancer.

If the cancer is first detected after it has metastasized to other parts of the body or has spread locally, there is no point in performing surgery. Early detection of cancer of the lung is the only possible means of effecting a cure by surgery.

GLOSSARY

Carcinoma   cancer; a malignant growth
Coin lesion   a white spot the size of a nickel or dime on an X ray of the lung
Cytology   the study of organic cells
Effusion   the escape of fluid into a part or tissue
Embolism   blockage of a tube or canal by an abnormal particle (embolus)
Emphysema   swelling caused by gas in body tissue
Metastasis   transfer of cancer from one part of the body to another
Periphery   outer edge or surface; region where nerves end
Rale   a crackling sound heard through a stethoscope during respiration
Tumor   an abnormal mass of tissue caused by inflammation

DEAFNESS

Cause and Nature

Deafness or loss of hearing is a relative condition varying from a slight loss of hearing to total deafness. There are many causes, some of which are repeated infection of the middle ear, earache, enlarged adenoid tissue, infection, and closure of the Eustachian tube. One of the most common of all causes of deafness is exposure to loud

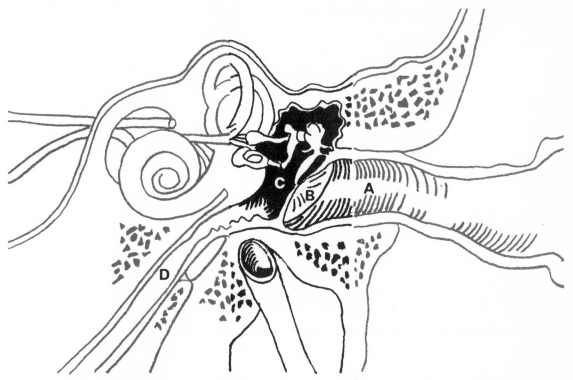

The ear: The external canal (A), the eardrum (B), the middle ear (C) (includes three small bones which transfer vibrations from eardrum to membrane over oval window and hence to nerve of hearing), and the Eustachian tube (D).

noises over a long period of time. This type is seen in men who work near noisy machines, trap shooters, and artillery men who are often exposed to loud sounds.

In a child or in an adult, the sooner deafness or partial loss of hearing is detected, the more chance there will be for improvement with the proper treatment.

Signs and Symptoms

A child may not hear when he is spoken to or an older person may find it difficult to understand a conversation that is carried on in a normal tone of voice.

In case of chronic infection of the ear with a running ear which persists, deafness in one ear may be total, while in the other ear the hearing may be normal.

There are many ways to test the ability to hear. The most accurate of these is the audiometer test. Measuring the distance a person can hear the whispered voice is a rough way of testing for loss of hearing.

Treatment

Any person who has a loss of hearing should be referred to an ear specialist who will test the hearing, determining what causes the loss of hearing and the steps to correct it. In some cases the use of antibiotics or medicine to clear up an infection of the middle ear will help. In the case of small children, an operation to remove enlarged and infected adenoids may be of great value.

In a certain number of cases operations

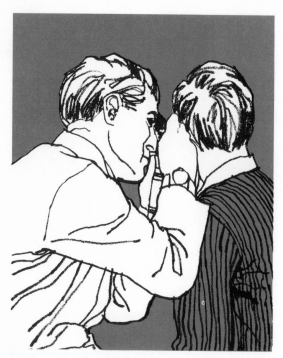

Ear examination by doctor.

on the ear will correct the loss of hearing. The so-called fenestration operation has been improved lately and people who have been hard of hearing for years are aided by this surgery. In other cases, the use of a hearing aid is indicated.

The choice of treatment should be in the hands of a good ear specialist who will determine the exact cause and use the proper methods to correct the deafness.

EARACHE

(*Otitis Media*)

Cause and Nature

Earache can follow measles, scarlet fever, influenza, or most any kind of an infection which involves the upper respiratory tract. The most common cause in children is the ordinary cold. Inflammation of the throat may cause the adenoid tissues around the end of the Eustachian tube to close it off and a collection of fluid occurs in the middle ear which cannot drain through the Eustachian tube and this causes pain. Sometimes this fluid is clear, sometimes it is pus. If the Eustachian tube is not opened up so the fluid can drain out, the eardrum will either rupture and allow the fluid to escape or it will have to be lanced by a doctor. A ruptured or lanced eardrum nearly always heals without any loss of hearing.

Signs and Symptoms

A doctor can look at the eardrum and see whether it is red or bulging and even sometimes it may be drawn in or retracted. In the early stages there may be a feeling of fullness in the ear or pain with a loss of hearing. In very young children, the drum may rupture by itself and the mother will notice fluid, pus, or blood draining from the ear.

Treatment

Heat to the external ear, warm ear drops (glycerin with a small percentage of phenol), aspirin to relieve the pain, and most important, nose drops (1% ephedrine in saline) which are allowed to go from the nose down the back of the throat thereby shrinking the swollen tissues, allowing the Eustachian tube to open and drain out the fluid, may clear up the condition. Never put drops in the ear after the eardrum has ruptured or has been lanced.

Chapter 9

Diseases of the Heart and Blood Vessels

ANGINA PECTORIS

Cause and Nature

This disease is characterized by attacks of substernal (under the sternum or breast bone in the middle of the chest) discomfort, which is usually brought on by exercise. This discomfort may be pain, burning, fullness, heaviness, constriction, or numbness.

It is usually caused by coronary artery disease which makes it impossible for the heart muscle to receive an adequate supply of oxygen when unusual demands are made on it. Arteriosclerosis of the coronary vessels is one of the common causes.

Signs and Symptoms

Increased demands on the heart muscle, such as emotion, exercise, or distention of the abdominal viscera (organs) by food or gas, may cause pain in the anterior chest, in the middle part of the left arm, or in the head or neck. Sometimes the pain is felt only in the upper part of the abdomen. Many patients find that they can terminate an attack by remaining absolutely motionless for a minute or two.

Treatment

Rest and avoidance of excitement and exertion will do much to prevent attacks. Do not overeat or eat food which disagrees. The patient should reduce weight to lessen the work of the heart muscles. This loss of weight should be accomplished gradually.

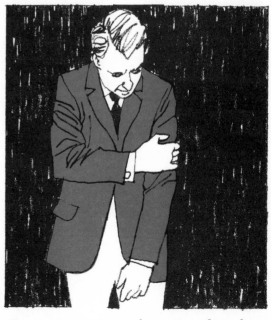

Heart pain starting in chest may radiate down arm. Sometimes the pain is only in the arm.

147

For the acute attack of pain, a nitroglycerin tablet (1/100 grain) held under the tongue will usually bring relief. These tablets should be carried in the pocket of persons suffering from angina. It is also wise to try to prevent an attack by taking a small dose of nitroglycerin (1/200 grain) held under the tongue before being subjected to excitement—as in making a speech—or anger which may be anticipated, as in the case of an undesirable interview.

Arterial dilators, of which there are many, should be taken indefinitely. Peritrate is a good one.

GLOSSARY

Anterior   in the front of or in the forward part of
Arteriosclerosis   thickening of arteries
Substernal   below the breast bone

CONGESTIVE HEART DISEASE

(Sometimes called "Dropsy")

Cause and Nature

The term "congestive heart disease," sometimes called congestive heart failure, is used to describe a condition which arises when the heart gets behind in its work due to some type of heart disease. In young people this congestive failure nearly always occurs in those who have some organic heart disease with a loud murmur or enlargement of the heart. In older people the condition may be caused by poor circulation to the heart muscle as in coronary insufficiency or arteriosclerotic heart disease.

In young people the condition is easily recognized, but in older people the onset may be slow and in some cases the diagnosis may be difficult.

Since the treatment of this condition may prolong life and certainly will make the patient more comfortable, it is very important to have a doctor examine and treat every case of congestive heart failure.

Signs and Symptoms

When the heart begins to get behind in its work of making the blood circulate through the body, certain signs and symptoms which are caused by the congestion of various tissues in the body always appear.

Dyspnea or shortness of breath is one of the most dramatic of these symptoms. This is especially true when the shortness of breath comes on while the person is at rest. A typical case of this symptom in a person with congestive heart disease is as follows. A person will awaken out of a sound sleep and be extremely short of breath. He will have to sit up in bed in order to breathe at all, and a dry cough may start which later may become productive of a blood-tinged sputum. This type of attack will require prompt treatment by a doctor and proper treatment will usually bring relief. In some cases the attack may pass off spontaneously, only to recur a few nights later. In any case this type of symptom should be treated by a doctor.

The heart may become irregular in its rhythm, so-called fibrillation, and the rate may be rapid. Sometimes if the congestion affects the gastro-intestinal tract there will be nausea and vomiting. Instead of waking from sleep with shortness of breath, the person may become short of breath with the slightest exertion.

A person with chronic congestive failure may present a swelling of both legs which disappears after a night's sleep. This is sometimes called "dropsy." In some cases of congestive heart failure there may be a slight fever, but this is not always the case. Most

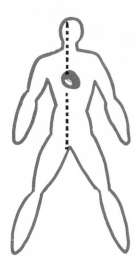

THE LIVING PUMP

The heart sits diagonally in the chest just behind the breastbone. If a line were drawn down the center of the body, slightly more of the heart could be seen to be on the left side.

The heart is a living pump of masterful design and function.

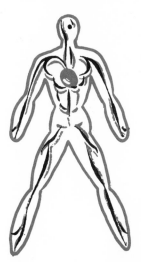

The heart pumps the blood out through tubes called arteries (indicated in red), into tiny tubes called capillaries, into tubes called veins (indicated in black) that lead back into the heart. All of your blood completes this cycle in 60 seconds or less.

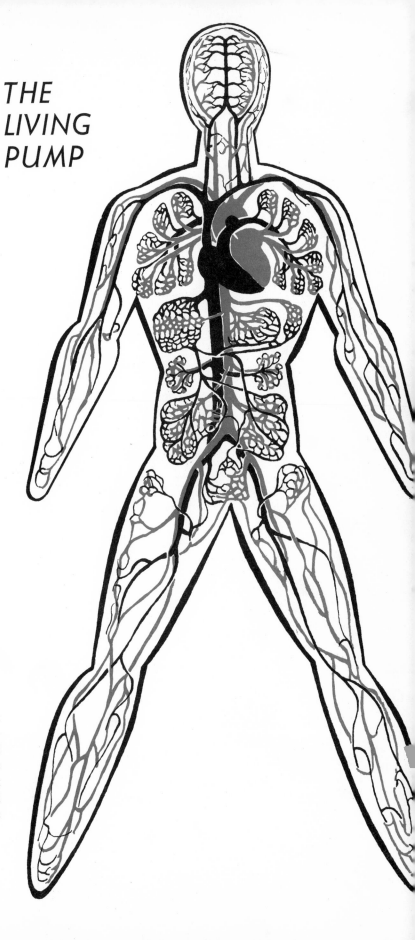

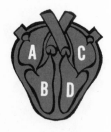

The heart is a muscle about the size of your fist. It has four chambers—right upper (A), right lower (B), left upper (C), left lower (D), and four valves that prevent blood from flowing in the wrong direction.

The blood circulates—follow it in diagrams below—like this: (1) Blood from your body flows into the right upper chamber of your heart. (2) When the right upper chamber is full, your heart contracts, and your blood flows through a valve into the right lower chamber. (3) Your heart contracts again, and the blood is forced through a second valve into the artery to the lungs. (4) Your blood eliminates waste gases through your lungs while absorbing oxygen, then flows into the left upper chamber of your heart. (5) The blood flow continues through a third valve into the left lower chamber of the heart. (6) Finally, your blood passes through a fourth valve into a large artery, from which it flows through smaller arteries all over your body.

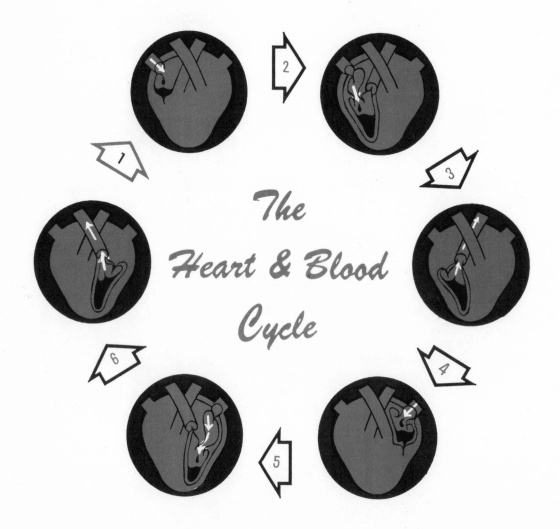

The Heart & Blood Cycle

cases do not have an elevation of temperature. Frequently there is high blood pressure, but this is not always so.

Treatment

The treatment of congestive heart failure must be in the hands of a competent physician. The doctor will see that the patient gets the proper amount of rest. He will probably give digitalis to strengthen the heartbeat and will restrict the use of salt in the diet. In some cases medicine will be given to stimulate the kidneys. If high blood pressure is present, medicine will be given to lower the blood pressure and take the extra work away from a failing heart.

The treatment of congestive failure is very important, for with the proper care many people can add productive and comfortable years to their lives.

It is imperative to seek treatment as soon as possible to ward off excessive damage to the heart and other parts of the body.

GLOSSARY

Congestion overfullness
Fibrillation muscular tremor

CARDIAC ARYTHMIAS

1. Extra Systoles

Cause and Nature

These are the most common of all heart irregularities, and are often spoken of as a dropped beat. Actually this irregular heart beating is caused by an extra or premature beat and then a long pause to pick up the regular rhythm. This pause causes the patient to think he has missed a beat.

The irregularity may be caused by eating a heavy meal, and often comes after exercise. Sometimes it is felt soon after going to bed at night.

Signs and Symptoms

The patient may notice a slight thump, or if he is feeling his pulse, may notice what he thinks is a dropped beat.

If there is no organic heart disease present, these extra systoles are of no importance and should be disregarded.

Treatment

No treatment is needed unless they become frequent enough to disturb the patient. Then quinidine sulphate, grains 3, taken three times a day will stop them. If this fails, see your doctor.

GLOSSARY

Organic pertaining to an organ
Systole contraction of the heart

2. Paroxysmal Auricular Tachycardia

Cause and Nature

This condition, popularly called palpitation, is caused by an abnormal stimulation in the auricles which causes the heart to beat rapidly, usually between 160 and 200 beats per minute. It is usually seen in young adults who have no organic heart disease and is not dangerous, although it will cause the patient and family to become apprehensive. It usually starts suddenly and stops suddenly.

Signs and Symptoms

An otherwise normal person will suddenly feel his pulse rate go up alarmingly. After speeding up, the rate does not vary. There is often a slight feeling of pain in the chest if the attack lasts for any length of time, and usually there is weakness.

Treatment

The patient may discover a movement or position that will stop the attack. Holding the breath, drinking ice water, or pressure over the eyeballs may be successful. If these do not stop the attack, a physician should be called. He may try carotid sinus pressure or administer a drug such as quinidine or digitalis.

GLOSSARY

Apprehensive   fearful
Auricle   chamber in the heart
Carotid sinus   nerves on an artery in the neck

3. Heart Block

Cause and Nature

This abnormality of conduction is usually caused by one of three things:

a. Digitalis, causing delayed conduction
b. Rheumatic fever
c. Chronic heart disease, such as arteriosclerosis

Its nature varies all the way from a slowing of the ventricular rate to forty a minute to complete ventricular standstill.

Signs and Symptoms

The pulse rate may be slowed to forty or fifty without any symptoms. On the other hand, slowing of the rate may cause fainting attacks. A complete standstill may cause convulsions or death.

Treatment

Treat the underlying cause. If the attacks of complete standstill (so-called Stokes-Adams syndrome) occur several times daily, the patient should be given epinephrine, ephedrine or paredrine. It is possible, however, for a patient to have a partial heart block—very slow pulse—and go on living a normal life. In such cases, where there are no symptoms, no treatment is necessary.

GLOSSARY

Arteriosclerosis   thickening of the arteries
Conduction   transfer of waves, sound, heat
Syndrome   a set of symptoms
Ventricular   pertaining to cavities of the heart

CONGENITAL HEART DISEASE

Cause and Nature

The cause is some defect in development of the heart, and the child is born with an inefficient heart. The most common forms are:

1. Patent ductus arteriosus
2. Coarctation of the aorta
3. Septal defects

Signs and Symptoms

A congenital heart lesion in a baby probably will be first diagnosed by a doctor who hears murmurs over the heart with his stethoscope. In addition, some types of congenital heart disease cause the patient's skin to have a bluish tint (cyanosis), and others cause the blood pressure to be elevated.

Treatment

In recent years great strides have been made in surgery of the heart, and many of these defects can be corrected by surgery if detected and treated early. Any child with a congenital heart lesion should be especially protected against infection.

GLOSSARY

Aorta   main artery
Congenital   occurring at birth

Cyanosis   bluish color of skin
Lesion   a local sore or change in tissue
Patent ductus   wide open duct
Septal   pertaining to a septum
Stethoscope   instrument for listening to body sounds

HYPERTENSION

(High Blood Pressure)

Cause and Nature

High blood pressure is really a sign and not a disease in itself. It is perhaps the most commonly misunderstood symptom with which man is afflicted. An understanding of this condition can save needless worry and discomfort.

In the first place, when a patient goes to a doctor's office his blood pressure is taken. If the patient is nervous or excited, the reading will probably be higher than it should be and the patient may go home with the idea that he has high blood pressure. This causes him to worry and the next time he comes to the doctor's office he is really concerned and his pressure is up a little.

One blood pressure reading taken in a doctor's office does not mean much. Repeated measurements must be made, uninfluenced by excitement, exertion, or fatigue, before a person's real level of blood pressure can be determined.

There are a great many factors which may cause high blood pressure. Roughly, they may be divided into three main groups:

1. Mechanical—i.e., when the arteries are small and their walls are hard, it takes a higher pressure to force the blood through.
2. Neural—this operates through stimulation of the vasomotor center—excitement, anxiety, etc

3. Humeral—this operates through substances which circulate through the blood and act directly on muscles of the small arteries.

Hereditary, emotional, endocrine, and other factors are probably concerned with elevating the blood pressure.

It should be remembered that in taking the blood pressure two readings are noted: the systolic, or high, and the diastolic, or low. For instance, in 190/80, the 190 is systolic, and the 80 is diastolic. Of the two, the diastolic is far more important. A few points change in this reading means more than larger changes in the systolic reading. It should be remembered that the readings, especially systolic, will vary greatly in the same person from time to time. I have seen the systolic pressure drop 50 points in twenty minutes in a healthy young man—from 170/80 to 120/80.

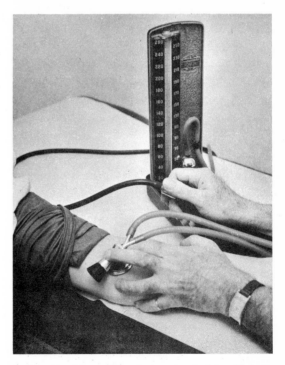

A doctor taking a blood pressure in his office. A simple and painless procedure.

Persistent high blood pressure will damage the heart, kidneys, and blood vessels. But always remember that high blood pressure can only be determined by an average of many readings, and not by one isolated reading.

Signs and Symptoms

There may be no symptom at first, but as the condition persists and organic changes take place, there may be headaches, usually worse early in the morning while still in bed, dizziness, flushing, nosebleeds, and cold extremities. As the condition progresses, heart symptoms may arise. The most common of these may be shortness of breath and fatigability. These may go on to congestive failure with swelling of the legs and irregularities of the heartbeat.

A certain number, about one-third, of hypertension cases develop cerebral hemorrhage or stroke. Minor strokes may occur which may be manifested by indefinite symptoms such as increased irritability, dizziness, fatigue, forgetfulness, ringing in the ears, anxiety states, disturbances of the vision, or speech disorders. Nocturia, or frequency of urination during the night, may accompany hypertension.

Treatment

The treatment of hypertension is that of the underlying disease, if possible. Excessive weight appears to cause an elevation in blood pressure and should be eliminated. Some patients with hypertension are helped by a low sodium diet. This diet is augmented by the administration of a diuretic or drug that causes an increase in the output of urine. There are many of these drugs; hydrodiuril is a good one. Mild sedation is helpful in allaying anxiety and tension. Surgery may be restorted to in certain extremely severe cases. There are powerful drugs that, if properly used by a physician, may give symptomatic relief. Many drugs are being advertised and used that do not help. It is very important, then, to have the advice of a competent physician in cases of hypertension. It is especially important to realize that one reading of an elevated blood pressure does not mean that the patient has hypertension.

GLOSSARY

Cerebral   pertaining to the brain
Diastolic   lowest pressure recorded in blood pressure recording
Endocrine   of the glands
Fatigability   susceptibility to being tired
Hemorrhage   bleeding
Hypertension   high blood pressure
Low sodium diet   very little salt in the diet
Nocturia   excessive urination at night
Systolic   highest pressure recorded in blood pressure
Vasomotor   controlling size of blood vessels

VARICOSE VEINS

Cause and Nature

Varicose veins are caused by a combination of factors. These may be: lack of supporting tissue surrounding the veins; high pressure within the vein when the person is upright; and, most important of all, incompetent or broken down valves within the vein itself. Sometimes a weakness of the valves appears to be inherited. Varicosities may be aggravated by prolonged standing, pregnancy, and heavy work.

These vessels appear usually along the medial (inner) and posterior (back) portion of the legs as tortuous, dilated vessels which become more distended upon standing.

Signs and Symptoms

After varicose veins have been present for some time, brown pigmentation of the skin of the lower leg is common. There is usually itching, and a heavy, tired feeling of the legs may persist. There may be an aching in the legs and swelling of feet or ankles. A combination of poor circulation and injury to legs may cause varicose ulcers, which are difficult to heal.

Treatment

An improvement of the circulation is the aim of treatment. Support to the leg may be accomplished by wearing elastic bandages or stockings. These must extend up as high as the distended veins. In the case of varicose ulcers, an antiseptic ointment may be used to clear up infection, then a piece of scotch tape may be applied directly over the ulcer. Over this tape a piece of sponge rubber is placed, and over all an elastic bandage (4 inch) is wound. This causes pressure over the ulcer preventing distention or slowing up of circulation.

Injection of the incompetent veins with a sclerosing solution will close the poor veins off, and cause the blood to return through the deeper, good veins in some mild cases.

Removal by surgery of the incompetent veins along with the perforating branches is the best treatment in persistent or extensive cases. Tests must be made to be sure the deep veins are in good condition before the incompetent veins are removed.

GLOSSARY

Distended   stretched
Medial   inner
Pigmentation   color
Posterior   behind
Sclerosing   closing off
Ulcer   a sore
Valve   fold in a canal or passage
Varicose   swollen

CORONARY OCCLUSION

Cause and Nature

Heart attack—coronary occlusion or coronary thrombosis—is extremely important and far too common. It is usually caused by coronary artery disease which narrows the lumen of the coronary arteries, and then one of them becomes completely closed off, thereby denying blood to a portion of the heart muscle. When the heart muscle is without blood to furnish it oxygen, pain occurs, and if any appreciable segment of the muscle is without oxygen long enough this muscle dies (myocardial infarction). The results may vary from sudden death to the other extreme where the patient, after proper treatment, recovers and lives comfortably for many years. The cause of narrowing of the coronary vessels has not been

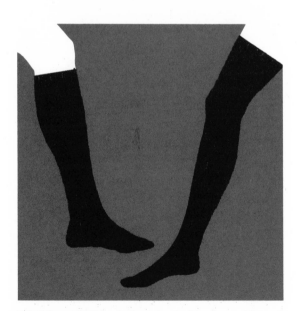

Elastic stockings help return the venous blood back up the leg.

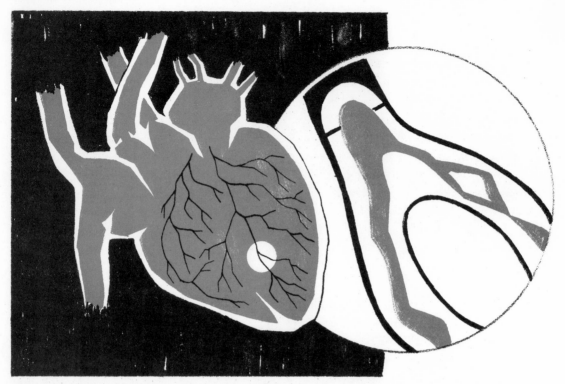

Heart Attack: A clot in the coronary artery which deprives part of the heart muscle of blood.

determined yet. It has apparently the same cause as narrowing of other arteries (arteriosclerosis) or hardening of the arteries.

Much work has been done recently on the theory that this calcification or hardening of the arteries may be caused, or at least influenced, by an overabundance of large, fatty particles in the blood. This has led to low cholesterol or low fat diets in an effort to prevent or to halt coronary artery disease before it becomes serious. While it has not been proven conclusively that this is the cause, enough evidence has been brought forward to convince many physicians that a low fat diet is important in prevention and cure of this serious condition.

A great deal of work has been done also in recent years to prevent heart attacks or coronary occlusion in young and middle-aged men. It has been determined that if a man is what is known as a Type B man, that is not the highly competitive, high pressure, high-strung, dead-line meeting type, something can be done about prophylaxis or prevention of coronary occlusion. This involves keeping his blood cholesterol down to about 200 and keeping the other fats or lipids in his blood down to a reasonable level. This objective can be obtained by diet and medication. These conditions will have to be attained by remaining under the supervision of a doctor.

Apparently the evidence to date points to the saturated fatty acids as the principal cause of trouble, while the unsaturated fatty acids apparently cause little harm and are, indeed, useful in our nutrition. A rough rule to follow in distinguishing between saturated and unsaturated fatty acids is that the saturated or dangerous fatty acids are derived from animals, as a rule, and the unsaturated ones are from vegetables.

As mentioned above, the work on this has not been completed yet, and the proof is not conclusive that these fatty acids contribute to coronary disease, but enough proof has been brought forward to make it worth while to be cautious about the amount and kind of fatty acids which you eat, and to find out from your doctor just what a low cholesterol diet is.

Signs and Symptoms

The patient will experience pain or a feeling of pressure below the sternum. This has been described as feeling as though a football were being blown up in your chest below the sternum. The pain may radiate down the left arm or in some cases down both arms. In other cases, it radiates to the jaw. Sometimes the pain is only felt in the left arm, and in other cases the pain is felt in the upper abdomen only. Shock is usually present, and the blood pressure drops. In many severe attacks there may be shortness of breath and a fear of impending death.

Treatment

This is one condition in which a doctor should be called immediately. The patient should not exert himself, and should remain in a semi-reclining position—that is, propped up so that the head and chest are slightly higher than the lower portion of the body.

These cases usually are hospitalized after an attempt is made to control the pain. An oxygen tent is used for this purpose. After the pain has subsided, the patient may feel that he is well and want to go home. This is very dangerous. Many deaths have

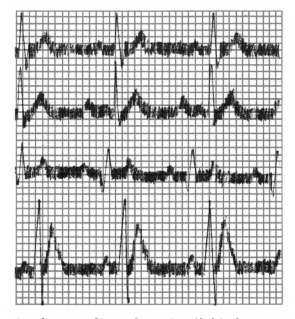 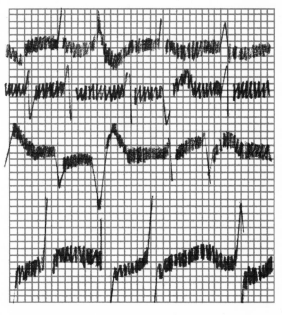

An electrocardiograph tracing (left) showing a normal heart beat. The tracing on the right shows an abnormal condition. These tracings must be interpreted by an expert.

occurred when patients have insisted on walking out of the hospital against the doctor's advice.

Prolonged and careful treatment is needed to allow the weakened and damaged heart muscle to be repaired. This can only be correctly supervised by a competent physician, and can best be accomplished by 100 percent cooperation on the part of the patient. Absolute rest is important at first. Loud talking, excitement, coughing, lifting, or even straining at stool must be avoided. The doctor will need certain laboratory tests such as electrocardiograms, blood counts, etc., to let him know how the case is progressing. For this reason, treatment in a hospital, where these tests may be made, is advantageous.

After the first effects of the attack are over, and the patient gradually resumes activity, it is extremely important to be guided by the advice of the doctor as to how much and how rapidly normal activity can be resumed. Medication for the rest of the patient's life may or may not be necessary. Certainly all excess weight must be removed and not regained in order to lessen the strain on the damaged heart. The diet is then doubly important—to keep off weight, and to avoid cholesterol or fats.

If the patient cooperates fully there is no reason why a person who has had one heart attack may not lead a long and useful life.

GLOSSARY

Cholesterol fatty acids
Coronary a term applied to vessels in the heart muscle
Electrocardiogram a graphic tracing of the heart contracture
Infarction any cutting off of blood supply which results in death or injury to tissue
Lumen channel within a tube or tubular organ
Myocardial pertaining to the heart muscle
Occlusion obstruction or closing of a passage
Sternum chest bone
Thrombosis formation of a clot

ARTERIOSCLEROSIS

(Hardening of the Arteries)

Diseases of the heart and blood vessels are the leading cause of death in the American people, and since this condition is one of the most common causes of death and sickness, it would be well for all of us to understand as much about it as possible.

Even doctors and research men who have spent their lives treating people with arteriosclerosis and trying to find out what causes it and how to prevent it, do not know all the answers.

A great mass of evidence has been produced and is being studied. It is to be hoped that sometime in the near future these studies will begin to pay off in the form of preventing the occurrence of hardening of the arteries.

Some of the possible causes that are now under study are: heredity, obesity, physical inactivity, rich diets, cigarette smoking (see chart on facing page), air pollution, the heavy use of coffee, and emotional stress.

There are three separate forms of arteriosclerosis and since each one is so important, it will be individually discussed. In order to understand the different kinds of arteriosclerosis it would be well to know the make-up of an artery.

Every artery in the body, large and small, is made up of three layers. The inner layer is called the intima, the middle layer is known as the media, and the outside covering is the serosa. Most diseases of the arteries are concerned with the inner and middle layers.

Arteriosclerosis

Hardening of the arteries is caused by a deposit of calcium in the middle layer or media of the artery.

Cause and Nature

This hardening and thickening of the middle layer of arteries is a common and almost universal result of the aging process in the human race, especially in the peoples of North America and Northern Europe. It is caused by deposits of calcium in the middle layer of arteries. In itself it does not cause a narrowing of the lumen or opening in the vessel; and hence by itself this kind of arteriosclerosis does not cause a diminution or decrease in the blood supply to the part affected. Thus, in older people, X rays may show a complete outline of the arteries in the legs. This outline is made by deposits of calcium and no decrease of the circulation to the feet can be noted. However, hardening of the middle layer may interfere with the nerve control to these vessels and account for some of the symptoms which go with the process of aging.

In many cases the calcium deposits in the media are accompanied by deposits of a fatty substance on the inner surface of the vessel called atherosclerosis (distinguish between the two names arterio- and athero-sclerosis). This deposit on the inner layer will cause the opening or lumen of the vessel to be narrowed and many symptoms including high blood pressure will occur. Remember that if the process is confined to the middle layer only, then the symptoms may be lacking or mild.

Signs and Symptoms

Generalized arteriosclerosis may be present for a long time without causing any symptoms if the inner layer is not affected.

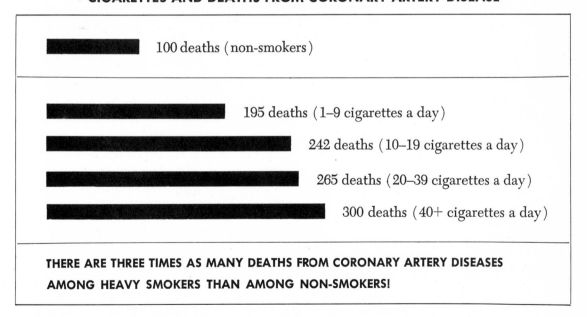

CIGARETTES AND DEATHS FROM CORONARY ARTERY DISEASE*

100 deaths (non-smokers)

195 deaths (1–9 cigarettes a day)

242 deaths (10–19 cigarettes a day)

265 deaths (20–39 cigarettes a day)

300 deaths (40+ cigarettes a day)

THERE ARE THREE TIMES AS MANY DEATHS FROM CORONARY ARTERY DISEASES AMONG HEAVY SMOKERS THAN AMONG NON-SMOKERS!

*Based on statistics released by the American Cancer Society for the age group 40 to 59.

Signs of hardening of the arteries may be detected by X ray or by feeling the hard arteries in the wrist, yet there may be no evidence of decreased circulation to the part. The blood pressure may be slightly elevated and the other signs and symptoms that always go with aging will appear. The parts most generally affected by hardening of the arteries are the heart, the brain, and the kidneys. These, along with the lower extremities, are usually affected only to the extent that the inner layer is also affected by atherosclerosis. Naturally, if the artery walls are hard they do not respond to the orders from the brain which are sent to

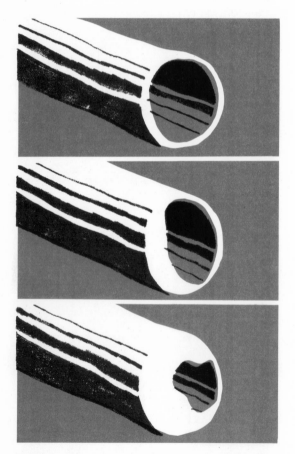

Deposits on the inner wall of an artery can gradually build up and close it off.

them by way of nerves as readily as a pliable artery would, but the only thing that happens here is a gradually slowing down seen in the process of aging.

Treatment

There is no known treatment for this form of calcium deposit in the middle layer of the arteries. Every person who attains old age is subject to this process and the only way to lessen the symptoms is to grow old in a sane and sensible way.

This applies to the mental as well as the physical part of aging. We should slowly decrease our activities as we grow older and try to make a sane mental adjustment to changes which eventually take place.

Symptomatic treatment may be used by a doctor to help make this adjustment easier. If there is restlessness, mild sedatives may be used. If there is pain, the use of aspirin or some other mild pain killing drug is indicated.

Atherosclerosis

Narrowing of the arteries.

Cause and Nature

This is a disease in which small patches of a fat-like substance are deposited beneath the inner surface of blood vessels. Although it may occur at the same time as senile arteriosclerosis, it is not to be confused with this natural process of aging which has just been described. The causes are different and the results separated from those caused by hardening of the medial portion of arteries. In older persons it is often hard to differentiate between the two processes, because they often go hand in hand. Do not forget that it is possible to have one without the other and many old people have calcium deposits in the middle layer without any symptoms because they do not have fatty deposits in the inner layer which narrow the vessel and cause symptoms.

The cause of atherosclerosis is not understood although there are many factors which seem to influence the degree or extent of its presence in any given individual.

Race seems to be a factor. The Jewish race living in the United States seems to be more susceptible to this condition. All white people may be affected by it more than colored people, and Africans living in their own country are less susceptible to this disease than Africans living in the United States. This also applies to Japanese living in Japan, who have this disease much less often than the members of their race who live in Hawaii or the continental United States.

Heredity and familial influences seem to play an important part in this disease. In other words, it may occur more often in one family than in another.

Sex seems to have something to do with it because women seldom suffer from this disease before the menopause. White men quite often are affected before the age of forty-five.

This brings up the question of age. It has been proven by post mortem examination that more than half the people in the United States who die before the age of fifty have atherosclerosis, and nearly all of the people who die after the age of seventy-five have atheromatous plaques or patches.

High blood pressure seems to increase the incidence although it is difficult to determine whether the atherosclerosis causes the high blood pressure or vice versa.

Since there have been no physical factors which can be absolutely blamed for the occurrence of atherosclerosis, the search for its cause has been concentrated largely on chemical causes. It is thought that the chemical content of the blood plasma in man may bring on this condition since man's plasma has different components than that of other animals which do not suffer from atherosclerosis.

Chief among the causes that have been studied to date is the fatty or cholesterol content of the blood plasma. Many forms of cholesterol are found in the plasma, and it has never been determined which ones are the causative factors. Some day we may know the secret and man will then be spared untold sickness and suffering.

For the present let us say that atherosclerosis seems to be affected by the chemical constituents of the blood plasma and that there may be a familial tendency.

Heavy smoking seems to be a contributing factor and gross overweight certainly has some bearing, for obese persons seem to suffer from the effects of this disease at an earlier age than do people who are not overweight.

Signs and Symptoms

The effects of atheromatous plaques which narrow a blood vessel will depend upon where the plaque is and how large it is.

Generalized deposits of this kind may cause easy fatigability and a gradual loss of capacity to perform physical or mental work. A localized deposit will cause symptoms in the part which has had its circulation disturbed. Atherosclerosis is the most frequent cause of heart disease, and since heart disease is the leading cause of death in the United States, it may be assumed that atherosclerosis is the "Captain of the Men of Death."

Decrease in blood supply to the heart causes pain, sometimes manifested in so-called angina pectoris, and cases of coronary occlusion or coronary thrombosis are nearly always the result of atherosclerosis.

When the atheromatous plaques are found in the blood vessels of the brain they cause strokes, which are due either to hemorrhage (the rupture of a vessel) or thrombosis, which is clot formation in a vessel which closes it off.

In cases where actual hemorrhage or closure does not occur, the vessels may become smaller and smaller, cutting off an adequate blood supply to the brain. This results in emotional instability and impairment of memory, especially loss of memory for recent events. The person affected may become irritable and hostile. This is the so-called cerebral atherosclerosis which may eventually lead to senile dementia.

Narrowing of the blood vessels to the kidneys will cause high blood pressure and contribute to other kidney diseases.

This lack of circulation in the extremities, especially in the feet, will cause many symptoms and may lead to gangrene.

Atherosclerosis of the peripheral arteries does not occur before the age of fifty-five, except in persons who have diabetes, and then it may occur at an earlier age. Therefore, if a serious disturbance in the circulation of the lower extremities occurs before fifty, it is probably not caused by atherosclerosis, but by Buerger's disease, or is contributed to by diabetes.

Treatment

Since the real cause of atherosclerosis is not known, a definite treatment cannot be suggested. However, enough is known about the disease to indicate that certain precautions, if taken early enough, may prevent its occurrence in a serious enough form to give symptoms. These precautions are:

1. Do not eat too much. Fat people are definitely susceptible to atherosclerosis.
2. Limit your intake of fat, especially animal fat. Corn oil can be substituted for animal fat.
3. If your blood pressure is high, take steps to keep it down. See a doctor who will prescribe proper medication. High blood pressure not only encourages deposits of plaques on the artery walls but increases the possibility of rupture of these walls with resultant hemorrhage.
4. People who have had coronary attacks caused by thrombosis or atherosclerosis should be under the supervision of a doctor who will advise them as to diet and medication.

Arteriolar Sclerosis

Cause and Nature

This third form of arteriosclerosis applies to the thickening of the small arteries found in the kidneys, the extremities, and other organs. These small vessels are called arterioles, and their walls are thickened by deposits of calcium in the middle layer and deposits of fats on the inner surface just as in larger arteries.

Signs and Symptoms

The signs and symptoms will depend upon which part of the body is affected.

In the legs, when the circulation becomes impaired, the first symptoms may be a numbness, burning sensation, and tingling in the toes. There may be cramps in the legs at night and a feeling of heaviness or weakness in the legs. One outstanding symptom—called intermittent claudication, which means a cramp-like pain—will occur in the legs after the patient has walked a block or two. Rest will cause the pain to go away, only to recur again after walking a short distance.

A slight blueness or discoloration of the toes may occur. This may progress to gangrene if the circulation is cut off entirely.

Treatment

Treatment of arteriolar sclerosis is not very satisfactory. A doctor will be able to help identify the early signs and give advice as to proper diet and exercises. In some cases medicine will help, but this must be prescribed by a doctor and usually is not very effective.

Proper care of the feet is important. Shoes must fit, corns and callouses should be treated with respect, and the patient should avoid exposure to dampness and cold.

GLOSSARY

Calcium   the basic element of lime, found in most tissue
Cerebral   pertaining to the main portion of the brain
Coronary artery   vessel to the heart
Dementia   insanity
Familial   affecting different members of a family
Fatigability   tendency to become tired
Hostile   angry
Medial   middle
Menopause   change of life
Obese   fat
Peripheral   situated near the surface
Plaque   patch or flat area
Plasma   fluid portion of blood
Pliable   supple
Senile   of old age
Stroke   hemorrhage or clot in a blood vessel in the brain
Thrombus   clot

BACTERIAL ENDOCARDITIS

Cause and Nature

This disease is usually caused by a streptococcus infection and can be divided in two classes—acute and subacute. Subacute bacterial endocarditis accounts for about ninety percent of the cases. Acute bacterial endocarditis is a rare disease.

This is a very serious disease and it usually lasts a long time. Before the discovery of penicillin and other antibiotics, the condition nearly always led to death. Now by the intensive use of the antibiotics most of the cases can be saved.

The word "endocarditis" implies an infection of the inner part of the heart, and the real disease process nearly always consists of an infection of the valves of the heart. The mitral and aortic valves are the ones most frequently involved. For some reason valves that have been previously damaged by rheumatic fever are the ones most often infected, and the ones which are slightly damaged are involved more often than badly scarred valves.

Bacteria are often found in the blood stream especially following minor surgical procedures such as the extraction of a tooth or removal of the tonsils. The bacteria are nearly always destroyed by the inner defenses of the body found in the liver, spleen, and bone marrow and hence very seldom cause much trouble. If, however, some streptococci circulating happen to lodge on the valves of the heart and start growing, then bacterial endocarditis results. This growth usually takes place in colonies of bacteria which cause irregular vegetation on the heart valve and it is a common occurrence for some of these small pieces to break off and go circulating through the blood. Often a small clump will get stuck in a small artery and become an embolism. These emboli are most dangerous when they occur in the brain, the extremities, and the mesentery. If they get stuck in a small artery and plug it up completely, this may lead to serious complications.

Signs and Symptoms

In some cases subacute endocarditis begins about three or four weeks after some other infection, or after a tonsillectomy or tooth extraction. In most instances the onset or beginning of the disease is so mild and insidious that the patient cannot tell exactly when he became ill.

The most common symptoms are fever, weakness, loss of weight, sweating, especially night sweats, malaise, joint pains, chills, and sometimes strong sensations in the hands and feet called paresthesia, or "needles and pins." There is occasionally paralysis in some part of the body.

There is a heart murmur which may change from time to time. As a matter of fact it has been said that any patient with a heart murmur and a persistent fever should be suspected of having subacute bacterial endocarditis. Bacteria can usually be found in the blood. The well known signs of congestive heart failure often appear, such as swelling of the legs and feet, shortness of breath, and cough.

Subacute bacterial endocarditis may last from one month to as long as two years. Before the discovery of penicillin and other forms of effective treatment of this condition, most of the patients who suffered from subacute bacterial endocarditis died within nine months of the beginning of the disease. Now most of them live.

Treatment

This should be in the hands of a physician, who will administer penicillin which is the most effective treatment for subacute bacterial endocarditis. Most often huge doses are employed—up to 75,000,000 units a day. The drug should be given over a long enough period of time to be sure that all the streptococci are killed. Sometimes the disease starts up again after penicillin is stopped, but if it doesn't recur within six weeks after stopping penicillin the disease is considered cured.

Other antibiotics such as erythromycin and streptomycin are often used in conjunction with penicillin. If the patient cannot tolerate penicillin, a combination of other antibiotics may be used, but these are not nearly so effective as penicillin.

GLOSSARY

Aortic valve   valve of main artery
Bacterial   caused by bacteria
Endocarditis   inflammation of the lining of the heart
Insidious   treacherous; more serious than it appears
Mesentery   a fold of tissue attached to the bowels
Mitral valve   valve of the heart
Paralysis   loss of motion
Paresthesia   an abnormal sensation

RAYNAUD'S DISEASE

Cause and Nature

Raynaud's disease or Raynaud's syndrome is named after the doctor who described it. The cause is not known but the signs and symptoms are caused by a contraction of the arteries in the extremities, usually the hands, and this contraction usually occurs in both hands. It is brought on as a rule by exposure to cold. Women are affected more often than men, and although it may occur at any age, it is not seen often before puberty or after the age of forty.

The attacks may be brought on by immersing the hands in cold water which will cause, for example, the first two fingers on both hands to turn blue; or if the vessels contract, as is most often the case, the fingers turn white.

Signs and Symptoms

A woman of twenty-five may notice pain in identical fingers of both hands when they are exposed to the cold. This pain may be preceded by a tingling in the fingers. When she looks at them she will see that the fingers have turned white and when they are warmed up they become red and painful. After proper treatment and care the attacks may disappear and the person may live to a healthy old age. However, if the attacks are severe and not relieved by treatment, they may lead to gangrene of the finger and necessitate amputation. Fortunately this is a rare disease.

Treatment

The patient should try to prevent exposure of the hands or feet to cold. Motorcycle riders have noted this phenomenon, but when they stop exposing the hands to cold the signs and symptoms disappear.

A doctor should supervise medication which will cause the vessels in the extremities to dilate. Prescoline is one drug that has been used successfully to accomplish this. Other drugs may be used to relieve the pain, but most important of all the patient should avoid exposure to cold. The body should be dressed warmly and the hands should be protected by warm gloves.

GLOSSARY

Amputation   surgical removal of a part
Contraction   a shortening or shrinking
Dilate   stretch beyond normal
Gangrene   dead tissue
Phenomenon   any remarkable appearance or unusual occurrence
Syndrome   a set of symptoms

TRENCH FOOT

Cause and Nature

This condition is caused by injury to the capillaries or small blood vessels in the feet when they are exposed to cold and dampness for a long period of time. Actual freezing does not occur. The soldiers who lived in the wet trenches over extended periods of time suffered from trench feet quite often.

Signs and Symptoms

The cold, wet feet become white and when they are warmed they become swollen and red because the capillaries have been damaged and cannot carry the blood off properly. Sometimes pain is present during the warming period.

If the capillaries have not been damaged too severely the feet may return to normal. If, however, the small vessels have been destroyed, small areas of gangrene may develop. When the damage has been moderate and healing or scarring takes place among the capillaries, fibrosis and neuritis may develop in the feet.

Treatment

The treatment is prevention of exposure to wet and cold. Dry socks should replace the wet ones when possible. After the feet have become white and cold they should be warmed in warm water but never rubbed, for the capillaries which are damaged may be further injured by rubbing.

GLOSSARY

Capillaries   minute blood vessels
Fibrosis   formation of fibrous tissue
Gangrene   dead tissue
Neuritis   inflammation of a nerve

BUERGER'S DISEASE

(*Thrombo-angitis Obliterans*)

Cause and Nature

This condition is brought on by a gradual closing off of the arteries in the extremities, usually the legs and feet. The cause of this obliterating or closing off is not known. Since it occurs in early life it is not arteriosclerosis, and the vessels do not have calcium in them which would show up by X ray.

The disease is seen most often in males between the ages of twenty and forty-five. It is most common among people who are heavy smokers and over half the cases are in young Jewish males.

After first being noticed in the feet and legs it may attack other parts of the body such as the brain, kidneys, or heart. If untreated or unrelieved by treatment, this disease may lead to gangrene of the extremities.

Signs and Symptoms

The first symptom noted may be pain in the calves of the legs or in one leg after walking a very short distance. This is called "intermittent claudication." As the disease progresses the pain may come on at night or when at rest. This pain may become severe and at times excruciating.

When a doctor examines the patient he will note a lack of pulsation in the arteries of the foot or leg. These have been closed off and the pain has been caused by lack of oxygen in the muscles. If the disease progresses to gangrene, amputation may be necessary. Sometimes the acute pain in feet or legs will be relieved by immersing the painful part in ice water for a short period of time.

Treatment

The first step a doctor takes in the treatment of Buerger's disease is the complete and instant stopping of the use of tobacco in any form. As a matter of fact, most doctors will refuse to treat this condition if the patient does not stop smoking cigarettes. Various drugs may be used to dilate the vessels of the extremities, but these must be prescribed by a doctor.

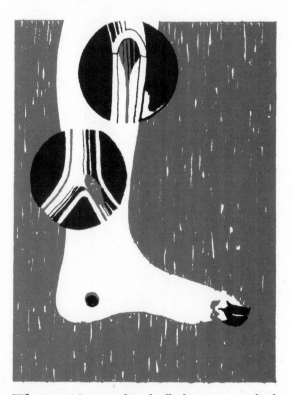

When arteries are closed off, the area supplied by them dies and becomes gangrenous.

Buerger's exercises are found to be helpful in some cases. They consist of:

1. Lying in bed and placing the feet and legs on a plank or some other inclined plane so they will be elevated to about forty-five degrees above the bed for five minutes.
2. Lying with the feet on the bed for five minutes.
3. Allowing the feet to rest on the floor while sitting on the bed for five minutes.

This takes fifteen minutes and should be repeated three times a day.

GLOSSARY

Amputation   surgical removal of a part
Arteries   blood vessels
Arteriosclerosis   hardening of the arteries
Dilate   enlarge
Excruciating   torturing pain
Gangrene   dead tissue
Pulsation   a throb or rhythmic beat

PHLEBITIS, THROMBOPHLEBITIS, PHLEBOTHROMBOSIS

Cause and Nature

The word "phlebitis" means inflammation of a vein. However, it is often used to describe a condition known as thrombophlebitis. When there is a clot in a vein and this is accompanied by inflammation we call it thrombophlebitis. If the clot is a simple non-inflammatory process we call it phlebothrombosis.

The causes of venous clotting are many.

1. Stasis or pooling of the blood in the vein caused by external pressure or by prolonged bed rest.
2. Local injury to the walls of the veins by stretching, by trauma, or by bacterial infection.
3. Any change in character of the blood which lead to coagulation or clotting.

Any condition which will tend to slow up the circulation of the blood will favor the formation of a clot. This is also encouraged by varicose veins, by old age, obesity, injury, and surgery. To prevent the formation of these clots is the reason that people are asked to get up and walk as soon after surgery as possible. This condition is frequently seen after childbirth. It has been called "milk leg."

The one great danger of this condition is that a piece of the clot may break off and circulate in the blood until it gets hung up in some of the small veins in the lungs. This is called a pulmonary embolism and is always dangerous. It can be fatal.

Signs and Symptoms

When there is no inflammation the condition called phlebothrombosis may be present without any symptoms and the signs of a swollen leg and blueness or cyanosis of the leg more often appear suddenly.

The onset of thrombophlebitis may be sudden and the symptom, that is pain, may be severe. If a small vein is involved the pain may be mild.

There is usually a redness over the skin at the site of the clot and a tender hard strand, which is the thrombosed vein, can be felt.

Sometimes there is a fever, a feeling of general malaise and loss of appetite. As mentioned above the danger of this condition lies in a pulmonary embolism. Sometimes the greater the pain and redness over the area the less chance there is of a clot breaking off. This does not always apply.

Treatment

As soon as the diagnosis is made the patient should be placed in bed with the leg elevated on a pillow and a cradle with electric light bulbs should be placed over the leg. This is to supply heat and to keep the weight of the covers off of the leg. The use of anticoagulant drugs will do no good once the clot has formed but they may keep it from extending. Medicine can be taken to relieve the pain, but the leg must not be moved either actively or passively.

If the clot seems to be extending upward the vein should be tied off high up in the thigh. This is a relatively simple operation and will often prevent serious complications.

The treatment of this condition should always be in the hands of a doctor.

GLOSSARY

Anticoagulant   preventing or opposing coagulating
Malaise   general feeling of discomfort or illness

ANEURYSMS

Cause and Nature

The term "aneurysm" is used to describe a ballooning out or swelling of an artery. This may take place in any artery, sometimes in the brain, at other times in the upper part of the aorta near the heart and, as described below, in the lower or abdominal aorta.

Anything that will cause the wall of the blood vessel to be weakened will result in an aneurysm. In the past there was a disease called syphilis which often caused an aneurysm in the arch of the aorta or in the upper part of this vessel. Now that syphilis can be treated effectively by penicillin we seldom see an aneurysm of the arch of the aorta.

An aneurysm of the abdominal aorta is nearly always caused by arteriosclerosis which weakens the walls of this large vessel and causes it to bulge out.

Signs and Symptoms

The signs depend upon where the aneurysm is located. If it is in the brain the signs will depend upon which part of the brain is affected.

Aneurysms of the arch of the aorta are usually detected by X ray or fluoroscopy.

Aneurysms of the abdominal aorta may sometimes be noted by a pulsated mass being felt in the abdomen, but this diagnosis must always be made by a doctor.

Treatment

In many cases no treatment is needed. However, when treatment is indicated it is

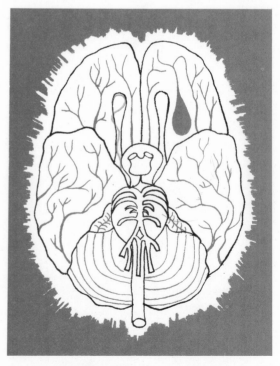

Aneurysm: The ballooning out of any artery in the brain or other parts of the body.

always surgery. The doctor must make this decision.

GLOSSARY

Arteriosclerosis a thickening of the middle coat of the arteries

ABDOMINAL AORTIC ANEURYSM

Cause and Nature

Abdominal aortic aneurysm is a term used to designate the enlargement or ballooning out of the large artery which runs down through the back part of the abdomen and supplies blood to all the lower part of the body.

This enlargement is usually caused by a wearing away of the two inner layers of the aorta while the outer layer stretches. When the two inner layers are destroyed they are replaced by clots which usually become arteriosclerotic and can be seen by X ray of the abdomen, which will reveal the walls of the aneurysm as an eggshell-like picture. The swelling usually starts at the point where the large arteries to the kidneys take off from each side of the abdominal aorta. This disease usually occurs in later life, nearly always after the age of fifty, except in rare cases. It is quite serious and should be treated by a doctor.

Signs and Symptoms

The first sign noted of an abdominal aortic aneurysm may be a swelling or mass in the abdomen which will pulsate with the heartbeat. This pulsating mass may be described by the patient and cause him to go to a doctor.

The mass may or may not be tender and it may be accompanied by abdominal pain. The pain is usually cramp-like or pulsating in character, coinciding with the beat of the heart which pushes blood through the aorta.

In some cases the pain may be excruciating when the layers of the aorta are being separated. This is called a dissecting abdominal aortic aneurysm.

At times there may be other diseases of the organs in the abdomen, such as a peptic ulcer, and the aneurysm may be discovered by accident since it may give rise to no symptoms.

Treatment

Surgery is the only active treatment for this condition and in recent years this operation has been perfected so that the hope for survival is greatly increased. Very few people die of the operation and some surgeons report that about sixty-two percent of the patients who are operated on live for over five years while only about ten percent of the patients who are not operated on live for over five years. It has been estimated that after the aneurysm has been discovered only about half of the patients live over two years if not operated on. Death usually comes from rupture of the swelling, which causes the patient to bleed to death.

The surgical treatment of choice is to take out the weak or ballooned part of the aorta and replace it with a plastic tube. The operation should not be considered safe in a patient who has another serious disease.

GLOSSARY

Aorta main artery
Aortic aneurysm a sac formed by dilation of aorta
Dissecting cutting apart
Peptic ulcer ulcer situated in stomach or duodenum
Pulsating throbbing
Rupture forcible tearing or breaking of a part

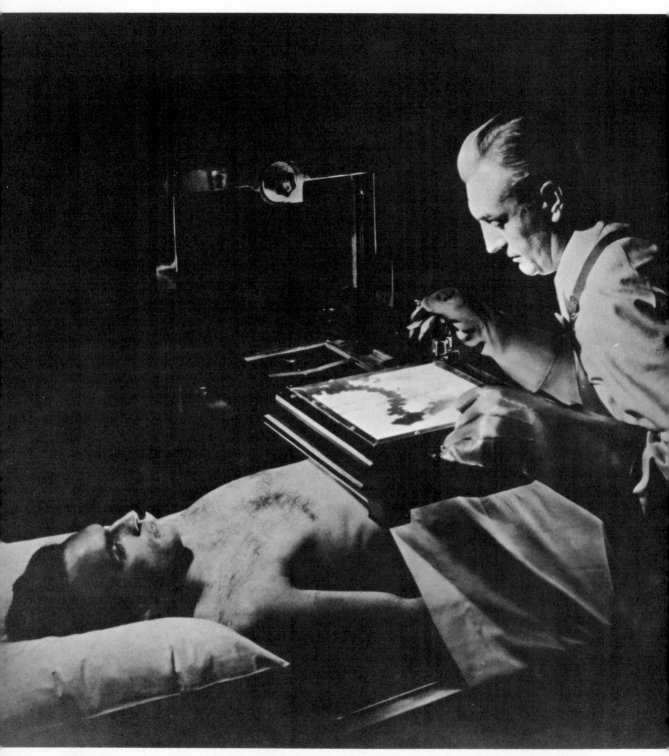

Radiologist examines patient's stomach through a fluoroscope. A contrast substance, Barium, has been taken. Ulcers and abnormal growth can be detected in this manner.

Chapter 10

Diseases of the Digestive System

MOUTH AND THROAT

Dental Caries

(Tooth Decay)

Cause and Nature

This is a degenerative disease of the teeth resulting in cavity formation and eventual destruction of the teeth. It is believed to be caused by acid-forming bacteria in the mouth which act upon carbohydrates such as are found in sugar and candies. This is augmented by nutritional deficiency of certain minerals and vitamins, poor dental hygiene, and lack of professional dental care.

Signs and Symptoms

The earliest signs are cavities which are present in the teeth of most children. These may progress into the pulp, causing pain and abscess formation.

Treatment

The treatment should start before decay begins. To prevent dental decay it is wise to start in early infancy with a well balanced diet and vitamin supplements—especially vitamins A, C, and D.

The amount of sugar and candy eaten should be limited, and dental hygiene should consist of thorough brushing of the teeth within ten minutes after eating. If the cleansing does not take place within ten minutes, the acid-forming bacteria have already started to work on the carbohydrates, and the damage has already begun. Regular visits, about twice a year, should be made to the dentist. Local application by the dentist of sodium fluoride to the teeth will cut down on the incidence of cavities.

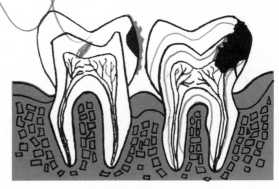

The start of a cavity (left). A toothache results when decay reaches the nerve (right).

171

Many cities are now using fluoridation of the public water supply and this, if done properly, has proven to be both safe and effective in decreasing the incidence of dental cavities.

GLOSSARY

Abscess   collection of pus
Carbohydrates   sugar and starch
Caries   death or decay of teeth; cavities
Degeneration   change of tissue to a less functional form
Hygiene   the science of health
Pulp   soft tissue inside the tooth

Halitosis

(Bad Breath)

Cause and Nature

There are many causes for bad breath and with a careful investigation the cause can usually be discovered and the condition corrected.

Offensive breath can be caused by some infection in the mouth, dental caries, infection of the gums, of the tonsils, or of the throat. In some cases it is simply some food which may be deposited between the teeth.

Some doctors think that bad breath is caused from some condition in the stomach or intestinal tract which prevents fats from being properly digested.

In some cases it may be an infection in the bronchial tree, or in the lungs themselves. Infection in some of the sinuses may contribute to bad breath.

Signs and Symptoms

At times a person may have offensive breath and not be aware of it. In these cases a friend or relative usually tell him.

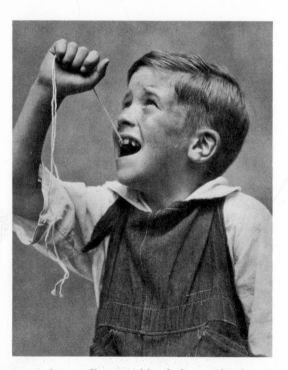

Brave boy pulls one of his baby teeth after it begins to wobble.

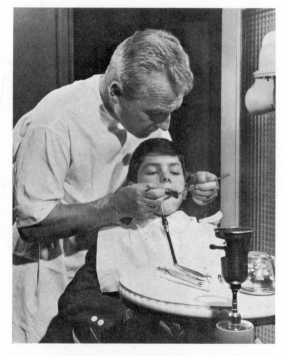

Modern dentistry can be performed with very little discomfort to the patient.

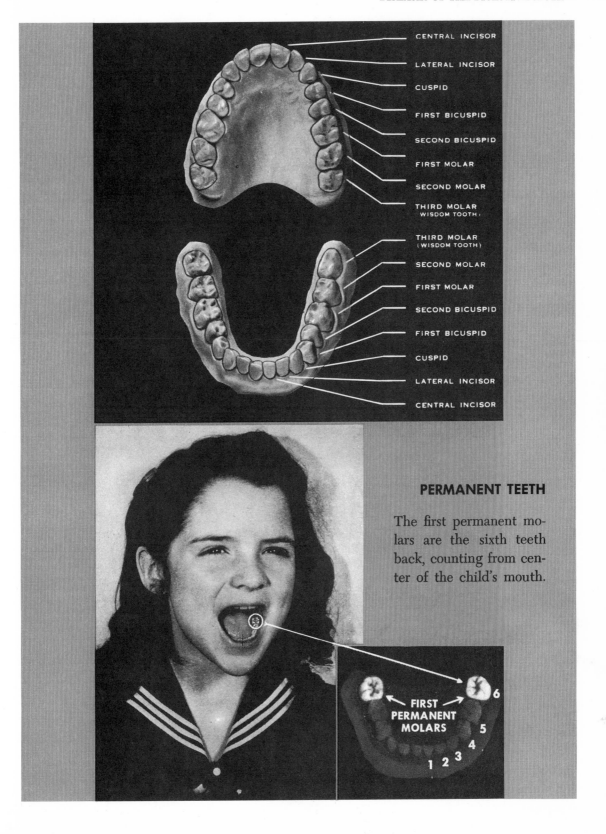

CENTRAL INCISOR

LATERAL INCISOR

CUSPID

FIRST BICUSPID

SECOND BICUSPID

FIRST MOLAR

SECOND MOLAR

THIRD MOLAR
(WISDOM TOOTH)

THIRD MOLAR
(WISDOM TOOTH)

SECOND MOLAR

FIRST MOLAR

SECOND BICUSPID

FIRST BICUSPID

CUSPID

LATERAL INCISOR

CENTRAL INCISOR

PERMANENT TEETH

The first permanent molars are the sixth teeth back, counting from center of the child's mouth.

FIRST PERMANENT MOLARS

6

5

4

1 2 3

In order to try and see if the bad breath comes from the mouth it may help to close the mouth and see if an offensive odor comes out of the nose.

Treatment

In order to treat bad breath successfully the cause should be found and corrected.

If the teeth and gums have been ruled out, then look elsewhere for some infection. If the causative organism can be identified, then sensitivity tests can be performed to see which antibiotic is the most successful against this particular infection.

If a mouth wash is needed, there are many of these on the market, but remember if it has an antiseptic in it, the antiseptic should be mild. The mouth wash should also be alkaline in nature to cut down on acidity in the mouth. Some times a mouth wash of ordinary baking soda will help.

In all stubborn cases your family doctor should be consulted and he can usually help.

GLOSSARY

Caries   cavities; decayed spots in the teeth
Sinuses   nasal cavities; passages

Pyorrhea

Cause and Nature

Pyorrhea is a common disease of the gums and membranes around the teeth. It is an inflammatory reaction which often results in the resorption of the bone of the alveolar process around the roots of the teeth. The cause is not known, but sometimes tartar around the base of the teeth is thought to interfere with the circulation and cause the teeth to become loose in their sockets.

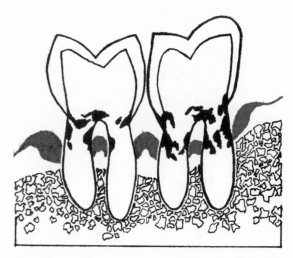

Pyorrhea: Gums are sore. Tartar deposits around roots. Teeth become loose.

Signs and Symptoms

The sign of resorption of the alveolar ridges can be detected by X ray. Soreness of the gums and the teeth becoming loose in their sockets are symptoms often noted.

Treatment

This is one of the common causes for young and middle-aged individuals to be forced to have their teeth removed and resort to dentures or false teeth.

The remedy is to have your teeth checked by a dentist. X rays should be taken and the tartar should be removed from around the base of the teeth. Once the sockets have become too large because the bone has been eaten away by resorption there is no remedy. Hence prevention is the only way to save the teeth.

GLOSSARY

Alveolar   tooth socket
Resorption   gradual destruction of the jawbone around the tooth root

Stomatitis and Gingivitis

Cause and Nature

Inflammation of the gums and mucous membrane of the mouth may arise from a variety of causes: poor dental hygiene; a specific infection (Vincent's infection) called trench mouth; or, as is most commonly the case, the condition may arise from a systemic disease such as pellagra, leukemia, or pernicious anemia. These conditions are also seen in chronic poisoning from lead, copper, silver, gold, or arsenic.

Improper care of the mouth during serious illness may lead to inflamed gums and mouth. This is especially liable to occur after prolonged fevers, if the mouth is not washed out after each feeding. A solution of one-half soda bicarbonate and one-half sodium chloride is good to use as a mouth wash—one teaspoon of each to a pint of warm water.

Signs and Symptoms

The gums become swollen and tender, the tongue and mucous membrane of the mouth may become red, and ulcers may appear.

Treatment

Proper mouth hygiene and proper diet is all important. The vitamins of B complex are very helpful in preventing or curing this condition. These can be secured in an economical form by taking two tablets of brewer's yeast three times a day.

GLOSSARY

Dental hygiene   clean, healthy mouth and teeth
Mucous membrane   the soft lining of the mouth and other body cavities; it secretes mucus
Systemic   affecting the body as a whole
Ulcer   an open sore

Vincent's Infection
(Trench Mouth)

Cause and Nature

This condition is presumably caused by the mixture of a fusiform bacteria and a spirochete. It usually has a sudden onset with sore mouth, swollen gums, fever, and general malaise. Children refuse to eat.

Signs and Symptoms

There may be swelling and redness of the tonsils with a grayish exudate or film over them. The gums are red, swollen, painful, and in some cases small ulcers appear.

Treatment

If untreated, the disease usually subsides in ten days to two weeks. However, penicillin given either by mouth or injection is almost specific, and will bring early relief. Soothing gargles of warm salt water and an ice collar will often help if the tonsils are infected. Aspirin may be given for comfort.

GLOSSARY

Exudate   discharge
Fusiform   spindle-shaped
Malaise   general discomfort
Spirochete   corkscrew-shaped organism

PEPTIC ULCER

Cause and Nature

This term is used to describe an ulceration of the stomach or duodenum; in other words, an ulcer located in the area bathed by the peptic juices. The area near the outlet of the stomach is the most frequently affected. The cause of these ulcers has never

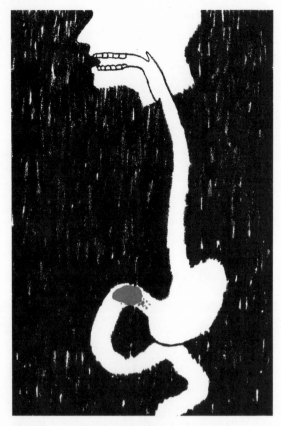

Ulcers are usually located near outlet of stomach.

been fully explained, but it has been shown that most of them are connected with or aggravated by emotional stress and tension.

The actual lesion is a small break or ulcer in the mucosa or lining of the stomach or duodenum (small bowel emptying from the stomach). They tend to be chronic, or recurring, and may heal in a short period of time, only to recur—just as an ulcer or sore on the leg may heal in a week, and break open again if injured.

Signs and Symptoms

The typical picture of ulcer is for the patient to complain of pain or distress in the epigastrium or upper stomach from one to three hours after eating. This pain is usually relieved by taking soda, or milk, or some food. The reason for increase in discomfort at this time is because when the stomach is empty the acid becomes concentrated and comes in contact with the ulcer or break in the mucosa. This causes pain just as placing salt or acid on a break in the skin of the hand will cause pain.

If the ulcer is near the pylorus, or outlet of the stomach, the swelling and spasm of this portion of the stomach may prohibit food from passing through, and the resultant vomiting may reveal undigested food that has been eaten one or two days before. The efforts of the stomach to force the food through the pylorus may sometimes be seen in the upper abdomen as waves passing from left to right.

Not all people with ulcers have pain, and the condition may go undetected for a long time, a so-called "silent ulcer." Most people with ulcers bleed a little from time to time, and about one in four exhibits visible signs of hemorrhage—vomiting old blood, coffee ground material, or passing blood by stool. The bowel movement is as black as tar. The so-called tarry stool and sometimes a severe anemia, accompanied by weakness, are the first signs the patient notices.

An ulcer may perforate through the stomach wall, allowing the stomach content to escape into the abdominal cavity. This is a very serious complication, and may cause death if untreated. The onset is usually sudden, with the development of excruciating abdominal pain which is present throughout the abdomen. The abdominal muscles become hard, almost boardlike, and shock rapidly sets in. The diagnosis may be confirmed by taking an X ray of the stomach with the patient in an upright position, and noting free air in the peritoneal cavity up under the diaphragm. This is a surgical emergency and should be operated upon as soon as possible.

Treatment

Since emotion and tension have been proven to be one of the causative factors, psychiatric treatment may get at the underlying cause. In the past, most of our treatment has been aimed at the relief of symptoms.

A few days rest at home or in the hospital may be a good way to start treatment. Coarse, highly seasoned foods should be left out of the diet. The bland diet meals should be small. In between meals feedings should be taken, such as a glass of milk, in order to keep the stomach from becoming empty.

In the past, the so-called Sippy treatment was very popular. For the first week the patient was given a glass of one-half milk and one-half cream every hour on the hour from 7:00 a.m. to 7:00 p.m. Every hour on the half hour he was given an antacid powder. This diet was gradually liberalized and smooth foods added.

The present day treatment is not so exacting. A smooth diet, small amounts at frequent intervals, and milk in between meals are used. There has been an improvement in antacids so that they are longer lasting, and are less likely to cause alkalosis. Most of them contain aluminum hydroxide, and they are put out under various trade names, such as Amphojel and Gelusil.

When under a doctor's supervision, drugs such as banthine and probanthine are very effective in decreasing the motility of the stomach and thereby promoting healing. These drugs may cause side ef-

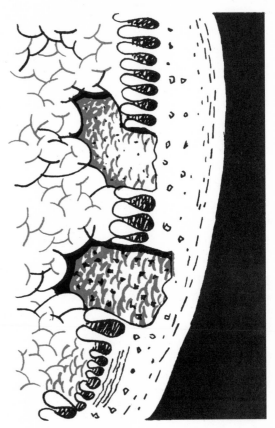

Duodenal ulcers: Acute (top), chronic (middle), and healing (bottom).

fects, such as dryness of the mouth and temporary blurring of vision, and should be taken only under supervision by a doctor.

Bleeding and hemorrhage from a peptic ulcer should be treated by bed rest and proper diet, transfusions, and some form of hematinic containing iron. Hemorrhage from peptic ulcer is seldom fatal if treated properly.

Surgical treatment is indicated in:

1. Pyloric stenosis
2. Failure of relief after a reasonable trial of conservative treatment
3. Perforation

When a gastric ulcer is large and persistent, it may become malignant—that is, turn to cancer. This is only true of ulcers of the stomach (gastric); the duodenal ulcers very seldom progress into cancer. It has been the opinion of some doctors that a persistent, large stomach ulcer should be excised because of the high percentage of cancer in this condition.

It is well to remember that medical treatment will cure most ulcers, that they may recur and be cured again, and that there is a definite connection between emotional strain, either recognized or unrecognized, in all peptic ulcers.

The most common symptom pointing to a peptic ulcer is pain when the stomach is empty. The diagnosis is confirmed by X ray.

If I Had an Ulcer

(Dr. Thorek, the famous Chicago surgeon, in a speech before the California Academy of General Practice, told what he would do if he had a peptic ulcer and I am inclined to agree with him.)

First of all, a peptic ulcer means an ulcer which is bathed by the digestive juices. It may be in the stomach or in the duodenum, which is the small bowel that empties out of the stomach.

When in the stomach, it is called a gastric ulcer, and when in the small bowel it is called a duodenal ulcer.

Gastric ulcers or stomach ulcers often turn into cancer—about one in every four becomes malignant. A duodenal ulcer rarely turns into cancer.

So, if I had an ulcer, I would ask the doctor its location. If in the stomach, I would consider going to a good surgeon, and having the ulcer and that part of the stomach cut out—a partial gastrectomy. This would cure the ulcer, and at the same time would lessen the danger of having cancer.

If my ulcer were in the duodenum, I would stay away from surgeons, and get a good internist or medical doctor to treat me by diet and medicine. In most cases, duodenal ulcer can be cured in this way, and there is very little danger of cancer.

GLOSSARY

Alkalosis excessive alkali in body tissues
Anemia deficient blood
Bland mild
Diaphragm partition separating abdomen from thorax
Duodenum first part of small bowel as it leaves the stomach
Episgastrium upper stomach
Excised cut out or off
Hematinic tonic to build up blood
Hemorrhage bleeding
Lesion sore
Malignant wild growing as in cancer
Perforate rupture; break through
Peritoneal inside abdomen
Pyloric stenosis narrowing of the outlet from the stomach to the intestine
Sodium chloride common salt
Spasm sudden contracting or cramp
Stool bowel movement
Ulcer a sore

CANCER OF THE STOMACH

Cause and Nature

This form of cancer causes an appreciable number of deaths. It usually occurs after forty, and is more common in men than in women.

Indigestion, persistent and of varying intensity, may occur; or the condition may not offer many symptoms until too late. This is the reason why periodic visits to the doctor are advisable, and also why a gastro-intestinal series or X ray of the stomach may be wisely included as part of the examination, even though there are no symptoms referable to the stomach.

Signs and Symptoms

Indigestion which persists, pallor, anemia, and perhaps pyloric obstruction are the commonest signs. Often there is no pain. Weight loss is usually present, and all persons over thirty-five who have these symptoms should have thorough examinations including X rays of the stomach, gastroscopy if the X rays are inconclusive, and gastric analysis.

Treatment

The only possible hope for successful treatment is early detection and operation for the removal of the cancer. Medical treatment is entirely ineffective.

GLOSSARY

Anemia   deficient blood
Gastric   pertaining to the stomach
Gastroscopy   looking into the stomach with an instrument introduced through the mouth and throat
Pallor   pale color
Pyloric   pertaining to the pylorus, the outlet from the stomach

APPENDICITIS

Cause and Nature

A bacterial infection of the appendix is the cause of acute appendicitis. This is one of the most common and most serious of abdominal disorders. The bacterial infection is usually aggravated by an obstruction in the lumen (inside) of the appendix, and perforation or rupture of the acutely inflamed appendix is one of the serious complications. This can be prevented by early diagnosis and prompt surgical removal of the appendix. If performed early in the course of the disease the operation is relatively simple. If the diagnosis is not made early and surgery is delayed, it becomes more complicated and more dangerous. Whenever the diagnosis of acute appendicitis is made, surgery should follow at once unless there is a mass in the abdomen which indicates that the appendix has ruptured and an abscess has formed. The abscess in this case will have to be drained, but there is not so much urgency in per-

forming the operation. This disease occurs most often in young people, but elderly people do have it.

Signs and Symptoms

The onset of acute appendicitis is usually sudden, with general malaise, abdominal pain, and nausea, and sometimes vomiting. There is generally a slight elevation in body temperature—very seldom a high temperature in early cases. The pulse is usually rapid, and the white blood count shows an increase.

Some hours after onset the pain localizes in the right lower quadrant of the abdomen, pressure over that point will produce pain, and guarding or tightening of the abdominal muscles will be noted. A physician should always be called, and under no circumstance should a person with pain in the abdomen be given a cathartic. The giving of cathartics for abdominal pain aggravates the condition and may precipitate perforation or rupturing of the appendix.

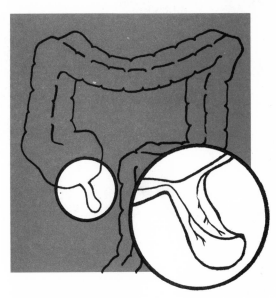

The appendix protrudes from the cecum (the beginning of the large bowel).

Treatment

The only treatment is early operation with removal of the appendix. Any reasonable suspicion of acute appendicitis justifies an operation.

GLOSSARY

Abscess   collection of pus
Cathartic   something taken by mouth to make the bowels move
Lumen   channel within a tube or tubular organ
Malaise   general discomfort
Nausea   tendency to vomit
Quadrant   any one of the four quarters of the abdominal surface
Rupture   forcible tearing or breaking

CONSTIPATION

Cause and Nature

This is one of the most common ailments from which civilized man suffers, and perhaps one of the least understood.

To begin with, constipation is not a disease but a habit. This habit is formed largely because our civilization does not permit us to have a bowel movement whenever and wherever we feel like it. Hence, people working in offices put off the urge to have a bowel movement, and gradually develop the habit. This also is true of others who do not obey the impulse, and who have not developed the habit of having a bowel movement at the same convenient time every day—say just before retiring.

Another common cause of constipation is faulty eating habits. We eat in such a hurry and in such a manner that there is often not enough bulk in the bowels, and not enough moisture because we do not take enough fluids.

A final consideration is the fact that people vary in their need to have bowel movements. One person may need to have one after each meal, and his neighbor may be perfectly normal and not constipated if he goes two or three days between movements. Another type of person who may have trouble with constipation is the tense, nervous individual who cannot relax enough to have an evacuation.

This habit, constipation, is further complicated by many old wives' tales such as "eliminating poisons by having a bowel movement," and terms like autointoxication. There is very little beside water and salt that passes from the colon to the blood stream, and the blood going from the colon passes through the liver, which is a very effective filter.

Many mothers are worried because they think their babies are constipated, when as a matter of fact, the little baby's colon has not had time to attain its full activity. The peristalsis, or wave-like movements of the colon which empty it, have not become perfected yet, and the baby is not constipated at all.

Signs and Symptoms

Any change in the bowel habit should be observed, and attempts should be made to correct the change. However, one should keep in mind that this is a natural function and we must aid nature by removing the causes of constipation, if possible.

Treatment

Living habits are important. A regular time for evacuation should be developed, if possible, and strictly adhered to. This is the most important single factor in preventing constipation. Another good rule to follow is to never deny the bowels an opportunity to move if there is a desire to go to stool.

Fluid intake is important. Every person should take as much as two quarts of water daily. Most of us do not drink enough water. Lack of sufficient fluids leads to a dryer, harder bowel movement. A good way to start correcting this is to drink a glass of warm water upon first arising, and drink several glasses during the day—preferably after meals.

Enemas and laxatives do no great harm if taken occasionally to help out the normal movement. Small doses should be taken, for instance, one or two teaspoons of milk of magnesia or twenty to thirty drops of fluid extract of cascara. If enemas are preferred, they are just as helpful and no more beneficial than drugs. Only small amounts of water should be used—for instance, one pint of warm water with one teaspoon of salt added is a good enema. High colonic flushes should never be used, except in very unusual cases of stubborn constipation, and the frequent use of enemas or cathartics should not be allowed to become a habit, because they dull the normal mechanism of a regular bowel movement.

Mineral oil should not be used as a regular aid every day, for there is some proof that if taken after meals it will delay or hinder the absorption of the fat soluble vitamins. Mineral oil mixed with agar is a better combination. This is sold in one form as Petrogalar. Violent purging is harmful.

Diet is all-important. Vegetables—at least two, to be eaten at the noon and evening meal. All fruits should be used if they agree with the individual. Meat, fish, eggs, and poultry are important parts of the diet, but they do not furnish bulk, which is made up by vegetables and fruits. A pint of milk a day is desirable. Whole grain cereals and bread are preferable because they contain vitamins and minerals. Oils and butter may help a person gain weight. Too much animal fat or saturated fatty acids is not considered advisable because of cholesterol content, but vegetable fats such as olive oil help correct constipation.

Artificial bulk has received a great deal of attention in correction of habit constipation. Bran should never be used alone, as roughage or artificial bulk, because it tends to become dry and packed. Various drugs are on the market which may be used to produce artificial bulk if the patient does not eat enough fruit or vegetables to furnish natural bulk. Methyl cellulose (celothyl) is one of the better of these.

GLOSSARY

Cholesterol   fatty acids
Colon   large intestine
Enema   flushing out the rectum
Laxatives   mild cathartics
Peristalsis   intestinal movement

IRREGULARITY OF THE BOWELS

Cause and Nature

Worry, tension, and irritants to the bowels such as bad food or medicine in the form of laxatives or cathartics, cause the bowel to go into spasm and this causes constipation. Sometimes due to advanced age the muscle of the bowel loses its tone and this results in so-called habit constipation. If the bowel moves too fast and does not go into spasm or become too lax, this is called diarrhea. In infrequent cases, or rare cases, the constipation and diarrhea alternate—that is, for a few days the patient will be constipated and then for a few days without taking a laxative he will have diarrhea. If this alternating diarrhea and constipation persists a doctor should be seen, for this condition could be caused by a polyp or growth such as cancer in the lower bowel. Sometimes poor habits cause constipation.

Signs and Symptoms

There is absolutely nothing to the belief that a daily bowel movement is essential or necessary. Down through the ages we have been taught by our families, sellers of patent medicine, and over radio and television, that we must have a daily movement in order to feel good and be healthy. Nothing is further from the truth and these advertisements for laxatives are simply a method used by these companies to try and make money. It has been estimated recently that Americans spent one hundred and twenty-eight million dollars in one year for laxatives and cathartics. Doctors know that people do not need to have a daily bowel movement to feel good and be healthy. In spite of some of the advertisements we see there is no such thing as autointoxication caused by constipation. Some small children and older people do not have a movement except every two or three days and this does not interfere with their health. If constipation persists over a long period, the person will feel full and over-distended, and should see a doctor.

Treatment

Habit formation is the single, most important way to get rid of constipation. Of course exercise and proper diet also play a big part. Many people, especially young female office workers, become constipated because they do not heed the urge to go to the bathroom, and pretty soon the urge stops coming. If the bowels go for too many days without moving the resultant stool may be hard, dry, and large. This may be difficult to pass and at times painful.

A good habit should be developed, such as going to the bathroom at the same time every day and giving the bowels a chance to move whether they want to or not. This habit may take weeks or months to develop but will eventually become a regular thing. Sometimes a conditioned reflex is set up by taking a warm cup of water or coffee on first getting up and then having a bowel movement.

The diet should have fruit juices, such as prune juice, and there should be sufficient bulk and roughage which can be furnished by green vegetables in the form of salads. Habitual taking of laxatives and cathartics makes the bowels lazy and causes constipation. They should not be taken except on rare occasions. Especially is it true that they should not be given to babies and young children. "Let the bowels take care of themselves."

GLOSSARY

Autointoxication   internal poisoning from the body itself
Diarrhea   frequent loose bowel movements
Distended   stretched
Laxatives   mild cathartics
Polyp   a growth
Reflex   a reflected action or movement
Spasm   sudden cramp

DIARRHEA

(Gastroenteritis or Enterocolitis)

Cause and Nature

Diarrhea is one of the most common ailments from which we suffer. It is not a disease, but is just a symptom indicating irritation or inflammation of the intestinal tract. This can be caused by many things which will be listed below. Usually acute diarrhea is caused by some simple dysfunction and will correct itself within a day or two. Occasionally it requires instant treatment, and on rare occasions it may be a manifestation of a more serious condition.

Acute diarrhea in infants should be quickly controlled, because an infant may become quickly dehydrated. Acidosis or starvation may intervene if the condition is allowed to persist for too long.

Signs and Symptoms

The attack has a sudden onset, beginning from two to five hours after eating, with nausea, vomiting, diarrhea, and sometimes cramps and prostration. If several people have an attack at the same time, a common source of food should be suspected. Recovery within twenty-four to forty-eight hours should result.

A few of the causes of acute diarrhea may be the eating of unripe fruit, spoiled foods, large amounts of roughage or cellulose, alcohol—in other words, anything that will inflame the intestinal tract.

Chronic diarrhea may result from many types of diseases, such as:

Lack of acid in the stomach
Cancer of the stomach
Acute gastritis

Intestinal causes include:

Bacillary dysentery caused by bacteria
Amebic dysentery
Intestinal parasites
Intestinal tuberculosis
Regional ileitis
Diverticulitis
Cancer of the colon (this usually results in alternating diarrhea and constipation)

Ulcerative colitis
Prolonged use of laxitive
Pernicious anemia
Allergy
Hyperthyroidism

Last, but not least, emotional and nervous states may cause diarrhea.

A common cause of acute food poisoning is improper refrigeration. As an example, a cream pie is purchased from a bakery where one of the bakers has a boil on his finger. The pie is placed in the trunk of a car or other warm place, and allowed to remain for hours before being eaten. This allows the staphylococci to multiply rapidly, and when the pie is eaten an acute case of food poisoning with diarrhea results.

Treatment

In acute diarrhea it is not advisable to take a laxative. A warm salt enema may give some relief.

The cramps may be relieved by aspirin and codeine, ½ grain, in simple cases. Pepto-Bismol will aid, and in bacillary infections certain of the antibiotics such as erythromycin or terramycin are of benefit. Food should be omitted for a short time and fluids should be taken to prevent dehydration. Warm tea, toast, and soft-boiled eggs may be taken after ten hours. This should gradually be increased to a regular diet.

Sometimes a simple remedy may help—fifteen drops of iodine in two ounces of water, taken three times daily will often help in a cure.

If the diarrhea persists, extensive study should be made to determine the underlying cause, and this should be treated.

One rare cause of diarrhea that is often overlooked is abscessed teeth.

GLOSSARY

Allergy   reaction against
Anemia   deficient blood
Colitis   inflammation of colon
Dehydrated   lacking sufficient fluid
Dysentery   inflammation of the intestines with frequent bowel movements
Hyperthyroidism   overactive thyroid gland
Parasites   organisms living upon or within another organism
Prostration   extreme exhaustion
Staphylococci   parasitic bacteria

DIVERTICULITIS

Cause and Nature

Diverticula are small pouches sometimes found in the intestinal tract, usually in the descending or lower colon. Irritating ma-

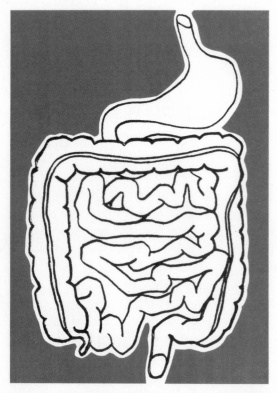

The gastrointestinal system: The stomach, small bowel, and large bowel (colon).

terial retained in these pouches will cause symptoms and require treatment.

Signs and Symptoms

Pain is the outstanding symptom. It is usually on the left side in the lower abdomen. This may be accompanied by nausea, diarrhea, and fever. The diagnosis may be confirmed between acute attacks by taking X rays of the colon following a barium enema. A complete gastrointestinal series of X rays of the upper and lower intestinal tract may be necessary.

Treatment

Rest in bed, with application of external heat to abdomen. Codeine with aspirin, such as Empirin compound with ½ grain codeine, may be taken for comfort. Do not take a laxative or an enema.

The diet should consist of warm liquids and soft foods.

Antibiotics such as neomycin, terramycin, aureomycin and sulfasuxidine may be helpful. A drug called salicylazosulfa pyridine when combined with tranquilizers or sedatives has been found to be quite effective in relieving the symptoms in this distressing condition.

To prevent recurrence of acute attacks, that is inflammation of the pouches which are there and will always be there, the following steps are advised: A bland, non-residue diet; mineral oil, one-half to one ounce daily (this is the one condition when daily mineral oil is advised); new antispasmodic drugs on the market now, sometimes help. Avoid fatigue and emotional stress.

GLOSSARY

Antispasmodic   relieving spasm
Bland   mild
Colon   large intestine

DIAPHRAGMATIC HERNIA

(Upside Down Stomach or Hiatus Hernia)

Cause and Nature

The peritoneal cavity or abdominal cavity in which the stomach is located is separated from the thoracic cavity which houses the lungs by a muscular partition called the diaphragm. The tube leading down from the mouth to the stomach is known as the esophagus. The hole or opening in the diaphragm through which the esophagus passes as it enters the stomach is found at the junction of the esophagus with the upper part of the stomach. If this opening or hole is enlarged either by injury or by a birth defect, the stomach may slide up out of the abdominal cavity into the thoracic cavity. This is a relative situation in which either a small part of the stomach may enter the lung cavity or in some marked cases the entire stomach may slide up into the thoracic cavity. These infrequent marked cases have been called "upside down" stomachs.

There are two main types of diaphragmatic hernias:

1. The sliding hernia in which just the upper end of the stomach slips up through the diaphragm into the lung cavity
2. The so-called paraesophageal hernia in which the top of the stomach stays fixed and the whole body of the stomach slips up through the opening in the diaphragm into the thoracic cavity

Signs and Symptoms

Most of these diaphragmatic hernias do not cause any symptoms. Even some of the larger hernias in which the whole stomach may slide up into the thoracic cavity may cause very little distress.

A small sliding hernia may cause a feeling of irritation at the lower end of the esophagus. There may be heartburn and sometimes difficulty in swallowing. The signs and symptoms usually appear immediately after eating. The person will have a feeling of pressure and will belch frequently. He may get up and walk around in an effort to get rid of this feeling of pressure. There may be irritation and some slight bleeding from these hernias, but as a rule the bleeding and subsequent loss of blood is not very great. X rays of the stomach and esophagus will usually confirm the diagnosis. The small or sliding hernias are very common, especially in older people, and as a rule do not cause any distress. The paraesophageal hernias are rare.

There may be a tendency to regurgitate

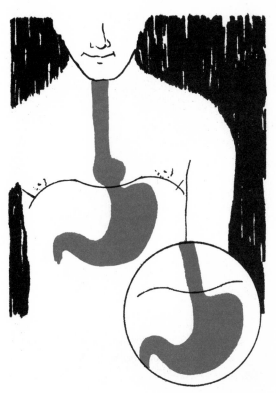

Hiatal or diaphragmatic hernia: The upper part of stomach bulges into the lung cavity.

food which has been recently eaten, especially if the person lies down soon after eating.

Treatment

The treatment for diaphragmatic hernia is usually medical and aimed at the symptoms. If there are no symptoms then treatment is not needed. The diet should be watched carefully. Small amounts should be eaten and there should be little roughage. Highly spiced foods and carbonated beverages should be avoided. Antacids should be taken often enough to prevent discomfort. The person should not eat just before going to bed but should have the evening meal three or four hours before retiring. In some cases it helps to elevate the head of the bed.

Surgical correction of these hernias is resorted to only if the symptoms cannot be controlled by medical treatment and if the symptoms are severe.

In cases where the entire stomach goes up into the lung cavity and embarrasses the breathing, surgical repair is nearly always successful. In the small sliding type of hernia, the symptoms may persist after an attempt is made to repair the hernia by surgery.

GLOSSARY

Antacid   correcting acidity
Diaphragm   partition separating abdomen from the thorax
Embarrasses   hinders or makes difficult
Esophagus   the gullet; the food canal to the stomach
Hernia   protrusion of a loop through an organ or tissue
Hiatus   a gap or opening
Paraesophageal   around the esophagus
Peritoneal   inside the abdomen
Regurgitate   flow back
Thoracic   pertaining to the chest

ESOPHAGEAL VARICES
(Varicose Veins of the Esophagus)

Cause and Nature

Esophageal varices are varicose veins in the esophagus. These large veins are usually found in the middle or lower part of the esophagus and may be present without causing any symptoms. They are usually caused by some back pressure in the veins, such as is seen in cirrhosis of the liver. These varices are a common finding in cases of cirrhosis of the liver.

Signs and Symptoms

Varicose veins in the esophagus or esophageal varices show no symptoms as a rule and may be unrecognized or found accidently when an X ray examination of the esophagus is made.

They often rupture and are a very common cause of hemorrhage. In many cases the hemorrhage is profuse and this is often the cause of death in people with cirrhosis of the liver; or they may be the cause of repeated hemorrhage without causing death.

Treatment

When a person is known to be bleeding from esophageal varices, transfusions should be given at once and enough blood should be given to replace that which is lost, if this is possible. Sometimes a balloon can be passed down into the esophagus and blown up causing pressure on the bleeding vein and stopping the hemorrhage.

When a patient has recurrent attacks of bleeding from esophageal varices he should be operated on to relieve the back pressure on the veins in the esophagus. This operation is called a portacaval shunt and is a very complicated one. The patient should be in good condition before it is attempted, and if the operation is successful, this may prevent the person from bleeding to death from one of the esophageal varices at some later date.

Cirrhosis   chronic scarring
Esophagus   the food canal to the stomach
Hemorrhage   bleeding
Portacaval shunt   operation connecting the circulation from the liver directly into the vena cava or large vein in the abdominal cavity
Varicose veins   swollen veins

FISSURE-IN-ANO

Cause and Nature

This term is applied to a crack or ulcer in the skin of the anus. It may be caused by a break in the skin following passage of a hard stool. This crack may become infected and give considerable discomfort.

Signs and Symptoms

Sometimes a small amount of bleeding is present. Usually there is a large amount of pain. This is especially noted following a bowel movement.

Treatment

Warm sitz-baths (sitting in a tub of warm water) will aid relaxation of the sphincter muscle, and promote healing. Prevent hard stools by taking mineral oil by mouth, and eating a proper diet. Do not delay going to stool. If spontaneous healing does not take place, see a doctor.

GLOSSARY

Anus   outlet of the intestines
Sphincter   muscle controlling the anus
Stool   bowel movement

GALL BLADDER COLIC

(Cholecystitis)

Cause and Nature

Acute gall bladder colic is usually caused by something blocking the outlet of the gall bladder, causing it to become distended and inflamed on the inside. The blockage is most commonly from gall stones. On rare occasions it may be from kinking of the cystic duct, which is the gall bladder outlet, or from pressure on the cystic duct from the outside.

Signs and Symptoms

Chills, fever, prostration, sweats, pain over the gall bladder region (sometimes radiating to the right shoulder in the back), nausea, and vomiting are usually seen with an acute attack of gall bladder colic. Jaundice may be present at some time during the attack.

Treatment

If stones are known to be present, and if the patient does not improve after conservative treatment, surgery to remove the gall bladder is indicated. In cases where the patient's condition will not permit removal of the gall bladder, incision and drainage of the distended organ is done with the subsequent removal of the organ.

For the immediate attack, which may subside, morphine for the relief of pain is given. Atropine is given to relieve the spasm, and heat applied to the upper right abdomen often helps. The diet should be high protein, low carbohydrate, and low fat, with no condiments or irritating substances.

After the attack, if surgery is not performed, the patient should have gall bladder

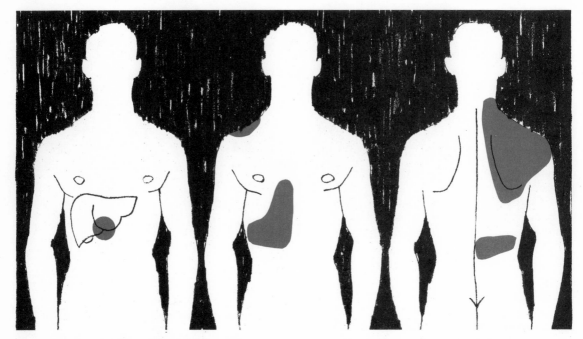

Location of pain in gallbladder colic—the most common site is in the upper right abdomen.

visualization X rays taken to determine the presence of gall stones and determine whether or not the gall bladder is functioning.

GALL STONES

(Cholelithiasis)

Cause and Nature

The cause of most gall stones is not perfectly understood. We know that about ten percent of all white adults have them, and that they are far more common in females than in males. Obesity seems to be a predisposing factor, as does age—they usually occur after thirty-five years of age.

Signs and Symptoms

A patient may have gall stones without knowing of their presence. They may be associated with indigestion, with vague discomfort, and mild pain in the right upper abdomen. There may be tenderness to pressure in the right upper abdomen. If one of the stones blocks the outlet of the gall bladder, there will occur an attack of gall bladder colic with severe symptoms as described above. There may be jaundice.

X ray of the gall bladder, after taking a special dye, will reveal presence of stones.

Treatment

Patients with gall stones can often be maintained without symptoms on a bland,

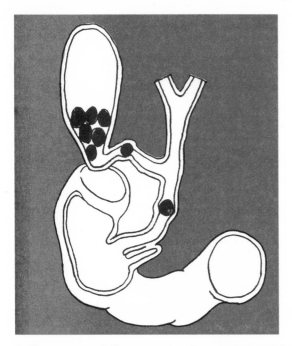

Gallstones may lodge in various locations.

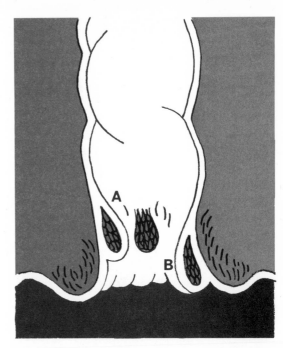

Hemorrhoids: Internal (A) and external (B).

simple diet without any condiments or irritants. Fats should be restricted, constipation should be avoided, as should obesity.

If attacks occur too often, the gall bladder and stones should be removed by surgery. There is no other way to remove the stones once they are present. They cannot be dissolved or made to disappear by taking medicine.

GLOSSARY

Bland   mild
Gall bladder   organ storing bile for digestion
Jaundice   yellow color of the skin due to the presence of bile pigments in the blood
Obesity   fatness; overweight

HEMORRHOIDS

Cause and Nature

Hemorrhoids are caused by straining at stool, lifting heavy objects, pregnancy, or any disease that blocks the portal circulation in the liver. They are distended veins of the anus, usually surrounded by congested and inflamed tissue. They may or may not protrude from the anal orifice. Hemorrhoids are described as external when they arise outside the junction of the skin with the rectal mucosa; or they may be internal when they rise above this juncture. They may be a mixture of both.

Signs and Symptoms

External hemorrhoids are small purplish masses which may protrude from the anus. These may itch, or they may give a feeling of fullness, or if irritated, slight pain. They may bleed if the skin is broken. If a clot forms they become very painful, and much harder and larger than usual. These thrombosed (with a clot in them) hemorrhoids may be corrected easily by having a doctor use a little novocaine, incise the hemorrhoid, and express the clot. This is a simple procedure and may be done in the office.

Internal hemorrhoids may be complicated by bleeding, swelling, protrusion, thrombosis (clot formation), or even ulceration or strangulation. They may cause a feeling of fullness, pain, a heavy dragging-down feeling, or just mild discomfort or itching.

Treatment

Hot sitz-baths (sitting in hot water), rectal salves, or suppositories. Correction of constipation may be sufficient. If, however, these do not aid, the internal hemorrhoids may be injected with a sclerosing solution— a solution which would close the vessel. Both external and internal hemorrhoids can be removed surgically.

Prevention of constipation is the single most helpful procedure. Manual reduction of a painful, protruding mass can be done by having patient lie on stomach, apply cold compresses, then gently push mass in.

Some doctors are using a technique in which they strangle, or destroy the hemorrhoid by placing a rubber band tightly around it. This is done by using an instrument that looks like a pistol.

GLOSSARY

Anus   outlet for the intestines
Hemorrhoid   a pile or enlarged vein in or outside the rectum
Orifice   entrance or outlet of any body cavity
Portal   entrance; portal circulation is in the circulation entering the liver

CRYPTITIS

Cause and Nature

This is an inflammation at the juncture of the skin and anal mucous membrane, usually caused by large hard stools or too frequent use of enemas. It is aggravated by spasm of the anal sphincter muscle.

Signs and Symptoms

Burning rectal pain, constipation, and heavy rectal feeling.

Treatment

Mineral oil every day, hot sitz-baths twice a day followed by instillation of warm olive oil.

ANORECTAL ABSCESS

Cause and Nature

A collection of pus in the anorectal region may be caused by infection following trauma (injury), by large, hard stool, enemas, or severe cryptitis.

Signs and Symptoms

An inflamed, hard painful mass in the tissues just back of the rectum can usually be seen. Walking, sitting, and bowel movements are painful. Fever may be present.

Treatment

Heat applied in the form of hot sitz baths is the first treatment. That is to just sit in a tub of hot water with the water level up around the hips. After the abscess has come to a head it should be opened and the pus drained out, just as in any other abscess. Local salves or ointments do very little good.

Aspirin can be taken to ease the pain, and in certain cases specific antibiotics can be taken by mouth to help kill the infection.

If the abscess goes for too long a time it

may rupture into the rectum or bowel and cause a chronic sinus tract which will have to be removed by surgery.

Abscess   collection of pus
Anal   pertaining to the anus
Cryptitis   inflammation at the juncture of the skin and anal mucous membrane
Enema   flushing out the rectum
Instillation   the act of dropping liquid into a cavity
Sinus   a cavity
Sphincter   a ring-like muscle that can close and open

FISTULA-IN-ANO

Cause and Nature

This is a canal leading from some place low down in the colon to the outside skin near the rectum. It usually discharges pus.

Signs and Symptoms

Abscess may form at the external opening, sealing it off. There may be pain and there is nearly always drainage.

Treatment

Heat, rest, and regular bowel habits are symptomatic treatments. The fistula nearly always has to be removed surgically.

Abscess   collection of pus
Fistula   abnormal passageway
Pus   an inflammation made up of white blood cells

INTESTINAL OBSTRUCTION

Cause and Nature

When the passage of the intestinal content is arrested, this is called intestinal obstruction. It may be caused by adhesions closing the bowel, by the bowel becoming twisted on itself, by a strangulated hernia with a loop of bowel in it, or by pressure from some tumor, either within the bowel or outside it. Sometimes it is caused by paralysis of the bowel following an operation.

Signs and Symptoms

The obstruction may be complete or incomplete, and the symptoms vary with the kind of obstruction. The location of the obstruction will also cause the symptoms to vary.

There is nearly always pain of a recurring, colicky character, which is accompanied by nausea and vomiting. The abdomen becomes distended with gas and it is impossible to pass gas or feces by rectum.

Treatment

Enemas are given in the hope that the obstruction is caused by a fecal mass and the lumen of the bowel can be opened by removing this mass. When this fails, surgery is needed to find the cause of the obstruction and to correct it. It is wise not to wait too long before resorting to surgery. Usually the upper part of the tract is emptied of gas and material by a tube into the stomach, to which suction is applied before the surgery is attempted. This tube is left in place until the function of the bowel is restored.

Adhesions   abnormal joining of one part to another
Feces   bowel movement
Gas   air in the intestines
Hernia   the protrusion or pushing out of a loop or knuckle of an organ or tissue through an abnormal opening
Lumen   canal within a tube or tubular organ
Tumor   an abnormal mass of tissue

AEROPHAGY

(Air Swallowing)

Cause and Nature

The causes of excessive air swallowing are numerous and the swallowing of too much air may lead to a great variety of symptoms.

In the first place, all of us swallow air when we eat, drink, or swallow saliva. However, under certain conditions we may swallow too much air and this may lead to distress.

It has been estimated that swallowed air accounts for about seventy percent of the air in the intestinal tract and stomach. Gases diffused from the blood stream may account for about twenty percent of intestinal gas and the other ten percent is caused by bacterial decomposition of food residue as it passes through the bowels.

All of us have known people who could belch whenever they wanted to but we do not realize that they are able to do this by deliberately swallowing large amounts of air. By the same token we do not realize that the feeling of fullness we experience after meals which is relieved by belching may have been caused by swallowing too much air unconsciously as we eat or drink; and this air added to the bulk of the food we have eaten causes discomfort.

Swallowing too much air, then, is a bad habit which may be caused by many things. It may be induced by emotional reactions to fear, anxiety, or tension. There may be some irritation of the stomach which causes pain and we have found that belching relieves this pain; hence, we subconsciously swallow air in order to belch and relieve the distress. We may swallow excessive amounts of saliva because of a chronic postnasal drip due to chronic sinus infection. The eating of food rapidly, gulping liquids, or excessive drinking of carbonated liquids and beer may cause the swallowing of air. The formation of too much saliva which is provoked by chewing gum, smoking cigarettes, sucking candy or mints, and subconscious sucking on poorly fitted dentures may also cause us to swallow an excessive amount of air.

Air which has been swallowed is not absorbed into the blood stream as are fluids or food, but must either be expelled through the mouth by belching or pass through the intestinal tract and the rectum as flatus. When swallowed air reaches the lower bowel it has picked up gases which are absorbed from the blood, together with gases resulting from bacterial decomposition of food.

When a person belches he does not get rid of as much air as he has swallowed (as a matter of fact, the mere act of belching is often followed immediately by unintentional swallowing of more air); so all of us have a certain amount of air in the gastrointestinal tract at all times.

It has been estimated that about half of the patients who go to a doctor complaining of discomfort in the stomach really have no organic disease but have symptoms which are said to be functional. A large number of these symptoms are caused by the retention of gas or swallowed air. In some cases the excessive swallowing of air may disguise some real organic disease of the stomach or bowels. For instance, a person with an ulcer may get some relief from belching and for that reason think that his trouble is gas on the stomach or indigestion and fail to go to a doctor for treatment.

Signs and Symptoms

The most common symptom caused by swallowing excessive amounts of air is a feeling of bloating or distention, especially after a meal. Other symptoms are frequent belching, audible or noisy movements of gas through the intestines, sometimes called "growling" of the stomach, and called by doctors "audible borborygmi." There may be excessive flatus or passing of gas by rectum, cramping pains or distress in the abdomen, sometimes called indigestion. A feeling of pressure or fullness coming on soon after a meal is usually a sign that there was air in the stomach before the food was added.

If the symptoms are relieved by belching, passing of air by rectum, an enema, or a bowel movement, they may be assumed to have been caused by air swallowing.

At times the pressure of trapped air may cause embarrassment to the heart, a rapid pulse, feeling of shortness of breath, and even pain on the left side of the chest which may lead the person to suspect a heart attack. Pressure on the diaphragm may lead to an attack of hiccups.

X rays of the stomach will show large gas bubbles and may lead to a correct diagnosis, especially if the X rays rule out any real disease of the stomach or bowels. The discovery that gas pressure is causing the pain on the left side of the chest often gives great mental relief to patients who had suspected that they had angina pectoris or heart trouble.

These symptoms may be increased by wearing belts or a girdle, slumping over in an easy chair after supper and watching television, or by lying down immediately after a large meal.

Treatment

The fact that most air is swallowed unconsciously makes it impossible to treat this condition by just telling the patient that this is the cause of his symptoms.

The underlying causes for excessive air swallowing must be corrected. Many of us who have this bad habit are nervous, apprehensive individuals, and as the symptoms increase the nervousness is increased. Therefore a very careful examination must be made including X ray, electrocardiograms, etc., to rule out any organic disease and thereby reassure the patient and decrease his apprehension.

The methods or courses of air swallowing, if understood, may be avoided. Some of them are eating rapidly, gulping fluids, smoking excessively, gum chewing, sucking candy or mints, drinking carbonated beverages or seltzers, or drinking through a straw or small-mouth bottles.

Foods which cause excessive gas should be avoided, or at least they should be eaten in small quantities. The gas-forming foods are beans, cabbage, brussel sprouts, cauliflower, broccoli, turnips, onions, cucumbers, and radishes. Excessive amounts of raw vegetables or fruits should be avoided.

Tight girdles or belts should not be worn after a large meal. In fact the consumption of only small meals is one of the treatments of this condition.

If some underlying cause such as an ulcer is found, it should be treated carefully by a doctor.

GLOSSARY

Apprehensive fearful
Dentures false teeth
Diaphragm partition separating the abdomen and thorax

Flatus   air in the intestines
Postnasal   behind the nose
Saliva   mouth fluid
Sinus   a cavity
Ulcer   a sore

INDIGESTION OR DYSPEPSIA

Cause and Nature

This is a very common symptom complex, characterized by belching, heartburn, upper abdominal discomfort or pain, and a feeling of fullness which usually occurs during or after eating.

Indigestion may be caused by serious systemic disease, but it is usually a result of the following simple causes:

1. Eating too much and too rapidly
2. Improper chewing or mastication, sometimes due to faulty dentures
3. Eating while excited or angry
4. Swallowing large amounts of air while eating
5. Excessive smoking or drinking
6. Eating poorly cooked foods
7. Eating foods with a high fat content
8. Eating certain kinds of food such as cucumbers, radishes, beans, cabbage, and onions

Indigestion as a rule results from altered activity of the stomach. Fats slow up the movement of the stomach and thus slow up its emptying. The same is true of overeating. Nervousness and anxiety tend to increase the stomach movements and cause it to empty too rapidly. Drinking increases, and smoking decreases peristaltic motion. Swallowing air in large amounts slows up the action and gives a feeling of fullness, with a desire to belch. Spasm of the pylorus, or outlet of the stomach may be slight in some cases—marked in others, and

may delay emptying and cause symptoms of indigestion. This spasm may be due to irritation of the area by an ulcer located nearby. Constipation will interfere with the normal passage of air and feces and slow the motion of the upper digestive tract.

Signs and Symptoms

NAUSEA may follow any condition which distends or stretches the walls of the stomach or small bowel. It may be accompanied by weakness, headache, dizziness, and sweating.

HEARTBURN usually is caused by distention of the lower end of the esophagus, or the retention of food particles in the esophagus. It is not caused by too much acid in the stomach, for the same symptom may occur in the absence of stomach acid. Even though this is true, doses of sodium bicarbonate (baking soda) or other antacids will usually cure heartburn.

FLATULENCE is caused by an excessive amount of gas in the stomach or intestine. If in the stomach, it may be expelled by belching. If in the intestine, it may be passed through the rectum as flatus. Nervous people who gulp down their food often swallow a large amount of air which causes a feeling of fullness. Sometimes, during the act of belching they will swallow more air. To prevent this, they should keep their mouths open after belching.

Treatment

The best treatment is prevention, in order to avoid indigestion. A person should eat a well-balanced diet, slowly, in pleasant surroundings, if possible. The food should be well cooked and all foods which disagree should be avoided. Smoking before meals should be discontinued, and the amounts eaten should be moderate. After a meal, a person should rest and avoid excitement.

Specific treatment after indigestion occurs may be as follows:

NAUSEA—washing out the stomach by drinking large amounts of water with soda bicarbonate (one teaspoon to the glass of water), and then vomiting the water and stomach contents will sometimes help. There are new drugs on the market which may help. These should be prescribed by a doctor.

HEARTBURN—usually helped by taking soda or an antacid.

CONSTIPATION—may be avoided by observing proper bowel habits, eating proper foods, and sometimes by taking small doses of a mild laxative.

GLOSSARY

Dentures   false teeth
Feces   bowel movement
Flatulence   gas or air in the intestines
Nausea   tendency to vomit
Peristaltic   of the nature of movement of the intestines
Pylorus   the lower opening of the stomach
Spasm   muscle contraction
Systemic   throughout entire body

IRRITABLE COLON

Cause and Nature

This condition is variously called spastic constipation, spastic colitis, mucous colitis, unstable colon, and nervous diarrhea. The many synonyms indicate that this condition manifests itself in multiple ways. It is caused by derangement of the autonomic nervous control of the colon, which may be brought about in many different ways. The most common form of irritable colon may be constipation, although diarrhea is some-

times encountered. Many causes, combined or alone, have been proven to cause irritable colon. These are:

1. Abuse of laxatives and enemas
2. Psychogenic stimuli in patients who are anxious, tense, worried
3. Faulty eating habits of long standing
4. Repeated failure to heed the urge to move the bowels
5. Chronic emotional tension seems to be the most common cause

Signs and Symptoms

Chronic constipation with dry stools covered with mucus is often noted. In some cases pure mucus may be passed. Diarrhea may alternate with constipation. A dull discomfort or pain in the lower and upper left side of the abdomen may be present.

The same cause which produces an irritable colon may result in loss of appetite in the morning, insomnia (inability to sleep), indigestion, a tired feeling, and headaches.

Treatment

The patient must realize that this is not a serious condition and effort should be made to relieve his tension and correct his faulty habits. He must realize that the tired feeling, headache, or indigestion is not caused by the constipation, but have the same cause.

Regular habits should be instituted. A bland diet is often helpful, and medication consisting of phenobarbital with belladonna will often give symptomic relief. Warm applications to the abdominal wall are at times found to be soothing.

GLOSSARY

Mucus   watery secretion of the mucous glands
Psychogenic   originating in the mind

INTESTINAL PARASITES

Intestinal parasites that cause symptoms when they live in the intestinal tract of humans belong to the class of animals without backbones (invertebrates) called metazoa. These invertebrate animals are very small but made up of many cells. They are much larger than bacteria and differ from animals of one cell which are called protozoa.

The metazoa may be divided roughly into the following classes:

1. Roundworms (Nemathelminthes)
2. Flatworms (Platyhelminthes)
   a. Tapeworms (Cestodes)
   b. Flukes (Trematodes)

In foreign countries there are many worms and flukes which cause infection, but only the ones which have been found to cause disease in the United States are listed here. Along with the name of the worm, the source from which a person becomes infected is named as well as the approximate number of known cases throughout the United States and Canada. This will give an idea of how common these infections are in our country.

We will consider first the roundworms as these are by far the most common. Trichinella spiralis or trichina, sometimes called "porkworms," are found in uncooked or poorly cooked pork, and there are about 21,100,000 cases in the United States and Canada. The disease caused by these worms is called trichinosis and as can be seen by the above number is a very serious health problem in this country. It can be prevented by cooking all meats, especially pork, well done.

The next most common roundworm is known as the pinworm or seatworm infec-tion. The technical name for this small worm is Enterobius vermicularis or Oxyuris vermicularis. There are 18,000,000 known cases in the United States and Canada, and these worms or their eggs are passed on from one person to another by contamination as they are found in the human feces, or bowel movements. Washing the hands before eating is a good way to prevent infection by seatworms.

The next roundworm to be considered is called the hookworm, of which there are two types known as Ankylostoma duodenal and Necator americanus. There are 1,000,-800 cases in the United States and Canada. The worm and its eggs are found in human feces, and the infection usually is acquired by going barefooted and stepping in human feces on the ground which contains the eggs of the hookworm. This worm causes severe anemia in the human.

The whipworm or Trichuris trichiura is found in human feces and there are 4,000,-000 cases in the United States and Canada. Since this worm is passed from person to person by contamination with human feces, good sanitation, that is, washing the hands before eating and the proper disposal of human feces, will help to prevent whipworm infection.

Strongyloides stercoralis is another small delicate roundworm that is passed on by human excreta or feces. It causes symptoms very similar to hookworm and is usually passed from one person to another by walking barefooted in the infested soil. There are fewer cases of this disease in the United States and Canada than of hookworm as there are usually only about 400,000 cases. Like hookworm, it is usually found in warmer climates such as the southern part of the United States. The way to prevent the disease is by wearing shoes and seeing to it that proper sanitary methods are used in the disposal of human feces.

The largest intestinal roundworm found in man is called Ascaris lumbricoides and this worm with its eggs may be found in the human excreta or feces which has been improperly disposed of. It may be contracted through the skin by going barefoot in infested soil or by eating improperly washed vegetables grown in soil fertilized by human feces. There are said to be about 3,-000,000 cases of this worm infection in the United States and most of them are found where the climate is moderate and there is a good deal of moisture.

This infection, again, can be prevented by proper disposal of human feces, by wearing shoes, and by washing the hands before eating.

The flatworm infections are not so common as roundworm infestations and they may be divided into two groups.

The first group is called the Cestoda or tapeworms. These consist of the beef tapeworm Taenia saginata, and there are about 100,000 cases of this disease in the United States.

The pork tapeworm, Taenia solium, is not nearly so frequently seen.

Dog tapeworm, Echinococcus granulosus, causes cysts in man known as echinococcus cysts and are infrequently diagnosed.

There is a small tapeworm called Hymenolepis nana which is found in soil polluted by human feces and there are about 100,000 cases of this in the United States.

The fish tapeworm, Diphyllobothrium latum, is contracted by eating fish which are infected and have not been thoroughly cooked.

The tapeworm may be present in man without any symptoms and may be detected by seeing the white segments passed in the stool. The head of the tapeworm remains clasped to the intestinal wall and as it adds new segments, or grows, these segments are passed off in the stool. They may look like a flat piece of noodle.

The tape worm may be prevented by (1) thoroughly cooking pork, beef, and fish, (2) protection of food from contamination, and (3) proper disposal of human feces.

One other form of flatworm infection is caused by flukes or Trematoda. These are not encountered in the United States and will not be discussed here.

Any form of intestinal parasite is dangerous to the health of the person infected or the host. The parasite can be identified by proper inspection of the stools and a doctor can prescribe the appropriate treatment once the parasite has been identified.

In the next few pages the intestinal parasites which are more commonly encountered in the United States will be discussed in detail.

GLOSSARY

Anemia   deficient blood
Larvae   young worms
Parasite   organism living within another organism
Segment   a piece cut off or marked off

TAPEWORM INFECTION

(Taeniasis)

Cause and Nature

There are three main types: the beef tapeworm (Taenia saginata); the fish tapeworm (Dibothriocephalus latus); and the pork tapeworm (Taenia solium).

The beef tapeworm is contracted by eat-

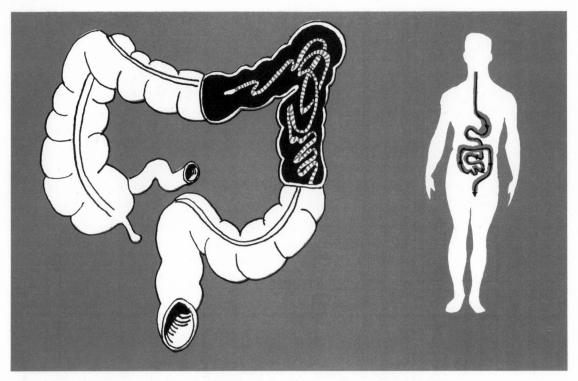

Tape worm fastened to wall of the colon—the long body extending downward.

ing poorly cooked beef which was infected when the beef animal ate food contaminated by human fecal material containing eggs of the tapeworm. In man, only one beef tapeworm usually develops. It passes out segments in the fecal material from time to time. The tapeworm is long and flat, and the segments can usually be seen in the stool.

Signs and Symptoms

The symptoms are usually nervousness and loss of weight, in spite of a good appetite. Very often there are no symptoms.

The fish tapeworm is caused by eating infected, poorly cooked fish. It usually causes no symptoms, but may cause diarrhea, weakness, and loss of weight.

The pork tapeworm causes symptoms similar to those of the beef tapeworm, but can be more dangerous. It is caused by eating poorly cooked, infected pork.

Treatment

Man is usually not a very good host for the tapeworm, and it may pass on without treatment. However, if the segments or eggs are found in the stool the use of atabrine tablets is quite effective. These should be given by a doctor who will usually give a saline laxative before and after the tablets.

HOOKWORM INFECTION

Cause and Nature

This infection is not seen as often as it formerly was, due to the efforts of the Public Health Service. It is still seen in warm climates, where the soil may be polluted with fecal material and the people go barefooted. There are two worms that cause hookworm disease—Necator americanus, and Ankylostoma duodenal.

The eggs, deposited in fecal matter on proper soil, will hatch in a few days. The larvae which result live near or on the surface of the soil. If a barefooted person steps on these larvae, they quickly penetrate the skin. They then go through the blood stream to the lungs, where they develop into worms which crawl up the throat and are swallowed. The mature worm attaches itself firmly to the lining of the intestine. Here it lays more eggs.

Signs and Symptoms

Sometimes a dermatitis or "ground itch," with severe itching, develops on the site where the larvae entered the skin. The itch disappears in about two weeks. The lung symptoms or cough are usually not severe, but the intestinal infection may result in symptoms ranging from vague digestive upsets to headache, dizziness, loss of appetite, pain in the abdomen, chronic fatigue, mental dullness, and anemia.

The diagnosis is made by a doctor, who finds the hookworm egg in the stool. Rarely is the adult worm seen in the feces.

Treatment

A doctor may use tetrachlorethylene, which has for many years been the best drug for killing the worms. The anemia should be treated with iron and a proper diet with vitamins should be prescribed.

Prevention should consist of not going barefooted, and taking the proper precautions to see that the soil is not contaminated with fecal material.

WORMS

(Pinworm, Seatworm, or Threadworm Infections)

Cause and Nature

This is one of the most common worm infections. It is seen often in warm climates and found quite often in children. The adult worm comes out of the rectum and lays its eggs, usually at night. These eggs are the cause of the disease being passed to other people by fingers contaminated with fecal matter, thus passing the infection on to food or water. The worms are small, white, and round.

Signs and Symptoms

Itching around the anus is the most common symptom. The child may be restless at night, nervous in the daytime, and may lose weight. The diagnosis is made by examining the stools for worms, looking at the rectum at night, or wiping the rectum with the sticky side of a piece of scotch tape. This can then be examined under a microscope by a doctor.

Treatment

Tablets of gentian violet, three-twentieths of a grain for children or one grain for adults, should be given—one tablet, three times a day, for one week. Then, rest a week, and take a second course of one tablet, three times a day for another week.

Another effective drug is piperazine citrate (ante par). This should be prescribed by a doctor.

Pinworm infections may spread through an entire family. It is very important to keep fingernails cut short and to wash the hands before eating. Children should wear cotton gloves and cotton underpants when they sleep, and a person who has a pinworm infection should sleep by himself. The sheets from the patient's bed should be handled carefully and never shaken.

ROUNDWORM INFECTION

(Ascaris Lumbricoides)

Cause and Nature

This worm is found in soil that has been contaminated by fecal material. The eggs are taken into the body by eating food contaminated by this soil. These eggs may be deposited in the lungs from the blood, where they develop into small worms which crawl up to the throat and are swallowed.

Signs and Symptoms

The adult worms are seldom seen because they remain inside the body of the sufferer. They are larger and longer than the pinworms. The condition must be diagnosed by a doctor, who has found the eggs in the stool of the patient.

The symptoms are a cough, nausea, fever, and at times the coughing up of blood.

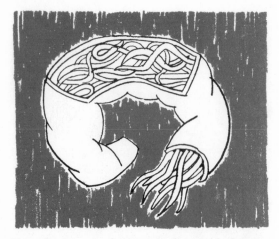

Round worms in the intestinal tract of a human. A rare, but serious, condition.

Treatment

For this condition the doctor usually prescribes crystalline hexylresorcinal, which is usually effective. Of course, care should be taken to wash the hands before eating as the eggs are found in the soil.

GLOSSARY

Anus   opening of the intestinal canal, at the rectum
Dermatitis   a disease of the skin
Fecal matter   excrement discharged through the bowels
Host   an animal or person infested by parasites
Parasite   an organism living within another organism

TRICHINOSIS

(Porkworm Infection)

Cause and Nature

This disease is caused by the invasion of the muscles of the body, (striated muscles), by larvae of the roundworm, called Trichinella spiralis.

It is usually caused by eating infected pork which has not been properly cooked. Sometimes in a large roast, the part in the center is not well cooked and those organisms are still alive when eaten. They are killed by thorough cooking or by freezing.

In spite of the knowledge we have on this disease, it is still very prevalent in the Midwest and to some extent, in the Deep South.

Any animal can harbor the Trichinella, as for instance, cases have been reported in people who eat bear meat which has not been well cooked. The bear had eaten a hog, which infected the bear, and the human beings who ate the rare bear meat became infected.

Some cases are so mild that they go unnoticed while others cause severe symptoms.

When the live worm is eaten, it attaches itself to the small bowel and a diarrhea may result. While in this position copulation takes place and the male dies, while the female works her way into the blood stream and eventually comes to rest in the muscle. Here she lays her eggs, as many as 1500 of them and these small eggs hatch into larvae, which in turn spread into the muscles where they eventually become encysted, that is surrounded by a shell, or cyst. They may live for years and eventually die. These cysts are often found in autopsies, in the muscle of a person who did not even know he had been infected.

These encysted larvae never cause a reinfection and the only way a person can become infected a second time is to eat some more poorly cooked pork which has the live organisms in it.

Signs and Symptoms

About a week after eating rare pork a person may have nausea and diarrhea. This may lead him to think that he has food poisoning.

If some of the pork that was eaten can be examined at this stage and the Trichinae found, doses of some drug to kill worms (such as Piperozin) may be taken and the infection may be headed off.

Once the organisms enter the muscle, nothing can be done to destroy them.

Depending upon how many Trichinae the person has eaten, his symptoms will vary. Pain, stiffness, soreness of the muscles, is usually accompanied by a fever which may go to 104°. At times there is swelling or puffiness of the eyelids.

The blood count will show an increase in the number of eosinophils and this, with the history of having eaten pork poorly cooked, will help make the diagnosis.

Treatment

There is no specific treatment unless the disease is diagnosed early as mentioned above. After about a week or ten days the larvae have begun to circulate.

Once the larvae become encysted there is nothing we can do about it.

The pain, fever, etc., can be treated by aspirin or aspirin and codeine. These symptoms gradually subside, leaving only a vague soreness of the muscles, which will also clear up.

Therefore the only treatment is prevention; that is, see that the pork or bear meat is well cooked.

GLOSSARY

Copulation   sexual union
Eosinophils   a structure or cell
Larvae   immature stage in insect life after it has emerged from egg—before assuming adult form
Striated muscles   striped markings; voluntary muscles because controlled by conscious effort

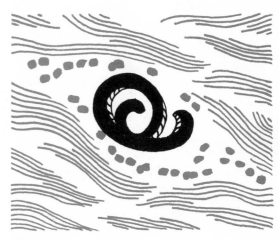

A cyst (shell) around Trichinosis that is embedded in muscles fibers.

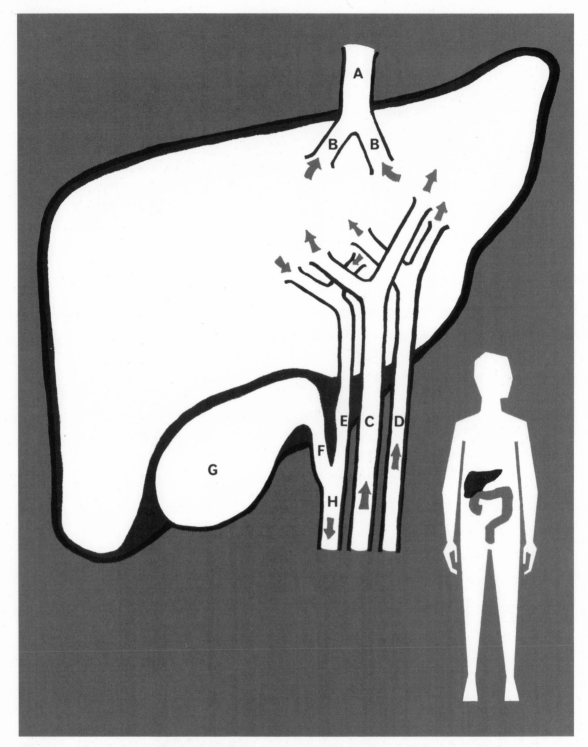

The liver: This diagram shows some of the circulation into and out of the liver—the inferior vena cava (A), the hepatic veins (B), the portal vein (C), and the hepatic artery (D). Also shown: the hepatic duct (E), the cystic duct (F), the gallbladder (G), and the common duct (H).

Chapter 11

Diseases of the Liver

THE LIVER AND ITS MANY FUNCTIONS

THE LIVER is the largest and one of the most useful of all the organs in the body. It is located in the upper part of the abdominal cavity just above the stomach and just below the diaphragm. The largest part of the liver—that is, its right lobe—is located below the diaphragm or just below the rib cage on the right-hand side of the upper abdomen; the smaller lobe, or the left lobe, is connected to the right lobe and lies on the left-hand side of the upper abdomen just above the stomach itself.

Attached to the lower surface of the right lobe of the liver is the gall bladder. This is located just about in the center of the right-hand side of the upper diaphragm just below the rib cage. The gall bladder is really a storage tank where the liver stores bile which it manufactures. This bile is kept in the gall bladder until it is needed and then it passes out through a tube called the cystic duct into a larger tube called the common duct which comes from the liver. From the common duct the bile goes into the upper part of the small intestine called the du-odenum. Then it mixes with the other digestive juices and helps in the digestion of fats. The bile comes out of the lower part of the liver in the hepatic duct and on up through the cystic duct into the gall bladder where it is stored until it is needed. The hepatic duct, which is called the common duct after it passes the cystic duct, is really just one large tube running down to the dou-denum or small bowel; and the gall bladder runs off of it like a pear would branch off of the main stem. This is the reason why a person can have the gall bladder removed when it becomes diseased or has stones in it. The person will remain as healthy as ever because the bile runs straight down the hepatic duct and common duct into the intestinal tract without stopping in the gall bladder or storage duct.

In a way, you could say that the liver is a big chemical factory. Particles or elements of food which are broken down into small particles before they leave the intestinal tract are carried to the liver by the blood in the "portal vein." Once they enter the chemical factory, or liver, these elements of raw material are manufactured into bile.

203

The sugar elements are stored in the liver in the form of glycogen until they are needed.

The liver also acts as a huge filter and strains out poisonous substances which are in the blood. This important function is called detoxification. In addition to manufacturing bile the liver takes different elements of proteins and manufactures a substance called urea.

Fatty acids are converted by the liver into body fats which may be stored. The liver also takes certain vitamins—A, D, and B complex—and stores them until they are needed. It takes vitamin K and changes it into prothrombin, which is essential to blood clotting.

To sum up some of the important functions of the liver, they are:

1. Detoxification (removing poisons from the blood).
2. Changing sugars into glycogen and storing this product until needed.
3. The manufacture of bile.
4. The formation of urea from proteins.
5. The storage of vitamin A, D, and B complex.
6. The digestion of fats which would be impossible if there were no bile.
7. The formation of prothrombin from vitamin K. This makes blood clotting possible.
8. Another function is the handling of cholesterol.

It can be seen from the above that a person could not live if his liver were removed. Fortunately, the liver has great recuperative powers. It has been proven that more than three-fourths of its cells can be damaged without causing serious symptoms and they will be rebuilt into new healthy cells. There are many tests which can be used to test the condition of the liver. These are the so-called liver-function tests.

GLOSSARY

Diaphragm muscular partition between the abdominal and chest cavities
Duodenum upper part of small intestine
Portal vein vein behind the neck of the pancreas

CIRRHOSIS OF THE LIVER

Cause and Nature

This is a chronic disease which has many causes. In most cases the cause is unknown, but any condition which causes destruction of liver tissue which is replaced by scar tissue is known as cirrhosis. This gradual replacement of active tissue by fibroid scar tissue alters the liver's function, and sooner or later causes symptoms. It occurs more often in males than females. Malnutrition, specifically the lack of proteins and vitamin B complex in the diet, is thought to be one of the causes, and this may account for its frequent occurrence in alcoholics.

Chronic poisoning with carbon tetrachloride or phosphorus will cause cirrhosis.

Signs and Symptoms

This condition may at first exist without symptoms. As the function of the liver gradually fails, gastrointestinal symptoms are seen such as loss of appetite, loss of weight, nausea, vomiting, and tenderness over the upper abdomen. As the scarring of the liver advances and the liver veins (portal veins) are blocked off, the signs and symptoms become more pronounced. Vascular spiders are seen on the face and upper body. Varicose veins, or distended veins, are noted in the form of hemorrhoids or esophageal varices. These varices, or distended veins in the esophagus, are very dangerous as a person may bleed to death when one of them ruptures.

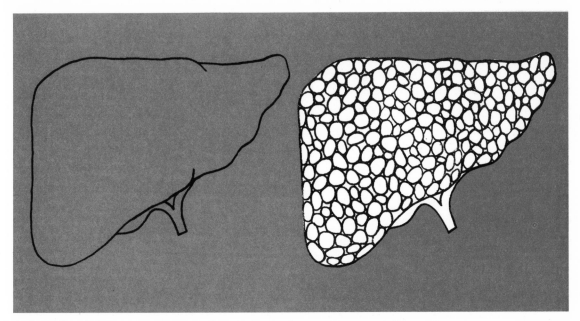

Cirrhosis of the liver causes scar tissue on liver (hob-nail liver) as shown above.

There is often jaundice, then swelling of the lower extremities with fluid (edema) and ascites (fluid in the abdominal cavity), followed by mental torpor and finally death.

Treatment

The diagnosis of cirrhosis is often not made until the disease has progressed to a dangerous state. If made early, the scarring of the liver can be slowed down by proper treatment, and many years of well-being may be added to a patient's life.

The treatment must be supervised by a physician and should consist of:

1. Bed rest for a part of each day.
2. A diet high in proteins and low in fats and carbohydrates.
3. Vitamin supplements, such as brewer's yeast, six grams or more daily, and injections of liver.
4. Transfusions to correct anemia.
5. In advanced stages, removal of fluid from the abdominal cavity by paracentesis, or tapping the cavity to let the fluid run out.
6. Large and dangerously distended veins in the esophagus can be reduced in some patients by an operation which partially relieves the portal pressure. This is called a porto-caval-venous-shunt.

GLOSSARY

Edema   swelling
Fibroid   of fibrous tissue
Jaundice   yellow color of the skin due to liver disease or presence of bile pigment in the blood
Malnutrition   imperfect food intake or assimilation
Torpor   sluggishness
Vascular   pertaining to vessels

ACUTE INFECTIOUS HEPATITIS

Cause and Nature

This disease has become quite prevalent throughout the United States and its causes and treatment should be understood by the general public.

Acute infectious hepatitis, or inflammation of the liver, occurs in two forms, each caused by a different virus.

The most commonly seen of the conditions is called viral hepatitis. This is caused by a virus "A" which is transmitted from person to person through the mouth and intestinal tract. It is seen in epidemic forms where many persons live together under crowded conditions and where sanitation is poor. It is passed from person to person.

The incubation period in this type, that is the time between exposure and the development of symptoms, is short—from twenty to forty days. When the acute symptoms subside the person is no longer liable to transmit the disease to another person.

The second form is caused by virus "B" and is called serum hepatitis. This is transmitted by transfusions with infected blood or plasma and may also be contracted by needles that have not been properly sterilized before an injection is given.

The incubation period in serum hepatitis is longer, requiring from sixty to one hundred sixty days. This type is not transmitted from person to person by contact with excreta but must be transferred into the bloodstream by needles. It became quite prevalent during the world wars when donated blood was not so carefully screened. This is the reason why hospitals ask a prospective donor of blood whether or not he has ever been jaundiced.

Signs and Symptoms

The onset of the disease may be slow or abrupt. Severe prostration and fever are said to be more common in type "A" or viral hepatitis than in serum hepatitis. If a person has never had a blood transfusion or injection while in a hospital and proves to have hepatitis it is most likely that he has viral hepatitis and not serum hepatitis. There are also many laboratory tests which will distinguish between the two.

During the period before the jaundice appears (this used to be called catarrhal jaundice) the person may have a loss of appetite, a slight rash may appear, and there may be pain or discomfort in the right upper part of the abdomen. The liver may be enlarged and tender, and laboratory tests will verify the diagnosis.

Treatment

During the prodromal stage, that is the stage before the jaundice appears, bed rest is important. After the jaundice appears the patient usually begins to feel better. There is no specific medicine for this disease, but the diet is important. The stools should be considered infectious during the early stages and the bed linens should be boiled. A person taking care of these patients should always wash his hands before leaving the room.

The patient should be encouraged to eat a bland diet and to do without alcohol. Any form of sugar such as hard candy or orange juice will help protect the liver.

When an epidemic occurs or when a person living in close contact with other members of a family is infected, the use of gamma globulin injections will give short-term immunity to exposed persons and in this way help to control the spread of the disease. This protection lasts for about six weeks. Usually a case of infectious hepatitis will produce lifelong immunity in the person who suffers from it.

GLOSSARY

Excreta waste material thrown off by the body

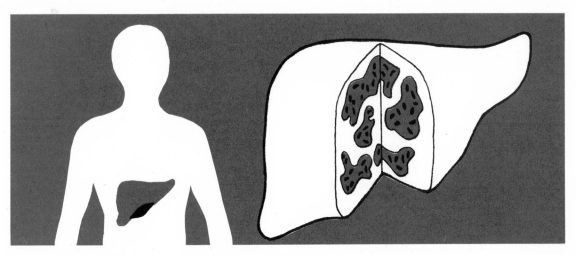

Liver cells throughout the liver may be injured by poisons or infectious Hepatitis.

Jaundiced   a syndrome characterized by deposition of bile pigment in the skin and mucous membranes resulting in a yellow appearance
Prostration   extreme exhaustion or powerlessness
Gamma globulin   a substance given by injection for the purpose of immunization

TOXIC HEPATITIS

(Liver Damage Caused by Chemical Agents)

Cause and Nature

Toxic hepatitis is different from infectious hepatitis in that it is not an infection but is caused by injury to the liver due to exposure to some toxic agent. These agents vary greatly in that some people may not be injured by certain drugs while others may receive liver damage from taking the same drugs. The sulfa drugs, para amino salicylic acid, and some of the antibiotics are examples of drugs which may cause toxic hepatitis in some individuals. Exposure to insecticides or cleaning solutions, or working in chemical factories may lead to toxic hepatitis. These poisonous agents may be breathed in, absorbed through the skin or swallowed.

Signs and Symptoms

Toxic hepatitis may come on slowly beginning with a loss of appetite, feeling of weakness, headache, pain in the upper abdomen, and finally fever and jaundice. History of exposure to the toxic agents named above and laboratory tests will be needed to distinguish between this condition and infectious hepatitis.

Treatment

The treatment consists of stopping the exposure to liver damaging substances and this includes alcohol. Injections of crude liver often help shorten the course of the disease, and bed rest and proper diet are important. The diet should be bland and high in carbohydrates or sugars.

Sometimes in severe cases transfusions of whole blood are helpful. The liver is one organ which has a great capacity for reproducing its cells and if given a chance will usually recover from injury if not severe.

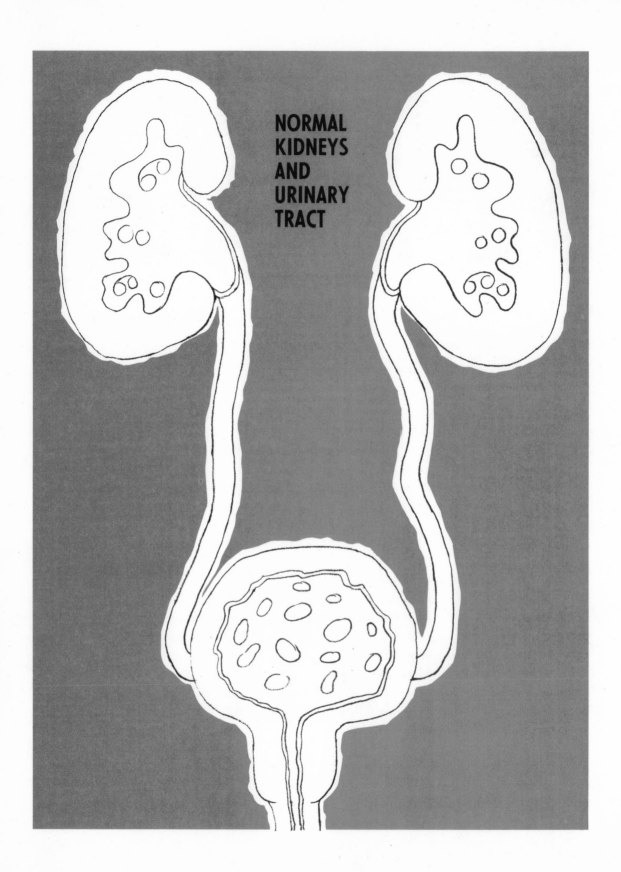

NORMAL
KIDNEYS
AND
URINARY
TRACT

Chapter 12

Diseases of the Kidneys and Urinary Tract

THE KIDNEYS are considered two of the most useful and important organs in the body. They work day and night and their functions are essential to life. The most important job the kidneys perform is the regulation of the body fluids. They do this by excreting fluids and the end products of metabolism and by conserving the correct amount of fluids and chemicals which are needed by the body. So the kidneys perform a highly specialized and complicated job.

The urinary tract is made up of the kidneys, ureters (tubes leading from the kidneys to the urinary bladder), the urinary bladder, and the urethra, or the tube leading from the bladder to the outside of the body. Since the prostate gland in man opens into the urethra, infections of this gland and its enlargement often help influence the condition of the urinary tract. Abnormalities of the prostate will be discussed in this section although strictly speaking the prostate is not part of the urinary tract but is part of the genital system in men.

Recent gains in understanding kidney disease and its treatment make the outlook better if it is detected and treated early.

DISORDERS IN THE URINARY TRACT

Signs and Symptoms

Diseases or disorders of the urinary system may result in the following clinical manifestations.

1. The act of urination may be changed in the following manner:
   a. Dysuria (painful urination)
   b. Nocturia (urinating during the night)
   c. Frequency (urinating often)
   d. Incontinence or dribbling (inability to control the flow of urine)
   e. Hesitancy (difficulty in starting urination)

The most often seen of these disorders is dysuria or painful urination. This is usually brought on by some irritation or inflammation of the lower urinary tract such as an irritation of the bladder or inflammation or enlargement of the prostate.

Frequency may be caused by the same thing which brought on painful urination, as well as anxiety and excitement.

Hesitancy may be caused by benign prostatic enlargement or by psychogenic causes such as anxiety.

Incontinence may occur in adults after a severe fright or in children as in bedwetting or enuresis.

2. Changes in the volume of urine.
   a. Polyuria (increased output of urine as in diabetes)
   b. Oliguria (decreased output of urine)
3. Changes in the composition of urine
   a. Albuminuria (protein in the urine)
   b. Hematuria (red blood cells in the urine)
   c. Pyuria (white blood cells or pus in the urine)
   d. Cylindruria (casts in the urine)

Albuminuria—Any infection of the urinary tract will usually cause albumin in the urine.

Hematuria—This may be caused by malaria, or by local disorders in the upper or lower urinary tract. Tumors in the bladder or of the prostate may cause red blood cells in the urine, as will chronic or acute nephritis. Kidney stones which are being passed down the ureter will often cause red blood cells to be found in the urine. Gross bleeding in the urine should be investigated carefully.

Pyuria—Pus in the urine can be caused by infection any place in the urinary tract.

Cylindruria or casts in the urine usually result from kidney disease.

4. Systemic signs of altered kidney function.
   a. High blood pressure (or hypertension)
   b. Edema (or swelling of body tissues)
   c. Uremia

GLOSSARY

Benign   mild character
Cast   a mold of a hollow organ such as a kidney tubule
Enuresis   bedwetting
Nephritis   inflammation of the kidneys
Prostate   male genital gland
Uremia   accumulation of poisons in the blood that should have been eliminated through the urine

ACUTE NEPHRITIS—BRIGHT'S DISEASE

(Acute Inflammation of the Kidneys)

Cause and Nature

Acute nephritis is caused by infection or by the action of some poison or toxic agent upon the kidney.

The infection of the kidney may follow some acute infection such as scarlet fever in which the streptococcus is the causative organism. Sometimes acute nephritis may follow a severe tonsil infection or boils. In some of these cases the toxin or poison manufactured by the bacteria may cause acute nephritis. Exposure to cold is sometimes followed by nephritis.

Toxic agents such as mercury, turpentine, and carbolic acid may cause an acute nephritis. Sometimes it occurs during pregnancy, and often following severe burns we encounter acute nephritis.

Signs and Symptoms

The most constant features of this condition are the urinary changes. The urine becomes very scant; sometimes only four or five ounces a day are passed. It is dark colored, may be called "smoky" urine, and when tested will show albumin, red blood cells, and casts.

When acute nephritis occurs in children following an acute infection, the onset may be slow, characterized by a paleness of the skin, and a puffiness or swelling of the tissues most noticeable, as a rule, in the face or ankles. There may be chills and fever in some cases but not in all. Pain in the back, vomiting, and nausea may be present, but these symptoms are not present in all cases.

In severe cases the edema or swelling caused by fluid in the tissues may be marked and the effusion of fluid may take place in the pleural cavity, affecting the lungs at times. Nosebleeds may develop during the course of the disease.

The condition may vary from a very slight, almost unnoticeable disease to a very severe one in which uremic symptoms may appear. Sometimes the swelling is so transient and slight that it may not be noticed, but on other occasions the swelling may be widespread and marked. In a few cases the symptoms may point to investigation of the stomach or digestive tract.

Treatment

Acute nephritis usually clears up and only about four percent of the cases result in death.

The treatment of acute nephritis should be in the hands of a doctor. The patient should be kept in bed until the symptoms have subsided; that is, the edema or swelling, and the high blood pressure has gone down.

Sometimes the urine will continue to show red blood cells and albumin for six to eight months after the onset. It is not wise to keep the patient in bed for this length of time.

The patient should be protected from exposure to people with colds, and should be kept warm and comfortable since exposure to cold or chilling may cause a flareup of the condition.

The diet should be watched carefully, and if there is much swelling the amount of fluid taken during the day should be limited. Foods containing protein and potassium should be avoided and large amounts of carbohydrates or sugar should be consumed. It is impossible to exclude protein entirely from the diet, but the amounts of protein taken should be severely restricted. Salt and sodium bicarbonate should be restricted drastically as they tend to increase the swelling.

Penicillin is much more effective than the other antibiotics and should be used.

The hemolytic streptococcus is usually one of the causative factors in acute nephritis. If penicillin is used early in a streptococcal infection, acute nephritis will seldom develop.

If infected tonsils are present, they should be removed between attacks of acute nephritis in order to prevent a recurrence of this disease.

GLOSSARY

Nausea feel as though you have to vomit
Toxic due to, or in the nature of, a poison
Transient moves from place to place
Uremic accumulation of poisons in the blood that should have been eliminated through the urine

PYELITIS AND PYELONEPHRITIS

Cause and Nature

Pyelitis is an inflammation of the pelvis of the kidneys usually caused by a bacterial infection. The kidney itself is rarely affected. When the kidney is also infected, the condition is called pyelonephritis. The disease is seen most often in females, especially in childhood, and may be caused by an ascending infection. That is, an irritation or infection of the urinary bladder (cystitis) may move up the ureters to the pelvis of kidney. Congestion may be due to pressure on the ureters as in pregnancy, or it may be caused by a kink in the ureter which prevents proper drainage.

The bacteria may be carried to it through the blood stream and it usually occurs when the resistance is lowered from any cause.

Signs and Symptoms

The most common sign is pus in the urine and cases of pyelitis may vary greatly in their severity from very mild to severe. Pain in the back, chills, high fever, and sweats are usually present. If the bladder is also irritated there may be frequency of urine and burning on urination. The urine will show albumin and white blood cells or pus.

Treatment

The patient should be kept in bed and fluids forced; that is, he should drink lots of water, and the diet should be light. Milk and fruit juices are good ways to obtain fluids and nourishment at the same time.

Aspirin should be given to lessen the discomfort and lower the fever.

There are several antibiotics which are quite effective in this condition. The most commonly use is gantrisin (one of the sulfa drugs). If this does not clear up the infection, furadantin, a very powerful urinary antiseptic, may be tried. The outlook in pyelitis is good.

GLOSSARY

Albumin   protein found in urine
Ureter   tube that conveys the urine from the kidney to bladder

NEPHROLITHIASIS

(Kidney Stone—Renal Calculus)

Cause and Nature

Kidney stones or gravel are caused by the formation in the pelvis of the kidney or in the kidney itself of concretions from the depositing of certain solid components of the urine. Why these concretions or stones are formed in some people and not in others has never been established. Men are affected more often than women.

It is the function of the kidneys to excrete certain chemicals or solutes through the urinary tract. The super saturation in the urine of some of these, such as calcium phosphate, magnesium phosphate, uric acid, and calcium oxalate, may lead to formation of stones under certain conditions. These conditions may be influenced by stasis, focal injury, infection, the alkalinity or acidity of the urine, and many other factors. The exact cause of this formation of stones is not entirely understood, but in order to treat them, that is, to prevent recurrence, the composition of the stone which is passed must be determined and then preventive steps may be taken. Quite often the patient may pass one stone or several small stones and never be bothered again.

Dr. William Osler gave a very descriptive account of the various signs and symptoms of renal colic (passing a stone) from personal experience. He describes attacks as resulting in three different kinds of pain:

1. A constant localized, dull pain, the area of which could be covered on the skin of the back in the renal region by a penny piece, and which could be imitated exactly by deep firm pressure on a superficial bone.
2. Paroxysms of pain radiating in the course of the ureter or into the flank, and as they increase accompanied by sweating, fainting, and nausea.
3. Flushes or rushes of hot pain at intervals, usually passing to the back, less often to the groin. Dozens of these flushes relieved the monotony of (2). The symptoms persist for a variable period. In short attacks they do not last longer than an hour; in other instances they may continue for a day or more with temporary relief. Micturition is frequent, occasionally painful, and the urine as a rule is bloody.

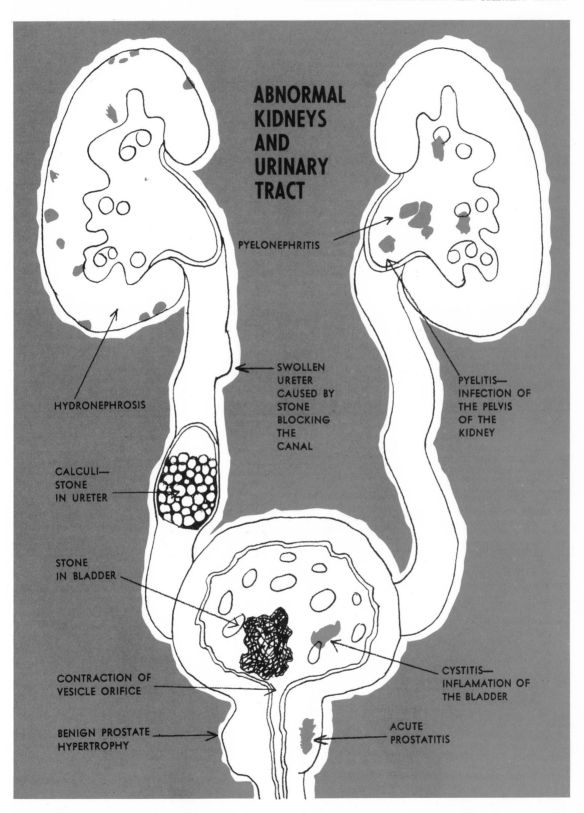

ABNORMAL
KIDNEYS
AND
URINARY
TRACT

PYELONEPHRITIS

SWOLLEN
URETER
CAUSED BY
STONE
BLOCKING
THE
CANAL

PYELITIS—
INFECTION OF
THE PELVIS
OF THE
KIDNEY

HYDRONEPHROSIS

CALCULI—
STONE
IN URETER

STONE
IN BLADDER

CONTRACTION OF
VESICLE ORIFICE

CYSTITIS—
INFLAMATION OF
THE BLADDER

BENIGN PROSTATE
HYPERTROPHY

ACUTE
PROSTATITIS

Signs and Symptoms

The patient may pass small gravel for years and never have an attack of renal colic or he may pass only one stone during a lifetime which may cause him to suffer excruciating pain.

The attack of colic begins when the stone enters the ureter. If the stone is the proper size and has ragged or sharp points on it, the pain may persist until the stone passes into the bladder. A feeling of soreness in the flank may persist for days and a few days after the cessation of pain the stone may be passed in the urine without any difficulty. The agonizing pain usually starts in the flank, passed down the side and into the testicle. It may at times pass, go down the inner side of the thigh or the affected side.

In severe cases there are nausea and vomiting, perspiration breaks out, and there may or may not be fever.

There is nearly always blood in the urine and white blood cells or pus may also be found. X ray and a urinalysis will usually confirm the diagnosis. Some stones show up in an X ray while others do not, depending on their chemical structure. Only about five or ten percent of the stones do not show up.

The composition of the stone should be determined in order to prevent other stones from forming.

Treatment

In treating the acute attack a doctor should be in charge. Often if the pain is on the right side this condition may be thought to be acute appendicitis. A urinalysis will help make the diagnosis, and X ray shows the stone in a majority but not all cases.

Medication for relief of pain and relaxing the smooth muscles should be given to encourage passage of the stone into the bladder. In some cases a larger stone becomes stuck in the ureter and a urologist or kidney specialist must remove it by cystoscopy. Once the stone passes into the bladder, the acute pain subsides and only a soreness remains in the flank.

Exact knowledge of the chemical composition of the stone must be known to minimize the chances of the formation of another stone by decreasing the supersaturation of the chemical involved by diet to combat stasis, and increasing the colloidal content of the urine.

If the stone is found to be made up mostly of urates, steps should be taken to keep the urine alkaline; and if the stone is composed of calcium phosphate, steps should be taken to maintain an acid urine. These things must be under the direction of a physician.

GLOSSARY

Concretions stones
Excrete pass on
Flank side of body
Focal center
Groin section of human body between lower part of abdomen and thigh
Micturition urination
Paroxysms sudden violent action
Ureter canal from the kidney to bladder
Solutes dissolved substances

PERINEPHRITIC ABSCESS

(Abscess about the Kidney)

Cause and Nature

Pus formation or abscess found in the connective tissue about the kidney may be caused by the following:

1. Extensive infection from a pyelitis or from an infection in the kidney itself.

2. Bacteria settling there having migrated from a distant focus of infection such as a boil or abscessed tooth.
3. Blows or injury to the kidney.
4. Perforation of the bowel, as in a ruptured appendix. The abscess formed in this way on certain occasions may extend up around the kidney.
5. Extension of pus from an infected spine, as in tuberculosis of the spine.
6. Extension of pus from an infection in the chest or thoracic cavity as in empyema.

Abscesses of the kidney do not occur as often now as they did before the discovery of the antibiotics. Since these powerful bacteria-killing drugs have been brought into use this type of abscess is seldom seen.

If infection is left untreated a perinephritic abscess may extend down to the groin and be seen as an abscess there, or it may rupture into the peritoneal cavity causing a peritonitis.

Signs and Symptoms

Pain in the back over the kidney region is usually present. This is aggravated by pressure over the kidney involved. In a few instances the onset may be slow and without pain. This pain, if present, may radiate down to the hip joint on the affected side. The patient feels less pain if he lies with the leg on the side of the abscess bent up at the thigh.

Pus may or may not be found in the urine. There are usually chills and fever with heavy sweats. A high white blood count is common, and the doctor may see or feel swelling in the region of the abscess.

Treatment

The abscess should not be allowed to form if the proper antibiotics are used early, and if it does form there is only one treat-

ment. The abscess must be incised or opened and the pus allowed to drain out.

GLOSSARY

Groin area between lower part of abdomen and thigh
Perforation a hole
Pyelitis inflammation of the pelvis of the kidney
Ruptured broken

UREMIA

Cause and Nature

Uremia is a poisoning of the body, or toxemia, resulting from poisons which build up when the kidneys are unable to act adequately. It may result from acute nephritis or from a long-standing chronic nephritis.

Signs and Symptoms

The symptoms are quite variable, but the signs which may be detected by examination of the blood and urine are easily interpreted. There is usually edema or swelling of the tissues; there may be acute headaches and loss of memory, followed by coma.

The coma may have a slow onset with shortness of breath, nausea and vomiting, and acidosis. Convulsions may be noted and signs of mental illness may appear. The convulsions may be followed or preceded by blindness. Headache is perhaps the most constant symptom. The vomiting may be profuse and there may or may not be diarrhea. Sometimes uncontrolled vomiting may set in before the presence of uremia or kidney disease is even suspected. There is usually high blood pressure.

Treatment

When uremia is diagnosed the treatment should be directed at the symptoms and at the disease or condition which has injured the kidneys.

The headache should be controlled with aspirin and codeine mixtures. Saline purgatives and hot baths to induce sweating sometimes help. The use of morphine to control or lessen the convulsions is quite helpful. All of this treatment must be under the direct supervision of a doctor.

In certain conditions patients do recover from the uremic state; one of these is a pregnancy which has caused too heavy a load on the kidney resulting in high blood pressure, blindness, loss of consciousness and convulsions, which is called eclampsia.

The termination of the pregnancy will cause all of these symptoms to disappear and the patient may live a long and healthy life thereafter.

If, however, the uremia results from chronic nephritis, that is a different story.

This requires careful and prolonged treatment by a doctor.

GLOSSARY

Coma   unconsciousness
Diarrhea   watery bowel movement
Nephritis   inflammation of the kidneys
Purgative   a purging medicine
Toxemia   intoxication
Uremia   accumulation in the blood of impurities that should have been eliminated in the urine

HEMODIALYSIS

For some time patients with chronic kidney disease (Bright's disease), have been able to receive a life-saving and life prolonging treatment called hemodialysis.

These people with worn out kidneys who would otherwise go into uremia and die, have been able to go to a hospital at regular intervals and have their blood passed

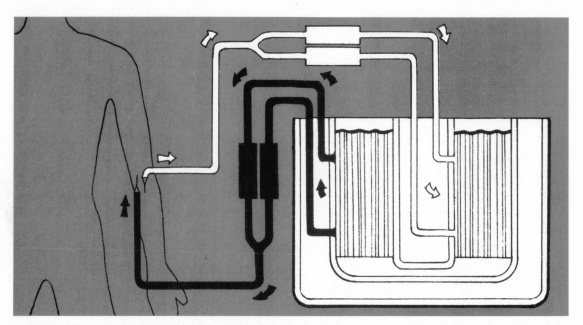

Artificial Kidney. Bad arterial blood passes through membranes and cleansing fluid and returns to body purified. This is life saving in acute conditions—renal failure after hemorrhage, poisoning, and transfusion reactions. It is life prolonging in chronic diseases where dialysis must be repeated time after time because kidneys are worn out.

through an artificial kidney which is called a dialyzer. This machine filters out all the impurities in the blood that the patient's kidneys have been unable to handle. The blood is returned to the patient's body in a purified condition that will allow him to return to work and be a fairly normal person for varying periods of time. Since this is a chronic condition, the treatment has to be repeated over and over again. The patient does not have to be admitted to the hospital, but when the treatment is finished he can put on his clothes and go home.

In large hospitals the load of patients rapidly becomes serious and a person has to make a date for his next treatment weeks ahead of time.

The machine, as you can imagine, is terrifically expensive. The procedure is not too complicated. The patient simply lies down and has one needle inserted into an artery and the other into a vein. The blood pumps out of the artery through the dialyzer and back into the patient's vein.

The number of patients requiring this treatment in large hospitals has become so great that a large machine, or dialyzer, has been invented which can take care of ten or fifteen patients at one time.

As mentioned above these machines cost a great deal of money, but modern science is advancing rapidly and soon they hope to have on the market a home machine that will cost only one or two thousand dollars.

In other fields, doctors have been able to successfully transplant a kidney from one person to another.

Surgeons have transplanted hearts on rare occasions and now are working on how to overcome the immune reaction which rejects some transplants; good progress is being made.

The time may come when most organs can be transplanted from one body to the other and continue to function.

CYSTIC DISEASE OF THE KIDNEY

Cause and Nature

The cause of cysts on the kidney is not clearly understood. There are various types of cysts, such as numerous small cysts which may result from obstruction of some of the tubules of the kidney. In other cases there may be numerous small cysts of unknown cause.

There may be a single very large cyst which in exceptional cases may become large enough to cause a swelling of the body in the kidney region.

A third variety of cyst is seen in the so-called polycystic kidney with great numbers of cysts of all sizes, from very small to large. This condition, when found, is usually present in both kidneys and the cause is not known.

Signs and Symptoms

Many people have cysts on the kidney and are not aware of it. Others have a large tumor of the kidney which may be felt and seen to increase in size. These tumors may involve both kidneys. One may be smaller than the other.

Blood in the urine may come and go at intervals for years, or the patient may present the picture of chronic nephritis if enough of the kidney tissue is destroyed. That is, the skin may be pale and the heart may be enlarged. The blood pressure is high, the urine shows albumin and casts, and the usual course of chronic nephritis is noted.

Treatment

As noted above, a large majority of people who have cysts on their kidneys are entirely unaware of the condition and may live a normal, healthy life.

If the cyst is large and only one kidney is affected, the cyst may be drained by operation. In some cases where one kidney is involved and there is one extremely large cyst present, the kidney may be removed and the person lead a long, healthy life thereafter. These treatments must be determined by the doctor.

GLOSSARY

Cyst   small sac
Nephritis   inflammation of the kidneys
Tubules   small tubes in kidney

HYDRONEPHROSIS

Cause and Nature

The term nephrosis or nephrotic syndrome is used to designate a disease of the kidneys which is not inflammatory in nature. An inflammation of the kidneys is called nephritis. When portions of the kidneys degenerate without inflammation being present it is called nephrosis.

The causes of nephrosis are varied. It may follow infections in children, or in adults it may be caused by syphilis. Thrombosis of the renal veins or chronic glomerulonephritis may result in the nephrotic syndrome.

Signs and Symptoms

Massive edema or swelling of the tissues of the body, albumin in the urine, and usually an elevation of the serum cholesterol are found. Pallor or paleness is present.

Treatment

The diet should be low in sodium and high in potassium. The steroids such as ACTH and cortisone are sometimes useful. Treatment usually extends over a long period and should be in the hands of a doctor.

GLOSSARY

Cholesterol   fatty substance in the blood
Degenerate   deteriorate
Glomerulonephritis   infection of a coil of blood vessels in the kidney
Renal   pertaining to the kidneys
Syndrome   group of signs and symptoms
Syphilis   venereal disease

CHILDHOOD NEPHROSIS

Cause and Nature

The nephrotic syndrome in children or childhood nephrosis is a long-lasting condition which may go unnoticed in its milder forms or may lead to protracted illness and sometimes death in the more serious forms. This condition can be treated or cured in comparatively short periods if recognized early and treated properly.

The causes are numerous. It may follow acute nephritis or may be caused by any number of toxins or poisons including drugs and heavy metals. It may even be caused by allergy to some substance such as immunizing agents or insect bites. The condition may follow an upper respiratory disease caused by bacteria or a virus. In childhood the most common time for it to occur is between one and five years of age. Two- and three-year old children are the favorite targets and we see the greatest number of cases in this age group. However, it may occur at any time during childhood. Boys are more often affected than girls.

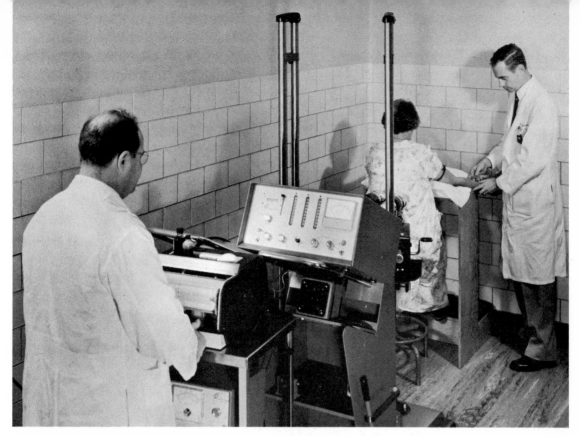

Renogram: a kidney function test. Doctor injects fluid containing radioactive iodine into vein. Assistant, left, adjusts count rate mete as blood goes through kidney.

Signs and Symptoms

This is usually a chronic illness. The first signs noticed may be a swelling of the eyelids in the morning, followed by a generalized swelling or edema of other parts of the body. The child may have a history of pus and blood in the urine. Sometimes, before the swelling appears, one of the common and distressing signs is a collection of fluid, called ascites, in the abdominal cavity. The child gains weight rapidly and the abdomen becomes larger. The urine may be scant.

Examination of the urine is important. A freshly obtained specimen will show albumin and sometimes red blood cells and casts. Blood chemistry is useful in establishing the diagnosis. Studies should be made to determine the ratio between albumin and globulin in the blood serum. A high blood cholesterol is a very common finding, and the blood pressure may be high.

Treatment

This condition must be treated by a competent physician who will usually hospitalize the patient at first for proper evaluation. He will hunt for possible foci of infection and use antibiotics, ACTH, or the adrenal steroids, urinary antiseptics, the proper diet and rest. Most cases recover.

GLOSSARY

ACTH a hormone: in full, adrenocorticotropic hormone
Ascites swelling in abdominal cavity caused by fluid in the peritoneal or abdominal cavity
Foci central points
Nephritis inflammation of the kidneys
Protracted long lasting
Syndrome group of signs and symptoms

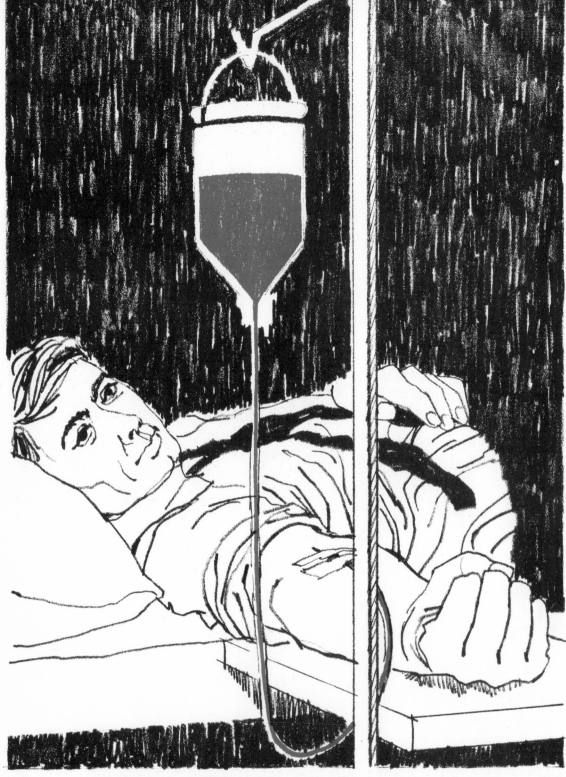

There are many blood banks throughout the nation where blood is stored to be used as needed. The above illustration shows blood being drawn from a donar and flowing into a vacuum flock. Some persons with unusual blood types make money by selling their blood.

Chapter 13

Diseases of the Blood

ANEMIA

Cause and Nature

When red blood cells are lost more rapidly than they can be restored, anemia is said to be present. There are several different kinds of anemia. In general, they may be divided into three main groups:

1. Macrocytic anemia (red blood cells are larger than normal)
2. Microcytic anemia (red blood cells are smaller than normal)
3. Normocytic anemia (red blood cells are average size)

The causes of anemia may be placed in two main classes, and under each class there are several subclasses.

Anemias caused by loss of blood

1. Hemorrhage
   a. Acute
   b. Chronic
2. Abnormal destruction of red blood cells
   a. Infections such as hemolytic streptococcus
   b. Parasites such as malaria
   c. Severe intoxications such as burns, lead poisoning

d. Unknown causes, such as sickle cell anemia and congenital hemolytic jaundice

Inadequate blood formation

1. Lack of the material to make new red blood cells
   a. Vitamins and proteins in nutritional anemia
   b. Iron in iron deficiency anemias
   c. Lack of a factor found in the liver which may cause pernicious anemia
   d. Lack of folic acid
2. Toxic States
   a. Chronic infections
   b. Cancer
   c. Chronic kidney trouble
3. Bone marrow, which helps form red blood cells, may be pushed out by some other tissue
   a. Cancer in the bone
   b. Multiple myeloma
   c. Hodgkin's disease
   d. Leukemia
4. Unknown causes, as in idiopathic aplastic anemia

Signs and Symptoms

The chief function of red blood cells is to carry oxygen. Therefore, most of the symptoms of anemia may be those caused by a lack of oxygen. These are weakness, fatigue, palpitation of the heart, dizziness, and fainting attacks. The signs are pallor, or pale skin, and edema (swelling) of the extremities.

Treatment

In general, the macrocytic anemias may respond to a large daily intake of liver, or to folic acid. The microcytic, hypochromic anemias will usually respond to iron, taken by mouth. The normocytic anemias require a different type of treatment.

If a patient is seen by his doctor and treatment is instituted, most of the anemias can be relieved—even pernicious anemia. But the treatment should begin early in the disease, and be faithfully adhered to. Transfusions of whole blood are helpful in most any type of anemia.

GLOSSARY

Congenital born with
Hemorrhage bleed
Jaundice yellowness of the skin and eyes
Myeloma tumor of the spinal cord
Palpitation fast beat
Parasite plant or animal living on some other living organism
Toxic poisonous

SICKLE CELL ANEMIA

Cause and Nature

This is a chronic hereditary anemia that can be called a hemolytic anemia. This type of anemia is seen almost exclusively in Negroes and it is found in about seven to nine percent of American Negroes; in other words about one in six hundred Negroes may have it. The blood stain shows a few red cells shaped like sickles or oat-shaped, and there is always an anemia present and an abnormal hemoglobin.

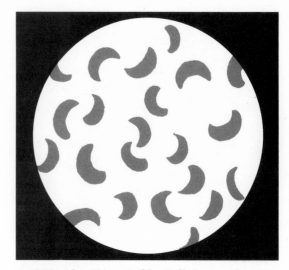

Red blood cells in Sickle Cell Anemia as seen under the microscope.

Signs and Symptoms

In most cases there are few symptoms but the patients may have long slender legs and in some cases chronic ulcers on their legs. The other symptoms are the same as those of any anemia.

There are sometimes serious complications, called crises, in which the patients have a fever and pains in their abdomen and legs. At times there are defects in the bones of the leg, especially the femur. The diagnosis must be made by a doctor.

Treatment

The treatment is mainly aimed at the crisis in these cases. About the only thing that will give relief is a transfusion of normal red blood cells which will not "sickle."

A doctor should always be in charge of the treatment of sickle cell anemia.

GLOSSARY

Anemia deficient quantity or quality of blood
Hemoglobin coloring matter of red corpuscles
Hemolytic breaking down the blood corpuscles

POLYCYTHEMIA VERA

Cause and Nature

The cause of this rare disease is unknown. Red blood cells are produced too rapidly, and the volume of red blood cells often becomes excessive. Fifteen million red blood cells per cubic millimeter of blood have been counted, although the average is about five million per cubic millimeter in a normal person.

Signs and Symptoms

The blood vessels and organs become distended and the rate of circulation is slowed down. The patient has a flushed look. There may be headache, ringing in the ears, dizziness, and weakness. Pain in the bones may be severe because of overgrowth of bone marrow.

Treatment

There is no cure, but the symptoms may be made less severe by withdrawing blood or bleeding the patient at intervals. Some doctors think that the use of radioactive phosphorus has been helpful.

LEUKEMIA

Cause and Nature

The cause is unknown, although it is thought to be similar to cancer in origin. An abnormal formation of white blood cells leads to a great overproduction of these white cells and their infiltration into body tissues.

There are three main kinds of leukemia, depending upon what type of white cell is found to predominate:

1. Myelogenous leukemia
2. Lymphoid leukemia
3. Monocytic leukemia

Each of these types may be divided into acute and chronic types of disease.

The disease may occur at any age, but chronic lymphatic leukemia may occur after sixty, while chronic myelogenous leukemia usually occurs before sixty. The acute leukemias usually occur before twenty-five.

Signs and Symptoms

These may vary with the type. Usually in acute leukemias the onset is sudden with fever, toxemia, and prostration. Bleeding of the gums may be present, with swelling. The white blood count, greatly increased, makes the diagnosis.

Treatment

Recent advances in medicine have improved the treatment of leukemia. The treatment of this disease, however, is very complicated and requires the best work on the part of the doctor as well as cooperation of the patient and his family.

No cure is known at this time, but symptoms may be alleviated, and remissions brought about by proper treatment in some cases.

GLOSSARY

Prostration   exhaustion
Remission   period of improvement
Toxemia   intoxication

AGRANULOCYTOSIS

Cause and Nature

This condition is characterized by an almost complete disappearance from the bloodstream and bone marrow of the granular leukocytes, or white blood cells. It is apparently caused by allergic reaction, usually to some drug. Drugs which are known to have caused agranulocytosis are: gold salts, aminopyrine, thiouracil, sulfonilamides and barbiturates. Only a very small percentage of people taking these drugs will suffer from the allergic reaction.

Signs and Symptoms

In some people the onset is sudden, with chills and fever, and sore throat. In other cases, the onset may be silent or slow. But in most cases there is weakness and fatigue. The white blood count gradually decreases to below two thousand white blood cells per cubic millimeter of blood. The normal is about five thousand per cubic millimeter.

Since the white blood cells are one of our most important tools in fighting infection, this condition should be treated before an infection gets the upper hand.

Treatment

The most important step is to discover and discontinue the use of the drug that has caused the condition. The second step is to use the proper antibiotic in adequate amounts to combat the infection.

If this disease is discovered soon enough and proper treatment started, the mortality rate is low; but if left untreated, it can be a very dangerous condition.

HEMOPHILIA

Cause and Nature

This is a hereditary disease occurring only in the male, but transmitted only by the female. The condition is one in which clotting, or coagulation, of the blood is greatly prolonged, and there is always danger of prolonged and dangerous hemorrhage even from a small injury.

Signs and Symptoms

It is usually first recognized in infancy, when the most noticeable sign is bleeding from a small injury that would not ordinarily cause bleeding. This bleeding may persist for hours or days, and is usually oozing in character. This may lead to severe anemia or death, if not stopped.

Treatment

Blood transfusions of fresh blood usually give the best results. Good results may be obtained by transfusions of plasma in some cases. For localized oozing from the nose or gums, bovine thrombin in gelatin form may be applied locally. A special form of plasma called "antihemophilic plasma" is very useful and should be used often enough by transfusion to stop bleeding attacks.

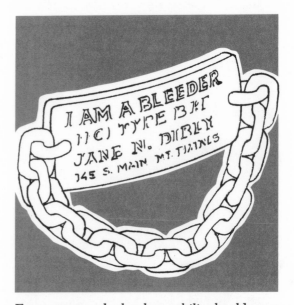

Every person who has hemophilia should wear an identifying bracelet in case they are unconscious from an accident.

Hemorrhage   bleed
Plasma   watery part of blood
Thrombin   clotting substance in blood

HEMORRHAGIC DISEASE OF THE NEWBORN

Cause and Nature

This bleeding in infants is caused by a deficiency in vitamin K. It usually occurs between the second and sixth days of life and may be seen in about one percent of newborn infants.

Signs and Symptoms

The oozing of blood may occur in the gastrointestinal tract, and result in vomiting of blood or passage of blood by bowels. There may be blood in the urine, or oozing from the umbilical cord, the nose, or mouth.

Treatment

The best way to prevent this condition is to give the mother injections of vitamin K before delivery. This should be routine procedure. The baby may be given a prophylactic injection of vitamin K at birth. The bleeding may be stopped promptly by giving injections of vitamin K in adequate doses. It can also be given by mouth.

Gastrointestinal   digestive
Deficiency   not enough
Umbilical cord   navel

HODGKIN'S DISEASE

Cause and Nature

This is a type of cancer involving the glands. The cause is not known. It is characterized by a progressive enlargement of the lymph glands of the body.

Signs and Symptoms

Enlargement of lymph glands on one side of the neck is frequently the first sign, although there may be other enlarged glands. As the disease progresses there is weakness, loss of weight, anemia, and sometimes a recurring type of fever. The diagnosis cannot be made by blood count, but should be determined by removing one of the glands for study under a microscope.

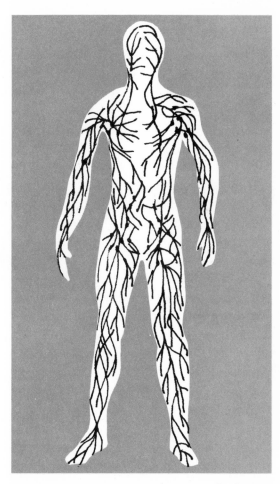

Lymphatic system: A protective fluid runs through the lymph channels. Note the lymph nodes which enlarge with infection.

Treatment

Early diagnosis and surgical removal of the glands is the best treatment, as in any case of cancer. However, there are many drugs which are used to palliate the symptoms. Local X ray often helps.

GLOSSARY

Anemia   blood deficiency
Palliate   to ease without curing

PERNICIOUS ANEMIA OR PRIMARY ANEMIA

Cause and Nature

The cause of this type of anemia is a defect in secretions of the stomach. The exact nature of this defect is not known, but the defect is permanent once it has become established. This lack in the stomach secretions causes a deficiency in the body of certain substances usually derived from food and this deficiency may lead to symptoms. The substance that is not absorbed has been identified as vitamin B_{12}, found in liver extracts. The cause for this failure is not known.

Another substance known as folic acid, when given along with vitamin B_{12}, to people with pernicious anemia, has produced an increase in blood formation and improvement in the general condition of the patient. The connection between vitamin B_{12} and folic acid has not been determined. People with pernicious anemia also show a lack of free hydrochloric acid in their stomach juices. This hydrochloric acid is a normal constituent in stomach secretions and its absence when detected by analysis of the stomach contents should lead to a suspicion of pernicious anemia.

This anemia is seldom seen in a person under thirty years of age. It is found in people with fair skins more often than those with dark skins. It is not inherited, as two people in the same family very seldom have pernicious anemia. The disease is seen as often in males as in females. People affected are found to be prematurely gray.

Pernicious anemia usually has a slow and insidious onset. One of the serious results of the condition is that in addition to anemia, it may lead to permanent damage of the nervous system. That is why the disease should be discovered early and treated adequately in order to prevent the nervous system from being damaged.

Signs and Symptoms

The symptoms most often seen in pernicious anemia are generalized weakness, a sore throat, and a numbness or tingling in the hands and feet. Other complaints are diarrhea, loss of appetite, and indigestion. The patient is usually pale with a light yellow tint to the skin, and the whites of the eyes show a slight jaundice. If the anemia is severe there will be shortness of breath, palpitation of the heart, sometimes dizziness, and occasionally pain over the heart. The tongue is usually red and slick in addition to being sore.

If the disease has progressed far enough to affect the nervous system, degeneration of the peripheral nerves will be noted in tingling or numbness of the hands and feet. There is a disturbed sense of position and on closing the eyes a person cannot stand erect without swaying to one side or the other. There is a loss of vibratory sense in the extremities—that is, if a vibrating tuning fork is held against the ankle bones, the vibrations cannot be felt.

The patient may become irritable, have a mild depression, and sometimes disturbances of the memory. Other signs which are quite distinctive are found in the blood count, and they can only be detected by a physician. Pernicious anemia is one of the macrocytic anemias.

Treatment

With proper care by a physician, the treatment of pernicious anemia has been quite successful since the discovery of vitamin B₁₂. It is no longer necessary to eat large amounts of liver. As a matter of fact, the treatment is relatively simple—adequate injections of vitamin B₁₂ will cause improvement in a few days, and a sense of well-being may be preserved indefinitely as long as the injections of B₁₂ are kept up. It is better taken in shots than by mouth as sometimes B₁₂ is not absorbed properly when taken by mouth. The shots of B₁₂ must be given indefinitely at periods from two to eight weeks.

If the nervous system has been damaged this damage cannot be repaired but it will not progress any further.

A very important word of warning is indicated here. Many people who have been taking multi-vitamins which contain folic acid over a period of years may develop anemia and not realize that they have it until severe and irreversible damage has been done to the nervous system. In other words, this is one disease in which long-sustained taking of vitamins which contain folic acid may mask the symptoms, and the disease will not be discovered until the nervous system has been damaged beyond repair. Therefore, examine the contents of your vitamin pills and stop taking those containing any appreciable amount of folic acid.

GLOSSARY

Folic acid   a vitamin
Jaundice   yellowness of skin and eyes
Palpitation   fast beat
Peripheral nerves   nerves near the outside of the body

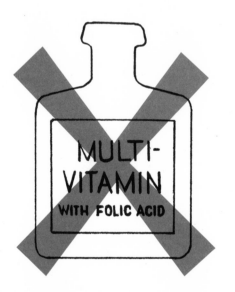

Vitamins containing folic acid should not be taken over long periods. This may mask damage to the central nervous system.

BLOOD POISONING

(Septicemia)

Cause and Nature

When live bacteria invade the blood stream, the person is said to have blood poisoning, or septicemia. This is a very serious condition and it usually follows an infection such as a tonsillar abscess, carbuncles, or bacterial endocarditis. The diagnosis is made when live organisms such as streptococci, staphylococci, and anthrax are found in the blood, and it has even been known to follow smallpox vaccination.

Signs and Symptoms

When a person is suffering from an infection of any kind and suddenly becomes a great deal worse, blood poisoning should be suspected and the blood should be examined for the living organisms. A sudden rise in temperature followed by a chill, is a suspicious sign. The common occurrence of red streaks up the arm or leg when a person has an infected blister is not blood poisoning. The red streaks are lymph channels that are carrying off the poison from the infected area and the infection is still in the lymph system and not in the blood. When the lymph glands become enlarged under the arm or in the groin this means that, again, nature is holding the infection to the lymph system and not allowing the bacteria to enter the blood. This is a protective mechanism and should be heeded by treating the infection carefully to prevent it from entering the blood stream.

In overwhelming infections with great numbers of bacteria in the blood stream, the patient may go into shock and even on to coma and death.

Treatment

With the advent of the antibiotics, such as penicillin and Ilosone, blood poisoning is no longer such a dreaded condition. The doctor will first find out what bacteria has invaded the blood stream and thus will determine which antibiotics are most effective in killing these bacteria. All big hospitals conduct sensitivity tests in the laboratories; when the antibiotic is found to be effective, large doses are given and the patient improves rapidly. The number of deaths caused by septicemia has greatly decreased since the discovery of antibiotics.

GLOSSARY

Abscess   a localized collection of pus
Bacteria   organisms which multiply
Carbuncles   inflammation of tissue with several openings
Coma   complete loss of consciousness
Endocarditis   inflammation of the inner lining of the heart
Sensitivity tests   experiments or tests made to determine which drug is most effective in killing certain bacteria
Shock   sudden vital depression
Tonsillar   of the tonsils

Chapter 14

Disorders of Nutrition and Metabolism

DIABETES MELLITUS

Cause and Nature

Diabetes is caused by an impairment of the body's ability to use foods—especially carbohydrates. A substance called insulin, which is formed in parts of the pancreas called the islands of Langerhans, is instrumental in the proper use of carbohydrates and the storage of glycogen in the liver. When there is a shortage of insulin or an improper use of insulin, the sugars are not used properly and they build up in the blood. Eventually, they show in the urine.

If the carbohydrates are burned in a normal manner, they break down the fatty acids to the end stage which is harmless. However, if they are not broken down all the way, fatty acids in the intermediate stage collect in the blood, giving rise to a ketosis, or diabetic acidosis, which finally leads to coma, if untreated. There is a tendency for diabetes to be hereditary. In arranging a diabetic diet, the amount of fats used is very important.

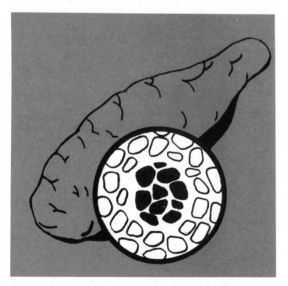

Pancreas: The inset shows an isle of Langerhans. These cells which produce insulin are scattered throughout the pancreas.

Signs and Symptoms

The onset of diabetes is usually slow and insidious. The most common symptoms are excessive thirst, excessive appetite, and the passage of an excessive amount of urine. There may be numbness and tingling of the extremities, recurring boils or carbuncles, and usually loss of weight and strength.

The diagnosis is made by finding sugar in the urine, and confirming this by testing the

229

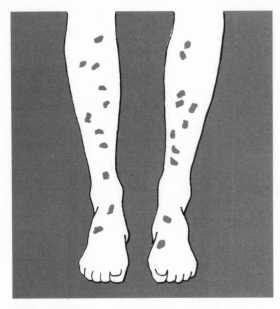

Brown leg spots are seen on some diabetics.

amount of sugar in the blood. In diagnosing diabetes mellitus there are certain danger signs which may point to the disease. These are 1) hypercholesterolemia, 2) obesity, 3) family history of diabetes and vascular disorders in the legs and feet.

Treatment

The management of diabetes mellitus should always be in the hands of a physician. With the proper diet, sometimes augmented by insulin or a new oral insulin-like substance called orinase, the diabetic patient can usually lead a perfectly normal life. Orinase can be taken in tablet form.

GLOSSARY

Carbohydrates   starches and sugar
Coma   unconsciousness
Glycogen   a sugar
Insulin   the substance which enables the body to use sugar
Ketosis   too many ketones in the blood
Ketone   combination of fatty and amino acids
Pancreas   the large gland which secretes insulin

HYPOGLYCEMIA

(Low Blood Sugar)

Cause and Nature

Spontaneous hypoglycemia or low blood sugar is called spontaneous to differentiate it from induced low blood sugar which may be caused by taking too much insulin.

Many patients are told that they may have low blood sugar, but this diagnosis should never be made before taking tests to determine the amount of sugar in the blood. Many of these tests need to be made before the diagnosis is confirmed. If the testing blood sugar remains below forty or fifty milligrams per 100 cc. of blood then the person may be said to be suffering from hypoglycemia.

This disease may have many causes. A great many cases are so-called functional hypoglycemia in which no cause can be found. In other cases tumors of the pancreas may cause the formation of too much insulin and result in low blood sugar. This condition is also found in patients with liver disease, with disease of the adrenal glands, such as Addison's disease, and sometimes it is seen in persons who have had part of their stomach removed resulting in poor absorption of sugar. Hypoglycemia may be associated with hypothyroidism.

Signs and Symptoms

The person who has hypoglycemia or low blood sugar usually has symptoms such as hunger, weakness, and anxiety which may come on several times during the day. In other cases these symptoms may persist and may even include sweating, "trembling inside," headache, and visual disturbances.

The signs and symptoms vary greatly from person to person, and since these symptoms may be experienced in other diseases it should not be assumed that low blood sugar is present until laboratory tests have proven this to be the case.

At times when a meal, some Karo syrup, orange juice, or sugar is eaten when the attack comes on, then a so-called presumptive diagnosis can be made. But since many of these cases of low blood sugar are functional, that is, no cause can be found, it is nearly always necessary to confirm the diagnosis by repeated blood sugar determinations in the laboratory.

Treatment

The treatment of spontaneous hypoglycemia may be divided into two forms: (1) the symptomatic treatment of functional hypoglycemia by eating candy or sugar in other forms, thereby relieving the acute symptoms, and (2) treatment of the underlying cause if one can be found. An example of this second form of treatment may be the use of cortisone in disease of the adrenal gland, or the use of thyroid in hypothyroidism. Thus when the underlying cause is helped the symptoms of low blood sugar may disappear.

GLOSSARY

cc. cubic centimeter (5 cc. equal about one teaspoon)

Hypoglycemia low blood sugar

Hypothyroidism deficient activity of the thyroid gland

DIABETES INSIPIDUS

Cause and Nature

Diabetes insipidus is a clinical condition caused by a deficiency of an antidiuretic hormone in the blood. This is a hormone that controls or decreases the amount of urine passed in a day. This hormone is not entirely understood but is thought to be controlled by the pituitary gland, which is located in the brain. The disease is relatively rare and may be inherited in a few cases. As a rule it is inherited by men only, although it can be acquired by women. Any condition which would affect the pituitary gland in the brain, such as injury, infection, or poor circulation, may result in diabetes insipidus.

Signs and Symptoms

This disease is characterized by a great thirst which leads to the drinking of copious amounts of water, and this in turn leads to the increase in urination because of increased production of urine every day.

The urine produced is normal. It does not contain sugar or albumin. Any person who urinates from five to twenty quarts of urine every day over a long period of time should be suspected of having diabetes insipidus.

Treatment

Diabetes insipidus is a disease that can be controlled readily by taking posterior pituitary substance. This medicine cannot be taken effectively by mouth, but posterior pituitary powder, if sniffed into the nose several times a day, will control the thirst and frequent urination. A water solution of pitressin can be injected several times a day, but this is painful and expensive. One other form of pitressin is available for injection. This is called pitressin tannate in oil and since it is released slowly, an injection under the skin every two or three days will control the symptoms of diabetes insipidus. Since there is no known cure for the disease these medicines which control it must be taken indefinitely.

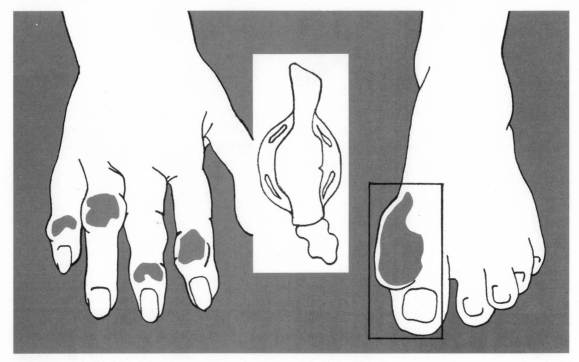

Tophi or collections of uric acid crystals around joints as seen in gout.

GOUT OR GOUTY ARTHRITIS

Cause and Nature

Gout is a result of the improper handling of uric acid by the body. There is usually an increased concentration of uric acid in the blood which is abnormal. There may be a deposit of sodium urate crystals around the joints and under the skin.

Gout appears almost exclusively in men, usually after the age of thirty. It is hereditary—it seems to run in families.

Signs and Symptoms

The onset of gouty arthritis is usually sudden, with acute swelling, pain, and inflammation of a joint. One of the most common places for this disease to strike is in the joints of the great toes. The acute attack may last from two days to two weeks, if un-treated, and has a habit of recurring from time to time.

After the disease has been present for some time, lumps which are sodium urate crystals may be seen around the joints under the skin or in the bursae of the elbow or knee. These can be felt with the hand.

Treatment

When there is an acute attack, the patient should rest in bed and be seen by a doctor. A drug called colchicine is almost specific, and if begun early and taken in proper amounts, will give early relief from pain. This drug, if taken in excess, will cause diarrhea or sometimes nausea and vomiting, but if taken properly will have no deleterious effects. In order to prevent future attacks, a strict diet is necessary. Alcohol is absolutely forbidden. The diet should

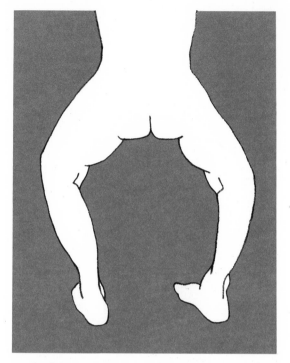

Lack of Vitamin D may cause bow legs.

be high in carbohydrates and low in fats and purines. The foods that contain purines in large amounts are: liver, sweetbreads, kidneys, sardines, beans, peas, and spinach. These should be avoided. Drugs are now on the market to prevent recurrence of gout.

RICKETS

Cause and Nature

A vitamin D deficiency in children predisposes to rickets. There may be other factors such as depletion of calcium and phosphorus reserves, usually due to an improper diet. Rickets is most likely to occur in premature infants, and during the period of most rapid bone growth.

Dark-skinned races do not absorb as much of the sun's ultraviolet rays as white races, thus are more susceptible to rickets.

Signs and Symptoms

Soft areas may be felt in the skull. There may be an enlargement of the places where the ribs join the cartilage, giving rise to a series of lumps—the so-called "rachitic rosary." The ends of the long bones, radius and ulna, tibia and fibula, may be enlarged. Flattening of the back of the head is common. Bow legs, knock knees, and flat feet are among the common manifestations.

Treatment

Rickets may be arrested by proper doses of vitamin D, along with an adequate diet, and lots of sunshine. In most cases, it may be prevented by the use of these same treatments.

GLOSSARY

Depletion   emptying or unloading
Fibula   outer and smaller of the two bones of the leg
Predisposes   makes receptive
Radius   larger bone or forearm on side of thumb
Tibia   inner and larger bone of the leg
Ulna   outer and smaller bone of forearm on side of the small finger

SPRUE

Cause and Nature

The cause is unknown. The disease is characterized by diarrhea with foul, bulky, fatty stools, severe stomatitis (sore mouth), loss of weight, anemia, and distention of the abdomen. There is usually a history of improperly balanced diet.

Signs and Symptoms

Many stools, gray in color, full of gas bubbles, and very voluminous. The abdomen is distended. There is a sore mouth and anemia. Gastric secretions are reduced.

Treatment

Folic acid, ten to twenty milligrams daily, sometimes combined with injections of crude liver extract, ten to twenty units daily.

The diet should be high in protein and low in carbohydrates and fats. Bananas are especially well tolerated. Vitamin B complex should be given. Ferrous sulfate is indicated for the iron deficiency and anemia. Other vitamins and minerals should be supplied in ample quantities.

GLOSSARY

Carbohydrates   starch and sugar
Distention   stretching
Folic acid   a vitamin
Stomatitis   sore mouth
Stools   bowel movements
Voluminous   large

BERIBERI

Cause and Nature

Beriberi is caused by a severe vitamin deficiency. The vitamin that is most often needed is vitamin B$_1$ or thiamine chloride. This disease often follows drastic restrictions in diet.

Signs and Symptoms

Mental depression, uncertain memory, irritability, sleeplessness, apprehension, constipation, epigastric distress after meals, easy fatigue, swelling of the lower extremities, and polyneuritis, or pain in several nerves, are often seen. All of these are found in beriberi to a greater or less extent.

Treatment

Large doses of vitamin B$_1$, thiamine chloride, an adequate diet, and doses of multi-vitamins will cure the condition, as a rule. Vitamin B$_1$ should be injected.

GLOSSARY

Deficiency   not enough
Epigastric   of the upper stomach
Extremities   end parts, such as hands and feet
Polyneuritis   inflammation of many nerves

PELLAGRA

Cause and Nature

Pellagra is a multiple vitamin deficiency disease with a special lack of niacin, one of the B complex vitamins. The advanced disease gives rise to dermatitis, dementia, and death, but this is rarely seen any more. The milder forms of the condition, though, are seen often and go unrecognized. The onset is slow and insidious.

Signs and Symptoms

Weight loss, irritability, and forgetfulness are accompanied by a dermatitis, usually on the exposed part of the skin, hands, face, and neck. This dermatitis is red at first, but the skin gradually becomes dark. When seen on the hands it is often spoken of as a glove-like dermatitis. The mouth may become sore, the tongue red and swollen. The patient is often depressed, and if left untreated, dementia may occur.

Treatment

Vitamin B complex in large doses should be given. Nicotinamide is the most important, and should be given daily by injection until improvement results. The general diet should be adequate.

GLOSSARY

Dementia   mental illness
Dermatitis   skin disease

PYRIDOXINE (Vitamin B$_6$) DEFICIENCY IN INFANTS

Cause and Nature

The heat used to sterilize canned baby formula destroys vitamin B$_6$ in the milk. The baby may develop irritability or recurrent colic.

Signs and Symptoms

Usually at about two and a half months, the baby may develop wakefulness, abdominal colic, and regurgitation after feeding.

Treatment

The best treatment is prevention, by adding B$_6$ vitamin to the formula after it is heated. The baby's formula should have two milligrams per day of vitamin B$_6$ added to it.

Treatment may be carried out by changing to powdered milk formula, and adding two milligrams of vitamin B$_6$ daily.

GLOSSARY

Colic pain
Regurgitation throwing up; vomiting
Sterilize to kill bacteria, usually accomplished by heat

SCURVY

(Vitamin C Deficiency)

Cause and Nature

Scurvy is caused by prolonged deficiency in vitamin C. It is rarely seen in infants who are breast fed, but may be seen after six months in bottle fed babies who are not getting sufficient vitamin C. In adults, it is seen in people on very restricted diets, such as alcoholics—people who are dieting over a long period without proper vitamin intake.

Signs and Symptoms

Babies with this disease fail to gain weight. They become irritable, lose their appetites, and have vague abdominal complaints. They cry when handled. Hemorrhages into the gums may be seen.

Adults have weakness, loss of weight, and various aches and pains in their joints and muscles. They develop hemorrhages in their gums, and may have large black and blue marks in the skin when they receive a light blow.

Treatment

Ascorbic acid or vitamin C is specific, given in adequate doses. Orange juice is a good source of vitamin C, and should be used as a preventive measure.

GLOSSARY

Hemorrhage bleeding

VITAMIN A DEFICIENCY

Cause and Nature

This condition is characterized first by faulty vision in dim light, and may progress to conjunctivitis (inflammation of the eye). The skin may be dry, rough, and scaly. It is caused by a deficiency of vitamin A.

Signs and Symptoms

First, difficulty in seeing at night, then burning and itching of the eyes. The skin then becomes rough, the hair dull and brittle, and the person has an increased susceptibility to any infection.

Treatment

Vitamin A (20,000 to 100,000 units) should be given over a period of months.

VITAMIN K DEFICIENCY

Cause and Nature

The deficiency of vitamin K may depress the clotting mechanism and cause spontaneous hemorrhages. For all practical purposes, this is only seen in newborn babies who do not have a good source of vitamin K in their diets. Most adults eat vegetables in which vitamin K is abundant.

If a newborn baby hemorrhages from the gastrointestinal tract, umbilicus, or mucous membranes, there is a likelihood of vitamin K deficiency.

Signs and Symptoms

Throwing up of blood in an infant, or passing blood by stool or urine. Then there may be small hemorrhages in the mucous membranes of the mouth.

Treatment

The best treatment is prevention—by giving the mother an injection of vitamin K shortly before the baby is born. If the baby presents signs of hemorrhage, usually injections of vitamin K will correct this condition—if it is caused by vitamin K deficiency.

GLOSSARY

Gastrointestinal tract   digestive tract
Hemorrhage   bleeding
Mucous membrane   smooth, moist covering of a
   body cavity
Stool   bowel movement

SIMPLE GOITER

Cause and Nature

Colloid, or simple goiter, is due to a lack of iodine. It is seen in localities where there is not enough iodine in the soil or water.

Certain inland areas of the United States have been found to have insufficient iodine in the soil, and are known as the "goiter belts."

Signs and Symptoms

The thyroid gland is enlarged (the so-called goiter). This enlargement may be relatively slight and cause cosmetic embarrassment, or it may be quite large, and give rise to embarrassment in breathing or swallowing. These goiters are not toxic.

Treatment

Surgery for the removal of large, unsightly goiters is the treatment of choice. An adequate intake of iodine, in such products as iodized salt, in known goiter areas, is the preventive action of choice.

GLOSSARY

Cosmetic   pertaining to appearance; beauty
Toxic   poisonous

HYPOTHYROIDISM

Cause and Nature

The cause is usually a depression in the function of the thyroid gland. There are many grades of hypothyroidism, varying from slight symptoms to myxedema, which is present when the thyroid ceases to function altogether.

Signs and Symptoms

The patient with mild or moderate hypothyroidism is not necessarily obese. He may be thin. There are chronic fatigue, lethargy, cold hands and feet, constipation, and intolerance to external cold. Irregular menstrual periods may be noted in women. The patient should take his pulse in the morning, and if the pulse rate before arising is 72 or more, it is unlikely that hypothyroidism exists.

Treatment

Persons who suspect they have hypothyroidism should see a doctor. Usually, one grain of thyroid taken by mouth daily will cause an improvement in the symptoms. It takes about a week or ten days for the first medicine taken to show any effect. The morning pulse rate should be taken, and overdosage will be manifest by a very rapid pulse, nervousness, etc. The medicine should be taken for about six months, and then discontinued to see if the thyroid gland has resumed its normal function.

GLOSSARY

Lethargy   drowsiness
Myxedema   swelling of face, hands, and body
Obese   fat

TOXIC GOITER

(Hyperthyroidism)

Cause and Nature

This disease is brought about by the overfunction of the thyroid gland. The cause is not known. It may manifest itself in the following two forms:

1. When the gland is slightly enlarged, firm, and overactive, causing symptoms
2. When the gland has one or more small nodules or lumps in it which are said to be toxic—that is, producing a harmful thyroid secretion which causes symptoms

Signs and Symptoms

There is nearly always a loss of weight. The patient is sensitive to heat, wears less clothing, and uses less bedclothes than the normal person. This is just the opposite from the hypothyroid patient.

There is a fine tremor of the fingers, and the patient is highly excitable and nervous. Weakness, shortness of breath, and palpitation are common complaints. The pulse rate is rapid, and the eyes are usually prominent and sometimes protruding (exophthalmus).

Treatment

This disease must be treated by a doctor, who will usually give the patient antithyroid medication and iodine, along with rest and vitamins, until the symptoms are better. Then he will operate, removing part of the thyroid gland.

GLOSSARY

Exophthalmus   abnormal protruding eyeballs
Nodules   lumps
Palpitations   fast beat
Toxic   poisonous
Tremor   shake

BURNING FEET

Cause and Nature

The burning feet syndrome is caused by a deficiency in nutrition or diet. It is seen often among prisoners of war and other persons who do not have enough to eat, but since most of the people of the United States have had enough food to eat, this disease is not seen very often.

Signs and Symptoms

There is an intense burning of the feet making it difficult to sleep and very painful to walk.

Treatment

Large doses of vitamin B or of brewer's yeast will relieve this condition. The correction of undernutrition by eating a well-balanced diet will prevent this condition from occurring.

Syndrome a group of symptoms

LEG CRAMPS

Cause and Nature

The causes of painful cramps in the muscles of the leg and feet are numerous and a large percentage of all people will suffer from these cramps at some time during life. It is well to understand the causes of cramps, and after the cause is determined, to apply proper treatment.

Some of the common causes of leg cramps are:

1. lack of calcium (seen in some pregnant women and old people)
2. deficiency of salt
3. poor circulation in the legs
4. varicose veins
5. deformities of the feet
6. night cramps in the legs of unknown origin

In a few diseases, the first sign may be leg or foot cramps. These diseases are anemia, diabetes, vitamin B deficiency, lead poisoning, and poisoning from the bite of the black widow spider. Cramps caused by disease are much less frequently seen than the simple cramps.

Signs and Symptoms

In some cases walking a few blocks will cause painful cramps in the leg muscles. These are usually caused by poor circulation.

In the later months of pregnancy some women suffer from muscular spasm or cramps which are very painful and are usually caused by a disturbance in their calcium metabolism.

After working hard on a hot day, younger people may suffer a painful knot or spasm in the muscles of their legs. This may be caused by an excessive loss of sodium. Many others suffer from cramps and knots in their muscles which come on at night for no apparent reason.

Treatment

The treatment of painful leg cramps will depend upon their cause. In the most common or simple cases of leg cramps, dicalcium phosphate tablets taken twice a day will give relief.

Cramps caused by excessive sweating and loss of salt can be helped by taking salt tablets or eating more salt.

In some cases there is a weakened arch in the foot which may cause cramps. The correction of this deformity will help.

In cases of varicose veins which result in poor circulation and muscle cramps, treatment of these veins by surgery will cure the cramps. In the large number of healthy people who have nocturnal leg cramps of unknown origin, five grains of quinine sulfate taken at bedtime will prevent the cramps quite often. Sometimes a dose of Benadryl, fifty milligrams taken at bedtime, will help those who do not get results from quinine.

Anemia deficient blood
Diabetes a disease
Nocturnal nightly
Varicose veins swollen veins

Chapter 15

Overweight

OBESITY

Cause and Nature

The cause for a person becoming overweight is practically always a matter of eating more food, or calories, than the person uses. Calories eaten and not used are stored up in the body in the form of adipose tissue, or fat. Glandular disturbances almost never cause overweight and will not be considered here. Heredity may play a part in obesity.

Signs and Symptoms

How much an individual should weigh is governed by his age, height, sex, and body build. Herewith is a table which gives approximately correct weights.

When a person is overweight, he is much more susceptible to heart disease, high blood pressure, diabetes, and gall bladder disease. The older a person becomes, the more important it is for him to refrain from becoming overweight.

Treatment

Essentially, the only way to lose weight is to eat fewer calories than are used in a day.

In this way, the body burns up some of its excess fat in the production of energy, and the person loses weight.

Exercise is a poor way to try to lose weight, as it has been estimated that an average person would have to walk thirty-six miles in order to lose one pound of weight. Exercise often increases the appetite—therefore, a person consumes more calories and puts weight on, rather than losing it. Eating less salt or drinking less water will not aid in losing weight.

A person must, therefore, realize that overweight is caused only by eating more food than he uses, and should correct his faulty habits of eating in order to lose weight.

Having determined what his ideal weight should be, a person (especially one over forty-five) should study calorie tables and figure out a diet of 1000 to 1500 calories per day. By staying with this diet, he should lose from one to five pounds a week until the ideal weight is reached. Then he should maintain his weight at this level by eating a diet which supplies just as much energy as he uses in a day. That is, he

239

TABLE OF NORMAL WEIGHTS

For Men of Ages 25 Years or More

| Height in Shoes | | | | |
Feet	Inches	Small Frame	Medium Frame	Large Frame
5	2	112–120	118–129	126–141
5	3	115–123	121–133	129–144
5	4	118–126	124–136	132–148
5	5	121–129	127–139	135–152
5	6	124–133	130–143	138–156
5	7	128–137	134–147	142–161
5	8	132–141	138–152	147–166
5	9	136–145	142–156	151–170
5	10	140–150	146–160	155–174
5	11	144–154	150–165	159–179
6	0	148–158	154–170	164–184
6	1	152–162	158–175	168–189
6	2	156–167	162–180	173–194
6	3	160–171	167–185	178–199
6	4	164–175	172–190	182–204

For Women of Ages 25 Years or More

| Height in Shoes | | | | |
Feet	Inches	Small Frame	Medium Frame	Large Frame
4	10	92– 98	96–107	104–119
4	11	94–101	98–110	106–122
5	0	96–104	101–113	109–125
5	1	99–107	104–116	112–128
5	2	102–110	107–119	115–131
5	3	105–113	110–122	118–134
5	4	108–116	113–126	121–138
5	5	111–119	116–130	125–142
5	6	114–123	120–135	129–146
5	7	118–127	124–139	133–150
5	8	122–131	128–143	137–154
5	9	126–135	132–147	141–158
5	10	130–140	136–151	145–163
5	11	134–144	140–155	149–168
6	0	138–148	144–159	153–173

Reprinted from Metropolitan Life Insurance Company, Stat. Bull. 40:1–12.

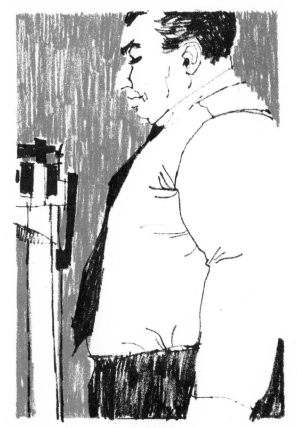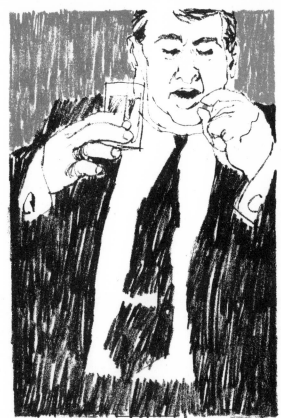

When dieting: Weigh often and take supplemental vitamins and minerals.

should weigh at least once a week, and if he starts gaining, the diet should be immediately reduced. It is easier to keep from putting on weight than it is to take it off.

If the person is under a doctor's care, it is sometimes helpful to take dexedrine, or a similar drug, to decrease the appetite. There is no substitute for will power, and this is what it takes to keep from overeating.

Any diet should include adequate protein for every meal in the form of lean meat, fish, poultry, eggs, or skimmed milk. Green and yellow vegetables may be eaten freely, but one should watch the intake of carbohydrates in the form of bread, potatoes, sugar, etc. The amount of fat eaten should also be restricted.

When reducing, it is important to take additional vitamins and minerals because the restricted diet may not furnish an adequate supply of these substances. A good vitamin for this purpose is mi-cebrin (Lilly)—one or two tablets daily. A list of different foods with their caloric values is included here, to enable the reader to figure out his own diet. Or by drinking four glasses of Metrecal a day, a person will be taking a good, well-balanced diet of 900 calories.

GLOSSARY

Adequate   enough
Calorie   a unit of measure used to express the heat-producing or energy-producing value of food
Heredity . traits transmitted from ancestors
Susceptible   having little resistance

CALORIE CHART*

Food	Calorie Count	Food	Calorie Count
Apple, raw, 1 medium	76	Lamb, leg, roast, 1 medium slice	103
Apricots, canned, in syrup, 4 halves	97	Lamb chops, broiled, 1 medium	178
Asparagus, 6 to 8 stalks	25	Lemonade, 1 large glass	104
Bacon, 2 crisp slices	97	Lettuce, 1 large head	50
Banana, 1 medium	88	Liver, 1 medium slice	120
Beans, baked, canned, 1 cup	295	Macaroni and cheese, 1 cup	464
Beans, green or snap, 1 cup	27	Mayonnaise, 1 tbsp.	92
Beef, steak, club, broiled 1 large piece	410	Meat loaf, 1 medium slice	100
Beef, rib roast, lean, 1 medium slice	96	Milk, skim, 1 glass (8 oz.)	87
Beef stew with vegetables, 1 cup	252	Milk, whole fresh, 1 glass (8 oz.)	166
Beets, canned, 1 cup	82	Muffin, 1 small	134
Biscuits, 1 medium	129	Noodles, cooked, 1 cup	107
Bouillon or consommé, clear, 1 cup	26	Nuts, mixed, 8 to 12 nuts	94
Bread, white, enriched, 1 slice	64	Oatmeal, cooked, ½ cup	74
Bread, whole wheat, 1 slice	55	Olives, green or ripe, 10 small	70
Broccoli, 1 cup	44	Onions, 2¼" diameter, 1 medium	45
Butter or margarine, 1 tbsp.	100	Orange, 1 medium	68
Cabbage, raw, shredded, 1 cup	24	Orange juice, frozen, after dilution 1 glass (6 oz.)	75
Cake, angel or sponge, plain 2" wedge	110	Pancake, 1 medium	59
Cake, chocolate layer, iced 2" slice	356	Peaches, canned, in syrup, 2 halves	79
Cake, coffee cake, 1 small piece	100	Peanut butter, 1 tbsp.	92
Cake, fruit, 1 small slice, 2x2x½"	106	Pears, canned, in syrup, 2 halves	79
Cantaloupe, ½ medium	37	Peas, canned, ½ cup	84
Carrot, 1 whole raw	21	Pie, apple or berry, ⅐ of 9" pie	331
Cauliflower, 1 cup	30	Pie, lemon meringue, ⅐ of 9" pie	302
Celery, 1 large outer stalk	7	Pie, mince, ⅐ of 9" pie	341
Cheese, Cheddar, 1" cube (1 oz.)	113	Pie, pumpkin, ⅐ of 9" pie	263
Cheese, cottage, ½ cup	107	Pineapple, canned, 1 slice and juice	95
Chicken, roast, average serving (¼ lb., no bone)	227	Popcorn, no butter, 1 cup	54
Chicken salad, ½ cup	185	Pork chop, 1 medium	296
Chocolate beverages (with milk), 1 cup	239	Potato, baked, 1 medium	100
Chocolate fudge, 1" sq.	116	Potato, sweet, baked, 1 medium	190
Chocolate malted milk, 1 average (13 oz.)	601	Potato chips, 7 large or 10 medium	108
Coffee, clear, 1 cup	0	Potatoes, mashed, 1 scant cup	159
Coffee, 1 tbsp. cream and 1 lump sugar	55	Rice, white or brown, cooked, ½ cup	100
Cola beverages, 1 bottle (8 oz.)	90	Roll, plain, 1 medium	118
Cookies, assorted, 3" diameter, each	109	Roll, cinnamon, 1 medium	178
Corn on the cob, 1 medium	84	Salmon, canned, red, cup	173
Cracker, graham, 2 medium	55	Sherbets, ½ cup	118
Cracker, saltine, 1 double	34	Shrimp, canned, drained, 3 oz.	108
Cream, whipping (35%), 1 tbsp.	49	Spaghetti with meat sauce, 1 average serving	396
Cream, coffee (20%), 1 tbsp.	30	Spareribs, roasted, 3 average ribs	123
Doughnut, cake or yeast, 1 average	136	Strawberries, raw, capped, 1 cup	54
Egg, boiled or poached, 1 medium	77	Sugar, granulated or brown, 1 tbsp.	50
Frankfurters, 1 medium	124	Tea, unsweetened, 1 cup	0
French dressing, 1 tbsp.	59	Tomatoes, fresh, 1 medium	30
Grapefruit, ½ medium	72	Tuna fish, drained, ⅝ cup	198
Gravy, medium consistency, ¼ cup	107	Turkey, 1 slice 4x2x¼"	100
Ham, smoked, cooked, 4½x2½x½" slice	119	Veal cutlet, breaded, 1 medium	217
Hamburger, medium patty (⅙ lb.)	331	Vegetable soup, 1 cup	82
Ice cream, plain, commercial, ½ pt.	294	Waffle, 1 medium with 3 tbsp. syrup	687
Ice cream, chocolate, ½ pt.	385	Watermelon, 6" slice 1½" thick	168
Jam or Jelly, 1 tbsp.	55	White sauce, medium, ¼ cup	107

*Caloric values based on the U.S. Department of Agriculture handbook No. 8. 1950.

Chapter 16

Vitamins

VITAMINS are organic substances which occur in many foods in small amounts, and are said to be necessary to the normal metabolic functioning of the body. They are present in most foods, and if a good, well-balanced diet is eaten, a person should obtain sufficient vitamins.

However, with the increased refining and processing of food today, it may be possible that inadequate amounts of vitamins are consumed, and it is usually wise to take a good multiple vitamin tablet each day just to insure against an unsuspected shortage of some particular vitamin. There are many of these vitamins on the market, and since the cost is often an important factor, one way of obtaining adequate B complex vitamins is to take brewer's yeast tablets—one, three times a day. These are inexpensive, and contain all the B complex vitamins.

In buying an all-around vitamin, one should be sure that it is manufactured or processed by a reputable drug company.

Symptoms of Deficiency

General nonspecific symptoms of a real vitamin deficiency may include dry skin, loss of weight, nervousness, irritability, headaches, easy fatigability, weakness, indigestion, loss of appetite, vague aches and pains, and a mild anemia. These symptoms may accompany many diseases, and as a matter of fact, with any disturbance of the body metabolism, there may be a shortage of vitamins.

A few of the specific vitamins and conditions caused by a lack of these vitamins are listed on the following pages.

VITAMIN A

VITAMIN A is found in all animals and salt-water fish. Another source of Vitamin A is the so-called Provitamin A or Carotene. It is found in green or in yellow vegetables and in fruit. Hence, some of these foods should be consumed every day in a normal diet.

Severe deficiency in Vitamin A leads to night blindness, thickening of the skin and mucous membranes, and may make a person susceptible to upper respiratory infections, bronchitis, and conjunctivitis. In cases of "A" deficiency, the hair becomes dull and brittle, and the skin becomes dry, rough, and scaly.

Treatment of this lack of Vitamin A may be accomplished by a proper diet, and by taking 25,000 to 50,000 unit capsules of concentrated fish liver oil daily. The use of mineral oil in excess will slow up the absorption of Vitamin A from the intestinal tract.

Overdosage of Vitamin A may lead to clubbing of fingers, sparse, coarse hair, anemia, bone and joint pains, and an oily, odorous skin.

VITAMIN B COMPLEX

There are many compounds in the Vitamin B complex, some of which are well known, others are not. The better known components will be described below.

VITAMIN B_1 (*thiamine chloride*). Occurs in yeast, lean pork, soy beans, bran, whole grain cereal, and egg yolk. Milling processes the Vitamin B_1-rich hulls of the whole grain cereals, and many products are now being fortified with synthetic Vitamin B_1.

Deficiency in thiamine, or Vitamin B_1, is characterized by mental depression, apprehension, inefficiency, poor memory, and clumsiness. There may also be loss of appetite, constipation, headaches, inability to sleep well, and easy fatigability.

When there is a severe deficiency of Vitamin B_1, the disease beriberi occurs. In this condition we have, in addition to the above symptoms, polyneuritis and swelling of the extremities.

Treatment is usually carried out by administering by mouth, tablets of Vitamin B_1 (*thiamine chloride*) of ten to fifty milli-grams, three times a day. It may be given by hypodermic, if medication cannot be taken by mouth.

VITAMIN B_2 (*riboflavin*). Occurs in liver, milk, eggs, nuts, yeast, seafoods, green, leafy vegetables, and lean meat.

Vitamin B_2 deficiency is probably the most clean-cut and prevalent vitamin deficiency we see. The symptoms at first may be vague, with some anxiety and below par feeling. This is followed by lesions in the corners of the mouth. These fissures or cracks have a crust on them that can be easily removed without bleeding. This condition is called "cheilitis." It may be accompanied by itching, burning, and excessive dryness of the eyes. The tongue may become smooth and purplish-red in color.

Treatment consists of the administration of Vitamin B_2 (*riboflavin*)—about fifteen milligrams daily.

NICOTINIC ACID. This is also a part of the B complex, and is found in lean meat, yeast, cereal grains, and peanuts.

A severe deficiency of nicotinic acid results in the disease called pellagra. This may be characterized by dermatitis, diarrhea, dementia, and may result in death. However, the severe cases of pellagra are rarely seen now. We do see milder forms which present a feeling of ill health, loss of weight, lassitude, irritability, and the tongue may become tender, inflamed, and swollen.

The dermatitis is usually the same on both sides of the body, and appears on the exposed parts of the body such as the hands and face. This dermatitis progresses from a redness, which resembles sunburn, to a dark tan pigmentation which, on the hands, is called a glove-like dermatitis.

Treatment is usually successfully carried

out by administering *nicotinic acid* or *nicotinamide.*

VITAMIN B₆ (*pyridoxine*). Occurs in lean meat, liver, fish, yeast, nuts, whole grain cereals, and molasses.

The role played by Vitamin B₆ in man is not entirely understood, but we do know that when babies are fed concentrated canned milk formula, which has to be heated, the Vitamin B₆ is often destroyed by the heat. A baby with Vitamin B₆ deficiency will become irritated, wakeful, have colic, regurgitate its feedings, and may go on to convulsive seizures.

Treatment for this condition is to change the formula from liquid to powdered milk. Administer Vitamin B₆ (*pyridoxine*)—two milligrams by mouth, at each feeding, until the baby is better. Many doctors think that all babies whose irritability is marked and unexplained should receive Vitamin B₆ (*pyridoxine*).

The other constituent of the vitamin B complex is called *pantothenic acid,* and its role in nutrition is not fully understood.

In summing up this important group of vitamins, the B complex group, it should be emphasized that an adequate supply of B complex can be taken by using brewer's yeast. These tablets are inexpensive, and two tablets taken three times a day will furnish more than enough of the B complex.

VITAMIN C

VITAMIN C, (*ascorbic acid*), occurs in citrus fruits, strawberries, and tomatoes. All newborn babies should have additional Vitamin C, if they are not breast fed. This can be given in their milk, in the form of ascorbic acid, or by giving them orange juice.

Serious deficiency of Vitamin C causes the disease called scurvy. The onset of scurvy is slow. Loss of appetite and weight, hemorrhage under the skin and under the gums, increased susceptibility to infection, and pains in joints are common.

Treatment for this condition is to administer *ascorbic acid* or Vitamin C pills. A large amount of orange juice and a proper diet will prevent the condition.

VITAMIN D

In nature, VITAMIN D is not widely distributed. Therefore, the ordinary diet may not furnish sufficient amounts of this vitamin. It is found in fish liver oils, milk and yeast fortified with ultraviolet irradiation, and Vitamin D is formed in the skin following exposure to sunlight.

The function of this vitamin is to maintain adequate supplies of calcium and phosphorous for the proper growth of bones. All babies should have additional sources of Vitamin D in their formulas. This will prevent rickets. Cod liver oil is a good source of vitamin D. Vitamin D in large doses may cause toxicity, shown in pallor, frequent stools, headache, loss of weight, and joint pains. This vitamin should, therefore, not be taken in too large doses.

VITAMIN E

VITAMIN E occurs in nature in wheat germ oil, peanut oil, corn oil, and cottonseed oil. The amounts of this vitamin in the above oils is considerable, and it is distributed to a lesser extent in many plants.

There has been no proof of a Vitamin E

deficiency in man. However, it is used to obtain symptomatic relief in such conditions as fibrositis, or muscular rheumatism. It also may be used in some of the muscular dystrophies to some advantage. When taken early, in large doses, it may prevent contracture of tendons of the hands and fingers, such as Dupuytren's contraction.

The components of Vitamin E are designated as tocopherols A, B, C, and D. They are more effective used all together or in mixed form.

VITAMIN K

The natural forms of VITAMIN K are not important as therapeutic agents. Synthetic Vitamin K is used when there is a tendency toward bleeding, which has been caused by a prothrombin deficiency. This deficiency may occur in liver disease or bile duct obstruction which prevents the absorption of Vitamin K.

Vitamin K may be used orally with bile salts or by injection. If the bleeding is caused by prothrombin deficiency, Vitamin K will often correct the condition. This is especially true when bleeding occurs from the intestinal tract or under the mucous membranes in newborn babies. A few injections of Vitamin K will often tide them over until their prothrombin level becomes normal, and their blood-clotting time is corrected.

OTHER VITAMINS AND FACTORS

There are a number of other vitamins which have been studied, but to date their use has not been proven to be of any partic-

ular value. In concluding the vitamin discussion, it may be well to emphasize the fact that if a person eats a good, well-balanced diet, there will be no vitamin deficiency. If a person wants to take one good multi-vitamin daily, just for safety's sake, there is no harm in doing this.

THE TRACE MINERALS

These minerals, found in traces in plant and animal life, are very important to normal nutrition. They are *calcium, iodine, sodium, potassium, magnesium, iron chlorides,* and *phosphates.* All of these are important to the growth and health of the body. But again, if a good, well-balanced diet is taken, there should be no shortage of these minerals.

Some of the present-day vitamin tablets contain small amounts of these minerals, and no harm will come from taking one of these vitamin tablets daily.

GLOSSARY

Ascorbic acid   vitamin C
Carotene   vitamin A
Complex   a group
Contracture   shrinking or shortening
Dementia   insanity
Dermatitis   rash
Dystrophy   faulty nutrition or growth
Extremities   end-most parts; hands and feet
Hypodermic   given under the skin; a "shot"
Irradiation   exposure to rays
Lassitude   a tired feeling
Metabolic function   changing food into energy
Polyneuritis   inflammation of many nerves
Prothrombin   a substance in the blood that causes clotting
Synthetic   artificial
Therapeutic   healing
Tocopherols   the E vitamins
Toxicity   poisonous action
Ultraviolet   invisible rays of light

Chapter 17

Diseases of the Nervous System

STROKES

(Cerebro-vascular Accidents, Apoplexy)

Cause and Nature

Cerebro-vascular accidents or strokes are classed about third in the most frequent causes of death and rank very high in causing disability, especially in older persons.

Since we are now experiencing a dramatic increase in the number of years a person may live, this condition becomes very important and an understanding of it may help in the early diagnosis and successful treatment in some cases.

Statistics have shown that in 1900, four percent of the population of the United States was 65 years old or older; in 1935, six percent was over 65 years old, and it is estimated that in 1980 about fifteen percent will be over 69. Therefore, the importance of strokes will increase with time.

There are many causes of a cerebrovascular accident, or stroke. But the three main causes are:

1. Hemorrhage in the brain
2. Thrombosis or clotting of some artery in the brain
3. Embolism or a small clot becoming stuck in an artery of the brain

In each case the brain tissue which is supplied with food and oxygen by the artery which is involved, will be destroyed. The location of the destroyed brain tissue and the size or amount of tissue destroyed will determine the signs and symptoms.

There are two main types of strokes: the so-called big strokes and the little strokes.

Signs and Symptoms

The signs and symptoms of these two classes of strokes will be described separately.

BIG STROKES. Depending upon the place in the brain where the injury occurs, the signs will differ. Usually the onset is sudden unconsciousness. At first there may be a weakness in one arm and one leg on the same side. One side of the face may sag or be smoothed out. The person may lose the ability to talk, and memory may be abolished.

There are many variations of these signs. Sometimes they are very marked, resulting in death without regaining consciousness; **247**

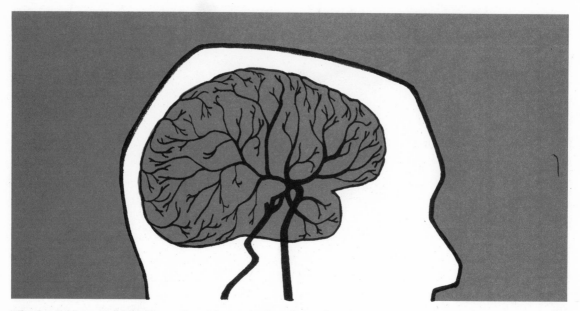

The brain's arterial blood supply is shown in the above drawing.

again they may be slight and clear up within days or months. All signs of paralysis may disappear and the person could live many years before suffering another stroke or dying from some other cause.

After a few weeks the arm and leg may remain paralyzed and indeed this condition may be permanent. If some of the motion returns to the paralyzed arm or leg, this is a good sign, and it may be possible by proper exercises to build the limbs back up to their former state of usefulness.

LITTLE STROKES. Dr. Alvarez has written at great length on "Little Strokes," and in one of his articles he says: "One of the commonest diseases of man is a slow petering out toward the end of life, and one of the commonest ways of petering out is that in which the brain is slowly destroyed by repeated thrombosis (clotting) of small sclerotic blood vessels." That is the plugging up by a clot slowly formed in a small vessel, which has a small opening anyway because the walls have been thickened by arteriosclerosis.

These little strokes are usually often repeated over the months and years. The only sign may be a temporary loss of speech or a fleeting weakness of an arm or leg, or of both, which clears up.

Sometimes the signs and symptoms may be apparently unrelated to the brain, such as repeated attacks of dizziness which clear up. There may be strange feelings of burning and itching over different parts of the body, or nausea, vomiting, belching, and gas. We must remember that these things all can and do occur to most of us without indicating that we have had a little stroke. The diagnosis must be confirmed by a physician.

One of the mental changes which occur with these repeated little strokes may be a complete change of character. A man who has been very neat, orderly, intelligent, and well-groomed may become slovenly, suspicious, profane, depressed, and self-centered. These slow, steady changes in mental attitude in older people may result from a repetition of little strokes.

Treatment

The best treatment, of course, is prevention, and it is to be hoped that medical science will discover some way to prevent thickening of the arteries or arteriosclerosis. In the meantime, we can help prevent these conditions by living a clean, healthy life, getting enough rest, good food, and fresh air, and by not punishing our bodies by overindulgence.

Once a stroke has occurred, the person should be kept at rest for ten days or so before attempts are made to see if the paralyzed arm or leg can be exercised. Then the exercises should be carried out under the instructions of a doctor, or a physiotherapist who is working under the direction of the doctor. A physician should be in attendance, as he will be able to determine the type of stroke. In rare instances surgical treatment may be indicated.

In all suspected cases keep the patient in bed and call a doctor.

GLOSSARY

Apoplexy stroke
Arteriosclerosis hardening of the arteries
Cerebro-vascular accident pertaining to blood vessels in the brain
Thrombosis clot

FACIAL PARALYSIS

(Bell's Palsy)

This is a paralysis of the muscles on one side of the face which are controlled by the seventh cranial nerve. It can occur in many conditions such as a stroke, but if it appears out of a clear sky with no other signs or symptoms, it is called Bell's palsy.

Signs and Symptoms

The onset is usually abrupt, that is a person may awaken in the morning with a relaxation of the muscles on one side of the face which causes a little difficulty in speech and a sensation of stiffness on one side of the face. In some cases this is preceded by mild pain, but not always. The patient cannot whistle and the eye on the affected side cannot be closed. The sense of taste on that side of the tongue may be lost.

Treatment

If the case is mild, it may begin to clear up within two weeks and will disappear

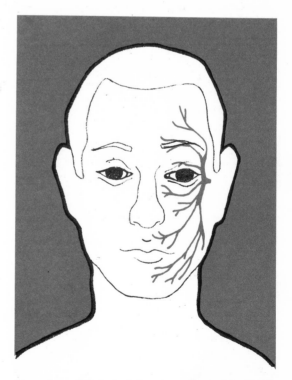

Branches of left facial nerve effected in Bell's Palsy. Ganglion is sometimes injected with alcohol in treating this condition.

completely in about two months. More severe cases take longer and if it lasts for over a year the damage to the nerve may be permanent. This seldom occurs.

The treatment cannot be direct, but is aimed at the affected muscles. The eye which cannot be closed should be carefully protected. It should be washed with warm boric acid solution morning and night. Glasses, (dark), should be worn to protect the eye from particles of dust.

The facial muscles should be massaged daily by the patient, always massaging upward. If the down sagging of the muscles is severe this can sometimes be helped by a V-shaped application of thin adhesive strips, with the point of the V on the cheek bone,

one strip going over the bridge of the nose and the other going to the side up to the temple.

In cases which do not recover as they should, sometimes surgical decompression of the seventh or facial nerve is resorted to but this has not been consistently helpful.

GLOSSARY

Cranial pertaining to the skull
Decompression removal of pressure

HEADACHE

Cause and Nature

Headache is one of the most common disorders suffered by the human race. This is

Headaches are often a symptom of a more serious disorder. Consult doctor if they reoccur frequently.

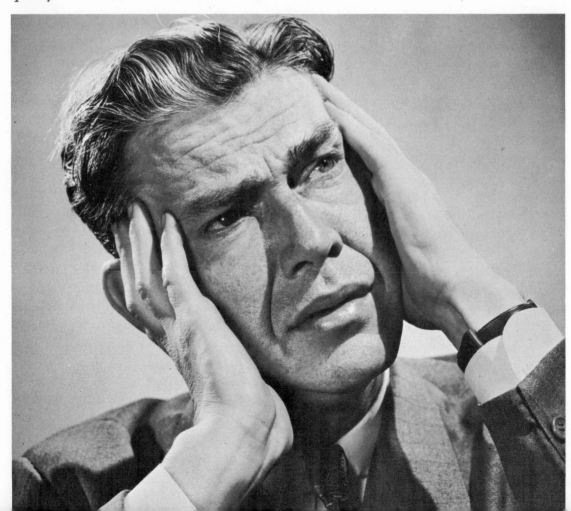

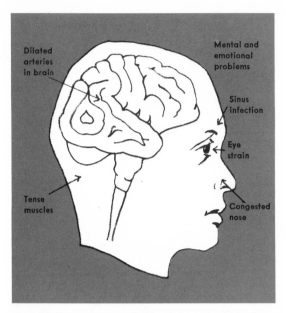

Headaches may result from various disorders.

not a disease but is a symptom, and while we do not know all that is to be known about headaches, there are certain types of headaches in which the causative mechanism is understood and for which treatment has been found to be fairly successful.

The physiology of the human body will give rise to the headache symptom when important mechanisms are out of order, thus establishing the main types of headache, which are:

1. THE VASCULAR MECHANISM: Migraine headache, usually affecting one side of the head only. In a great many headaches the blood vessels play a leading part, and we know that in migraine headache there is an initial contraction of the cerebral arteries. That is, arteries of the brain give rise to various prodromal or warning signs that an attack of migraine headache is about to start. Important among these signs are various lights and spots in front of the eyes. This

initial contraction of the cerebral blood vessels is followed by a dilatation of these same vessels, causing the pain of the migraine headache, which is often on one side of the head and may be quite severe.

We also know that drugs which cause the vessels to contract and do away with the dilatation of the vessels will cause the pain to subside.

2. HIGH BLOOD PRESSURE: Another form of vascular headache may be experienced by a person with high blood pressure causing the vessels in the brain to be stretched. This type of headache is most usually noted upon awakening in the morning and goes away after the person gets up and moves around for a while. It is nearly always noted first in the back part of the head.

3. EYE STRAIN. Headaches caused by eye strain are quite common. They are often caused by some error in refraction, meaning that the glasses worn by a person are not the proper glasses. These headaches tend to occur around the eyes and in the forehead or temple and seem to come on most often when a person is using his eyes during heavy reading or fine sewing. The eye strain headaches are mostly noticed in the late afternoon or evening after the eyes have been used for some time. Headaches of this type can be corrected by obtaining and using proper eye glasses and are usually relieved temporarily by resting the eyes or by taking a nap.

4. TOXIC HEADACHES. Any acute disease such as measles may be accompanied by headache caused by the toxins or poisons in the blood. Infection of the teeth or sinuses may result in a similar type of headache.

5. PSYCHOLOGICAL MECHANISMS: It is a well proven fact that many people with chronic headaches are plagued by emotion-

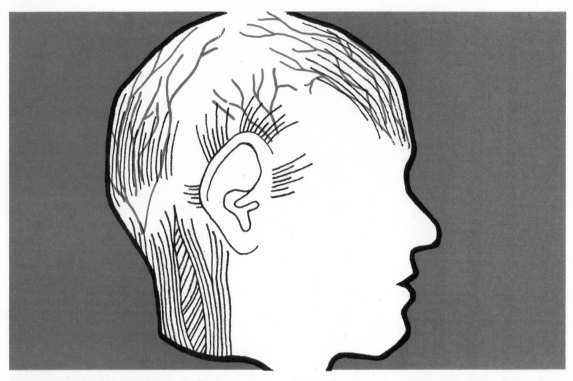

Tension headaches result when the posterior neck muscles become tight and pull on the places where they are attached to the scalp.

al distress and tensions which make themselves felt by headaches. In some, the headache may be caused by a conversion mechanism which is the patient's method of expressing mental unrest by converting it unconsciously into a physical symptom such as headache.

6. TENSION HEADACHES: This is probably the most common type of headache to which the human race is subjected in this day and age. In a way, the cause for a tension headache is simple. That is, the muscles in the back of the neck and on top of the shoulders (trapezius) are contracted and tight. This causes a pull on the back of the scalp where this muscle is inserted, or fastened, and a headache results.

The things which cause the muscles to tighten are far more complicated and hence successful treatment is most difficult in some cases.

These headaches may range in intensity from just worrisome to excruciating pain. The pain may be referred to the whole scalp, to the face, or it may remain in the back of the head.

People who suffer from this kind of a headache runs pretty much true to form. They usually hold themselves in with a tight restraint, do not express their anger or resentments, and sometimes are not even aware of them—that is, the resentments are subconscious. They are usually highly competitive and believe in having everything just so. In other words, they are perfectionists and are usually anxious to please other people.

A person who has recurrent headaches of

this nature should always see a doctor, for it is possible to have tension headaches and to have some lesion or growth in the brain at the same time. Both conditions can contribute to the headaches, but a doctor can usually tell the difference between the causes.

In the true tension headache the doctor can feel tension in these muscles in the back of the neck and on the shoulders. He can sometimes feel tender spots in the posterior part of the scalp. Most important by taking a careful history he may uncover some hidden anxiety or resentment of which the patient may not be aware. This does not require a psychiatrist as the family doctor can usually handle these cases successfully.

A physical examination is needed to rule out some physical cause and to determine if the muscles in the posterior part of the neck are indeed tense and tender. The doctor can then prescribe a tranquilizer such as Meprobamate or Equanil. He can advise hot towels to the back of the neck, massage to these muscles, and aspirin or aspirin and codeine to relieve the pain.

After the doctor has determined that there is no physical cause present, then the doctor-patient relationship becomes most important. The doctor will try to determine if the headaches usually come on Sunday when the patient is worrying about what is going to happen on Monday. He will see if the patient is capable of "letting off steam", now and then, or if he always holds a tight rein on his feelings and is always polite and smiling, although inwardly he may be quite angry.

The doctor will learn as much as he can about the patient's attitude toward school, his job, or his home life. In this way after several visits he may be able to explain to the patient the cause for this tension and the headaches may disappear after the patient corrects these causes.

7. HEADACHES DUE TO INJURY to the head are often quite severe. If these injuries result in intercranial hemorrhage, the pain may last for a long period. This type of headache is usually accompanied by dizziness.

8. HEADACHES USUALLY CAUSED BY ANEMIA: These headaches usually occur in people who have a severe lack of hemoglobin. These can be corrected by raising the hemoglobin content of the blood by proper treatment. These headaches usually occur in the front part of the head and may become generalized—that is, spread all over the head.

9. BRAIN TUMORS OR ABSCESSES: Many persons who are plagued by frequent headaches become convinced that they probably have a brain tumor. Such fear is usually unfounded as brain tumors do not occur too often and they can usually be ruled out by a doctor, thereby ridding the patient of undue apprehension.

Tumors of the brain usually cause a characteristic type of pain. This pain occurs in short spells or paroxysms lasting from a few minutes to a few hours—the average being about an hour. The pain may be mild or it may be almost unbearable.

There is usually a dull, deep aching pain which may be accompanied by nausea and vomiting.

As the tumor grows these attacks become more severe and occur more frequently, lasting longer as time goes on. Most often the pain is on both sides of the head and it may tend to occur in the front part of the head. However, this is not an ironclad rule, as the pain can occur in any part of the head and may be a clue as to where the tumor is located.

Any person with recurring attacks of headache which last only a short time and are accompanied by nausea and vomiting should see a doctor.

10. SUBARACHNOID HEMORRHAGE: This type of headache usually occurs when a small blood vessel ruptures in certain parts of the brain. The patient may be perfectly well and experience a sudden severe generalized headache and a few minutes later become unconscious. When the patient recovers consciousness the headache is still severe and may last for several days. There is no paralysis and the diagnosis must be made by a doctor.

One false idea which is quite prevalent should be corrected at this point. Many people think that a headache is the sign that they are going to have a stroke. This is not so. The kind of hemorrhage which occurs inside the brain and causes paralysis of one side of the body or one arm or leg is not preceded by a headache as a general rule, since there is no feeling in this part of the brain.

The headache of a subarachnoid hemorrhage occurs where the hemorrhage is in the subarachnoid space which is on the outside of the brain.

11. TEMPORAL ARTERITIS: The cause is not known. The temporal artery which is located in the region of the temple on each side may become inflamed and give rise to a dull headache. The pain usually starts over the inflamed artery and can be aggravated by pressing on the artery in the temple. It is often severe and lasts for a long time. People who are over the age of fifty-five usually are the ones who have this type of headache. The condition should be treated by a doctor in order to keep the eye on the affected side from being damaged.

Pain in temporal arteritis must be differentiated from pain around the eye which occurs in acute glaucoma, and this can be done by a physician. When the diagnosis is made, treatment with steroids such as cortisone should be started at once to prevent injury to the eyesight. Aspirin and codeine can be used to control the pain.

12. HISTAMINE HEADACHE OR HORTON'S HEADACHE: This is a type of headache which does not occur frequently but when it is experienced, can be very painful and disturbing to the patient's physical and mental health. The typical case can be diagnosed and treated properly because cer-

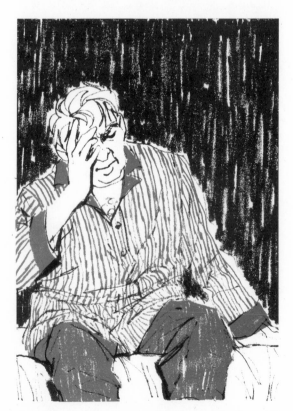

Arteritis and Histomine headaches both result in pain near one of the eyes.

tain specific conditions, or signs and symptoms, are nearly always present.

In the first place, histamine headaches occur nearly always in men over fifty years of age. The headache comes on at night after the patient has been asleep for a while and may recur night after night.

The pain starts in around the eye and is felt on one side only and when it recurs is always on the same side. This pain is severe and may extend over the cheek and forehead on the same side, but never crosses over to the other side, and never is felt below the lower lip.

There is nasal congestion on the side affected and the eye on that side may become red with tears flowing from it. These headaches disappear in the daytime but usually come on every night shortly after the man has fallen asleep.

When the proper diagnosis is made by a doctor, the histamine headache can be cured by repeated small injections of histamine sulphate, which will desensitize the patient to this substance.

This type of headache is often mistaken for tic douloureux or trigeminal neuritis; however, a doctor can tell the difference.

Treatment

The treatment of headache varies with the type of headache and its cause. Migraine headache should be treated with a drug which will cause the dilated vessels to contract. One such drug is ergotamine.

The tension headache should be treated with aspirin or aspirin and codeine compound until the underlying or causative disease can be brought under control.

Psychogenic headache may be successfully treated by a psychiatrist. Headaches caused by high blood pressure will subside when the blood pressure is brought down, and there are many medications which may be used to accomplish this.

Headaches due to allergy are relieved by finding the substance to which the person is sensitive and using injections of small amounts of this substance to desensitize the patient.

Headaches due to eye strain may disappear after the proper glasses are obtained.

In summary, it is well to know that headache is a symptom and that the underlying cause must be sought and treated. While this is being done, aspirin or a combination of aspirin and codeine should be used in sufficient quantities to relieve the pain. Fortunately, most headaches are transient affairs which can be relieved by taking the proper amount of aspirin or other pain relieving tablets containing aspirin in combination with other drugs.

A doctor should be consulted in any case where headache persists in spite of aspirin.

GLOSSARY

Anemia   lack of red blood cells or hemoglobin
Cerebal arteries   arteries of the brain
Contraction   tightening
Desensitize   to make immune, not sensitive
Dilate   enlarge
Dilatation   enlargement
Glaucoma   disease of the eye; increased pressure in eyeball
Intercranial   inside the skull
Hemoglobin   substance carrying the coloring matter and oxygen in the red blood corpuscles
Paroxysms   sudden violent action
Paralysis   unable to use or function
Posterior   dorsal or back of
Subarachnoid space   three membranes cover the brain and spinal cord—the pia mater next to the brain, the arachnoid, and the dura mater; the space between the arachnoid and pia mater is called the subarachnoid space
Tic douloureux   painful involvement of a nerve of the face
Toxic   poisonous

EPILEPSY

Cause and Nature

Epilepsy is classed among the convulsive disorders but it is characterized by repeated attacks of unconsciousness, with or without convulsions.

There are three main types of epileptic attacks:

1. Petit mal or small attacks in which there is an abrupt loss of consciousness, which may last from a few seconds to a half a minute. There is no convulsion, the patient may become pale and have a funny look in his eyes with a twitching of eyelids or sudden laughter. The patient usually recovers without any memory of the incident.

2. Grand mal or the common epileptic fit may have a certain warning sign, such as pressure in the head, noises in the head, or sudden outbursts of temper Following these warning signs the attack starts suddenly with a loss of consciousness and the body becomes rigid all over, with the jaws closed tightly. In the second phase there is an alternation between stiffening of the body and sudden relaxation. This gives a jerky appearance to the attack. This second phase usually lasts from two to five minutes and the patient may bite his tongue or injure one of his limbs during the thrashing about. There also may be involuntary urination or foam may appear at the lips. The attack is ended in a period of exhaustion and the patient drops into a deep sleep from which he may awaken without memory of the attack.

3. Jacksonian attacks of epilepsy result from some local injury which may be an old injury to the brain. They are characterized by sudden clonic (jerky) motions of alternating contraction and relaxation of the part affected. These motions may be limited to one arm or to one side of the body.

The cause of epilepsy is unknown.

Signs and Symptoms

There are certain tests that can be made by means of electroencephalograms, which give a distinctive picture. The diagnosis can be made with the help of these tests.

The attacks may be brought on by loss of sleep or extreme fatigue.

Treatment

People who have epilepsy should not drive automobiles or engage in any activities where a sudden loss of consciousness would prove disastrous. The diet should have an acid ash, and excess of salt or any alkali should be avoided, as should the use of alcohol. There are certain drugs such as phenobarbital and dilantin taken in the proper doses may cut down on or do away with the attacks in some cases. The epileptic person should always get lots of sleep.

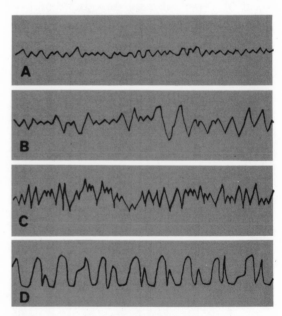

Electroencephalogram tracing as seen in three kinds of Epilepsy. (A) Normal, (B) Petit mal, (C) Grand mall, and (D) Jacksonian type.

During an attack, efforts should be made to keep the patient from injuring himself. His clothing should be loosened and a piece of wood covered with a soft cloth should be placed between the teeth to keep the patient from biting his tongue.

After the attack the person should be allowed to sleep until the feeling of extreme fatigue has been relieved.

GLOSSARY

Convulsions violent series of contractions of the muscles

Electroencephalogram a graphic tracing of the electrical activity of the brain

Involuntary not under control

MULTIPLE SCLEROSIS

Cause and Nature

The cause is not known. This disease is characterized by multiple widespread signs and symptoms, caused by multiple areas of degeneration of the myelin sheaths of nerves, followed by sclerosis or scarring in these areas.

Since these spots of degeneration may occur anywhere in the central nervous system, the clinical course may have many variations.

Signs and Symptoms

The onset is usually slow but may be sudden. Disturbances of vision, double vision, dizziness, cleavage in speech, and emotional instability are among the common signs and symptoms.

The intention tremor of the hands, scanning speech, and nystagmus, which are supposed to be the three signs that identify this condition are not always present. The disease may last from one to twenty-five years, the average being ten years.

Other signs, such as disturbance of the reflexes and weakness, are usually present sooner or later. Sometimes there is pain in various portions of the body.

This disease tends to go into remissions, that is, the patient may get a little better and stay that way for years or months; then the course of the disease is resumed.

Treatment

There is no specific treatment. A great deal of research and work is being done on the treatment and we hope that some day a solution will be found.

Histamine acid phosphate intravenously has helped in some cases. A low-fat diet is thought to be beneficial and good nursing care is all-important in the advanced stage.

A doctor should be seen and should supervise the treatment of this condition at all times.

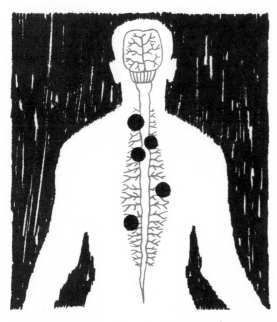

Central nervous system showing degeneration. These areas may be few or widespread in number.

PARALYSIS AGITANS

(Palsy or Parkinson's Disease)

Cause and Nature

This disease is caused by deterioration in parts of the central nervous system, usually the basal ganglia of the brain. When seen in young people, which is rare, it may be the result of encephalitis or inflammation of parts of the brain. In older people the deterioration may be due to lack of circulation resulting from arteriosclerosis. This is a slowly progressing, chronic type of disease characterized by slowness of movement, tremor or shaking of the hands, and usually, muscular rigidity.

Signs and Symptoms

The rapid tremor of the hands is usually characteristic and is spoken of as a "pill rolling" movement. The muscles assume a certain rigidity and the face becomes smooth and mask-like. The walk is characteristic in that usually the body is thrown in advance of the feet.

All of these signs and symptoms develop insidiously and slowly.

Treatment

Physiotherapy often helps improve the strength and certain drugs such as artane help relieve the tremor. A doctor should supervise the care of these cases.

NEURITIS

Cause and Nature

The word "neuritis" means inflammation of a nerve, and any nerve in the body may become inflamed or irritated. The condition is characterized by a sharp burning, boring type of pain along the course of the affected nerve.

The pain is increased by pressing on the nerve or going through a motion which stretches the nerve.

Herpes zoster or "Shingles" is a neuritis of an intercostal nerve. The cause is a virus.

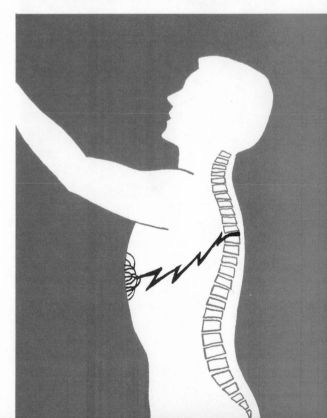

For instance, sciatic neuritis or sciatica, as it is sometimes called, is an irritation of the sciatic nerve which runs down the back of the leg. This pain can be increased by bending the trunk forward with the knees straight, because this stretches the inflamed nerve.

Inflammation of individual nerves may be caused by trauma or injury to the nerve, such as pressure from a herniated disc, or by the spread of local inflammation from the tissues surrounding the nerve to the nerve itself. The nerve may be irritated by a toxic or poisonous substance such as seen in lead poisoning or in diseases like typhoid fever. Deficiency states, caused by lack of vitamins, such as seen in beriberi, will cause neuritis. One of the common causes is consuming too much alcohol, which results in an alcoholic neuritis or polyneuritis, when many nerves are involved.

Sciatic nerve distribution: Inflamation of the nerve is called Sciatic Neuritis.

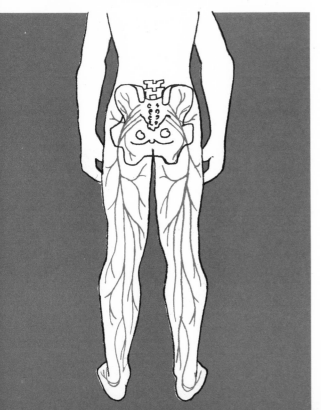

Signs and Symptoms

There may be a numbness or tingling along the course of the nerves, and where the pain comes it is distinctive, usually because of its boring nature and the tenderness to pressure which follows the course of the affected nerve.

Treatment

Treatment consists of curing the underlying cause. If the nerve is being compressed by a herniated disc or pressure from a fracture, the pressure should be relieved by surgery or traction. In the case of vitamin deficiency this lack of vitamins should be corrected. Aspirin and other drugs which relieve pain should be used.

When poisoning by a heavy metal such as lead caused the neuritis, special treatment for lead poisoning should be used.

GLOSSARY

Beriberi condition caused by a vitamin deficiency
Fracture broken
Herniated protruding like a hernia
Trauma injury or wound
Toxic poisonous

TRIGEMINAL NEURALGIA

(Tic Douloureux)

Cause and Nature

This is an irritation of one or more of the branches of the trigeminal (facial) nerve. The cause is unknown, but is usually comes in older people and almost always involves only one side of the face.

Signs and Symptoms

A sudden sharp pain strikes the temple side of the face, jaw or teeth. The pain

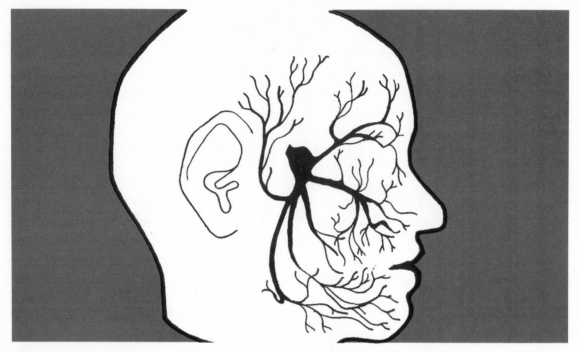

Trigeminal neuralgia and tic douloureux affect the facial nerve shown above.

comes without warning and usually lasts for only a few seconds. The frequency of these paroxysms gradually increases, although there may be long periods of freedom from pain.

Treatment

The medical management of this condition does not offer much help. Analgesics such as aspirin or aspirin and codeine may help lessen the pain, and large doses of vitamin B₁ have been used to cut down the severity of the pain. Surgical treatment by dividing the branches or injecting alcohol into the nerve may cause the pain to cease, at least for five or six months.

A recent advance in the medical field has led to the development of a drug called Tegretol, put out by "Geigy". It has performed very well in relieving the pain of tic douloureux, or trigeminal neuralgia. The people who take this drug are nearly all relieved of the painful attacks. The family doctor should prescribe the dosage and change it according to the response he gets from the patient.

GLOSSARY

Paroxysm a sudden violent action

MENIERE'S DISEASE

Cause and Nature

This is a disease of the inner ear which is due to a swelling of the tissues in the labyrinth or organ of equilibrium.

Ringing in the ear (tinnitus), dizziness (vertigo), and deafness occur.

These three symptoms usually appear together, but the deafness and ringing in the ear may appear before the dizziness or vertigo. The attacks of dizziness may occur in paroxysms which may be quite violent and may be accompanied by vomiting.

Signs and Symptoms

Deafness, ringing or buzzing in the ear, dizziness which occurs from time to time in violent attacks, and vomiting are the outstanding symptoms of this disease.

Treatment

Mild cases may be treated by a vasodilator such as nicotinic acid given in doses large enough to cause flushing. A salt-poor diet is often helpful and sometimes in severe cases, surgery is indicated. At any rate a doctor should treat this condition.

There is a new product called SERC proven to be helpful in some cases of Meniere's disease. The oral diuretics are also used now in the disease.

GLOSSARY

Equilibrium   balance
Paroxysms   sudden violent action
Tinnitus   a ringing noise
Vertigo   dizziness

MYASTHENIA GRAVIS

Cause and Nature

The cause is not known. It is more commonly seen in young females and old males but it may appear in either sex at any age. It is not hereditary.

The disease is characterized by weakness of the muscles and ease of fatigue. Often the first complaint is double vision and drooping of the eyelids, which may be followed by a difficulty in swallowing and in talking. This is all because of a weakness of the muscles, which is progressive. Then there may be difficulty in walking because of weakness, especially noted in climbing stairs.

Signs and Symptoms

Drooping eyelids may be noticed. After resting, the patient may feel strong but soon tires out when the muscles are used. There is usually no pain. Difficulty in swallowing, talking, and walking is common. By injecting a drug called tensilon, a doctor may be sure of the diagnosis in myasthenia gravis.

Treatment

Neostigmine is a drug that has been used in the treatment of this disease. The difficulty seems to stem from a failure of the nerves to transmit their impulses to the muscles, and this trouble seems to arise at the neuro-muscular junction. Neostigmine appears to help the impulse to jump this gap.

New drugs which are very much like neostigmine have just about replaced it in recent years. Two of these drugs are pyridostigmine (or mestinon), and mytelose. These drugs are given in sufficient amounts to keep the patient from feeling weak. This varies with different individuals. Some of the side reactions from taking too many mestinon pills might be excess salivation, rumbling of the stomach, pain in the abdomen, and, at times, diarrhea. Such side effects may be lessened by taking several drops of tincture of belladonna or by decreasing the amount of the drug taken.

This disease may be successfully controlled for many years with proper treatment, and there is no reason why a person so treated should not live his or her full span of life.

GLOSSARY

Neuro-muscular   pertaining to nerves and muscles
Salivation   excessive secretion of saliva
Tincture   a solution

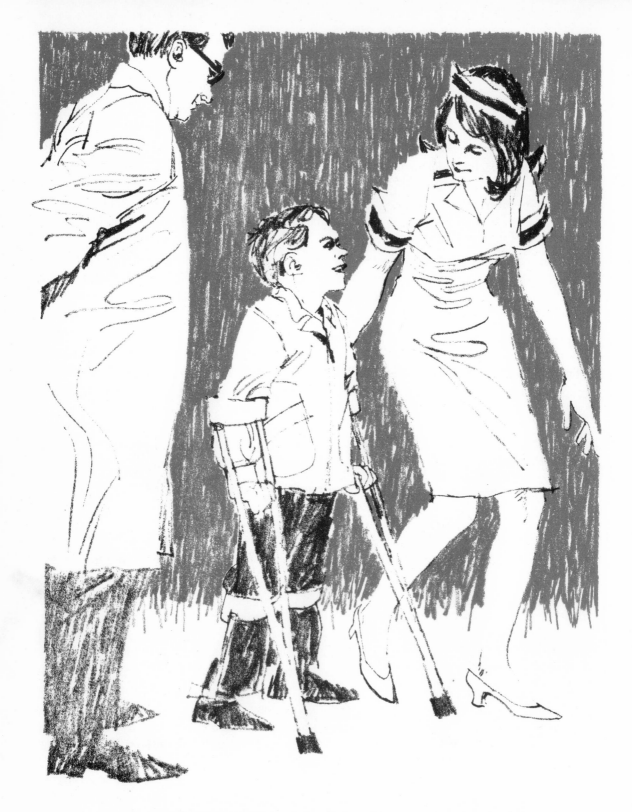

Cerebral Palsy victims, such as the young boy above, can be taught to walk again under the supervision of specially trained therapists and doctors.

CEREBRAL PALSY

We read and hear a good deal these days about cerebral palsy and it may be well to know just what the term means. The word "cerebral" means "of the brain," and doctors think of "palsy" as a weakness, or lack of control of the muscles. Hence, the two words together mean a weakness or lack of control of the muscles, due to some condition in the brain.

This is a general term and covers a number of conditions ranging from a slight lack of control of body movements, to trouble in speaking and walking, and even in eating, seeing, and hearing. There are some cases in which the child may be retarded mentally, but in most cases the mentality is not affected. It is difficult to tell this by just seeing the child, so we must assume that he has normal mentality. It has even been proven that some children with cerebral palsy may be brighter than other children who have perfect control of their muscles.

There are many causes for cerebral palsy and it is not always easy to determine the cause in any given case. The defect responsible for the condition may occur before birth, during birth, or after birth. Some part of the brain may not develop as it should before birth, or the mother may have a very difficult, hard labor, and the damage to the brain may occur during labor. This does not happen very often, and very few cases of cerebral palsy can be blamed on hard labor, since most babies that are born after a long, hard labor are perfectly all right. Cerebral palsy may be caused after birth by an accident which injures the brain, or by some severe illness which does the same.

The important thing for parents to know is that if their child has cerebral palsy it is not their fault. Once they are free from the feeling that something they have done has caused this condition, and know that they are not at fault, they can give more attention to improving the situation. They should get as much help as they can to allow their child to live as normal a life and one as nearly like other children as it is possible for him to do.

It should be understood by the parents that many children with cerebral palsy do well, and are able to make their way in life. In order to help the child, the parents must realize that they need assistance from doctors, nurses, physical therapists, occupational therapists, speech therapists, medical social workers, and teachers. These should all work hand in hand with the child and parents.

Unfortunately, the many services needed by a child with cerebral palsy cost a great deal. If there is no place in your town or county where these services are available, you should find out what town or state does supply these services, and make arrangements for the child to take advantage of them. They are always available somewhere. It is remarkable how much progress some of these children make with the proper care.

It must always be borne in mind that your child, if he has cerebral palsy, *is* a child and, like most children, he needs help and guidance. One of the most important things to remember is to treat him as nearly like any other child as you can. Encourage him to think, speak, and act for himself.

If the handicapped child has sisters and brothers, let him have his place in the group, for he can learn a lot from them. The parents themselves must be sure to adopt a proper attitude toward the handicapped child, recognizing his strength and limitations. In this way the brothers and sisters will take their cue from the parents, and will make the handicapped child feel that he is one of them. This will teach him to get along with people when he grows up. He should feel that he is a part of the family group.

ANOREXIA NERVOSA

(Complete Loss of Appetite)

Cause and Nature

The cause of this disease is not fully understood but it is thought to be some deep emotional disturbance, sometimes associated with anxiety, compulsive features, and at times, with depressive tendencies. The condition is seen most often in young women and sometimes follows a long dieting spell which has been initiated in an effort to lose weight.

There is not only a complete loss of appetite but there is an actual aversion to food in any form. The patient may nibble a little from time to time, but often feels that it is impossible to swallow food.

Signs and Symptoms

Anorexia nervosa in young women is often accompanied by a cessation of their monthly periods. If there is any sensation of hunger at all, it is satisfied by just one or two bites and the person cannot eat any more. There is an extreme loss of weight and the person becomes almost literally skin and bones. The patient may be confined to bed because of weakness or may be active and even restless. When the members of the family try to get them to eat they will resort to all kinds of deception to prevent compliance.

In some severe cases, if untreated, swelling or edema appears and the person may even go on to starvation and death.

Treatment

The treatment is not easy. First of all a complete examination with X rays and other laboratory tests must be done by a doctor to rule out any real disease which may be causing loss of weight and appetite.

Then an effort must be made to get the person to eat. This is often accomplished by a complete change of environment, by moving away from the family to some new climate and locality. Gentle persuasion and attemps to correct the cause of the emotional disorder are sometimes helpful. Treatment by a psychiatrist is not always helpful but may be tried in severe cases.

TICS

Cause and Nature

An irregularly repeated jerky movement which has no apparent cause is known as a tic. This may consist of a twitching of one side of the face from time to time, or shrugging of one shoulder, or making a face at regular intervals.

These compulsive acts may occur in children or in adults, and they may persist for a long time or be lost without any treatment. The person feels compelled to make this motion from time to time, and cannot refrain from doing it. This is caused as a rule by some emotional stress or strain. If the cause is not discovered and corrected it may last from childhood throughout the person's life. The milder tics usually disappear when the situation that has caused the stress has been corrected.

Signs and Symptoms

Overanxious parents who expect too much from a child, such as perfect grades in school, may build up in that child a certain amount of insecurity and stress which will cause him to develop a tic—which to him is a release of nervous tension.

Treatment

A doctor should be consulted, and if this nervous habit is found to have no physical cause, a simplification of the child's life is usually advised. Give the child lots of love and help him to lessen the fear or feeling of insecurity that is causing this habit. The same approach may help older people who have developed these compulsive movements. It has been found that medicines such as sedatives do not have any appreciable lasting effect on tics. Calling attention to the tic may make the act become more pronounced.

SLEEP WALKING

Cause and Nature

Walking while asleep is a very common occurrence and there are few people who have not walked in their sleep at one time or another. It has been estimated that there are over four million sleep walkers in America. It is more common in younger people and usually does not occur very often. The average person will awaken after he has walked a short distance—such as across the room.

The real sleep walker may go out of doors and walk for some distance before awakening. This condition is usually brought on by some disturbance or unrest in the subconscious mind which comes to the surface while the person is asleep and the sleep walker tries to act out the dream situation.

There are a great many false tales about the marvelous feats performed by sleep walkers, but as a matter of fact, a person walking in his sleep can do no more or no less than he could do if he were awake.

Another commonly accepted theory about sleep walkers which is false is that they should be awakened with great caution because if awakened suddenly they may harm themselves. This is not true. You may safely awaken a sleep walker if he is not in some precarious condition, like out on the limb of a tree or on the roof of a house. In this case, the fears which are absent while the walker is asleep may reappear and he may be afraid to descend from the roof.

One typical report of a sleep walker will tend to show how this condition usually arises. A pretty young married woman who had been known to walk in her sleep came out of the front door of her house one night without any clothing. She climbed up a tree in front of the house and began picking leaves from the nearby branches. A passerby saw her and went into the house to get her husband. The husband called the fire department and they sent some men with a net to stand beneath the tree in case she should fall. Then the husband climbed into the tree and awakened his wife. She was greatly embarrassed but able, with his help, to climb down out of the tree without falling.

When asked what she had been dreaming, she replied that she dreamed that she had been attending a dog show and had decided to turn all of the dogs in the show into French poodles with a tuft of hair on their tails. A close examination of the tree into which she had climbed showed that she had pulled the leaves off the branches of the tree, leaving a tuft of leaves out on the end of each short branch. Hence, she had been acting out her dream, thinking that the tree branches were tails of dogs in the show.

Signs and Symptoms

When a person is suffering from some form of anxiety or has hidden fears which he has suppressed or pushed back into the subconscious mind, he is more likely to walk in his sleep and act out some of the dreams he has at night. This is more common in younger people than in old and is especially common among teenagers or even younger children. There is no sudden shock when the person is wakened; therefore, they should be awakened as soon as possible.

At times this is only a temporary condition which may occur for only a few times, while in other people it may be a habit and these are the ones who should be treated.

Treatment

Since many sleep walkers can easily unlock windows and doors when still asleep, the most effective way in which to stop a person from walking in his sleep is to try and relieve the anxieties and fears which he keeps hidden in the subconscious mind. If he is nervous, depressed, or restless during the day, a good physical examination should be performed by a doctor in order that any physical cause for this condition may be ruled out. In some cases the use of tranquilizers during the day may help in calming the person.

Care should be taken in the case of a known sleep walker to see that he is not able to get out of his room while walking in his sleep. He should sleep on the ground floor if possible, for as explained above, the person who walks in his sleep may fall or be injured just the same as he would be if he entered a dangerous situation while awake. He has no supernatural powers, nor is he protected from injury by some mystic means.

If the sleep walking habit becomes troublesome and the family doctor cannot cure it, then the walker should be seen by a good psychiatrist who can in many cases find out the cause for this habit and correct it.

GLOSSARY

Psychiatrist   a specialist dealing with mental disorders
Subconscious   existing but not felt
Suppress   stop by force
Tranquilizer   drug having a quieting effect

Chapter 18

Diseases of the Skin

ACNE VULGARIS

Cause and Nature

A common, chronic inflammatory disturbance of the sebaceous glands, usually having its onset during adolescence, and terminating early in the thirties. It causes untold worry and embarrassment to young people of both sexes.

The principal underlying cause may be the endoctrine glands. (See page 268.) Contributing factors may be faulty fat and carbohydrate metabolism, or allergy to certain foods. Dandruff may be one of the exciting causes. Physical and emotional strain contribute to the condition, and infection of the lesions is often contributed to by the nervous habit of pinching or squeezing the lesions. Deficiencies in vitamins A, D, and B may aggravate the acne.

Signs and Symptoms

The primary lesion is the blackhead (comedo). The top of the blackhead is black not because of dirt but because of oxidation of the substance within the comedo. Inflammatory lesions, papules, pustules, no-

dules, crypt formations, and scarring follow as results of the initial blackheads. The face, shoulders, chest, and back are areas most often affected.

Treatment

Treatment should be aimed at prevention of complications, such as infections;

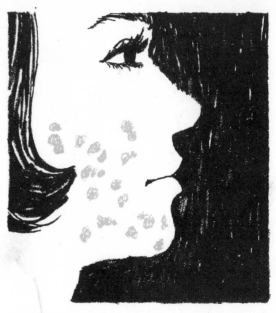

Unsightly acne lesions cause much unhappiness to both male and female teenagers.

267

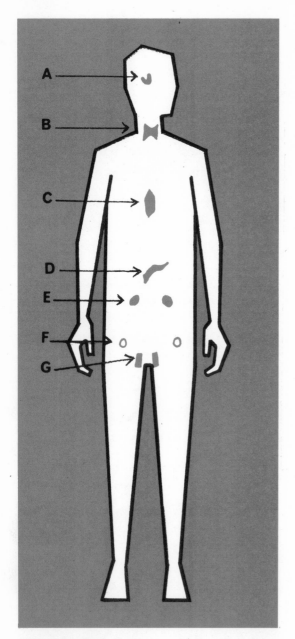

The **endocrine glands** or glands of internal secretion are located in various parts of the body. They manufacture and secrete hormones directly into the blood stream. Hence they have no ducts or out going tubes. Shown in diagram are: (A) pituitary gland in the brain; (B) thyroid and parathyroid glands in the neck; (C) thymus gland in the chest; (D) pancreas in the abdomen; (E) adrenal glands over the kidneys; (F) ovaries in women; and (G) testes in men.

these are followed by scarring. The patient should be assured that a cure is possible if absolute cooperation is given. Following are steps in treatment:

1. Absolute cleanliness of face and body. The scalp should be washed often, and the face four times a day, using soap and allowing the lather to remain on the face three or four minutes, then rinsing the face, first with hot, then with cold water.

2. After washing, the blackheads should be gently expressed. A comedo extractor can be used.

3. Never squeeze (pick or pinch the lesions excepting in the above manner.

4. Anemia should be corrected, if it exists. Large doses of Vitamin A—150 units daily —should be given for five or six months. A multi-vitamin tablet like micebrin should be given twice a day.

5. Small doses of thyroid may help.

6. The use of sulphur, lotion, or soaps is important to produce mild peeling of the skin.

7. Diet is most important. This should be low in fats and carbohydrates. Highly seasoned foods, chocolates, nuts, pork, cokes, and bananas should be forbidden.

8. If pus forms in one of the lesions, it should be released by a small incision— such as one made by a sterile needle. Do not squeeze.

Improvement should be noted in two or three months.

GLOSSARY

Allergy   oversensitivity to some substance
Anemia   deficiency of red corpuscles in blood
Crypt   pit-like depression
Endocrine   secrete internally
Lesion   wound or local sore
Metabolism   chemical changes within body
Nodule   small bump
Papule   small solid elevation of skin
Pustule   small elevation of skin containing pus
Sebaceous   fatty
Sterile   free from bacteria

IMPETIGO

Cause and Nature

The lesions of impetigo usually appear on the face, neck, or hands. They are contagious—can be passed from one person to the other. They are caused by infection of the superficial skin by streptococcus, staphylococcus, or both. The lesions are discrete, have a small red area around them, have a yellowish crust, or appear in the form of a pustule. New lesions may appear by spreading the pus to other areas.

Signs and Symptoms

The lesions first appear as a red spot. Then a small blister may appear which fills with pus, and when this ruptures the lesion is covered with a yellowish crust.

Treatment

After warm compresses have been applied to soften them up, the tops should be removed from the lesions, and one of the antibiotic ointments, such as neomycin and bacitracin should be applied.

Improvement and cure should take place in four or five days. Penicillin may be given by mouth to speed the cure. Cleanliness is imperative.

GLOSSARY

Lesion   wound or local sore
Staphylococcus   cause of infection
Streptococcus   cause of infection

SYCOSIS VULGARIS

(Barber's Itch)

Cause and Nature

This is a chronic infection of the hair follicles on the face due to an invasion by the staphylococcus. It is commonly seen in the beard, hence the name.

Signs and Symptoms

The pustular lesion on the bearded surface of the face is nearly always pierced by a hair. The lesions may spread slowly and may be accompanied by burning, itching, and pain.

Treatment

This condition is often chronic and resistant to treatment. Underlying causative factors, such as infected teeth, seborrheic dermatitis (dandruff), or diabetes should be ruled out. The patient should shave at least every forty-eight hours. Antibiotic ointments can be tried until an effective one is found. Neomycin with bacitracin or terramycin ointments are usually effective. They should be applied twice a day. When possible, the hair should be removed from the lesion.

The treatment must sometimes be prolonged. In order to affect a cure. Crusts should be removed before applying medication.

GLOSSARY

Chronic   of a long duration
Follicles   depressions or sacs
Incision   a cut
Infection   invasion of foreign organisms
Lesion   wound or local sore
Pustular   covered with pus

PARONYCHIA

(Whitlow or Infection Around Fingernail)

Cause and Nature

This inflammation around the fingernail may be acute or chronic. It may be caused by infection from bacteria or fungus (monilia). The infection may enter through an abrasion left when a hangnail is pulled off, and is seen often in people who have their hands in water a great deal.

Signs and Symptoms

Red, swollen, painful area around the fingernail is noted. This may become larger, until it points or comes to a head. The yellow pus can then be seen underneath the skin. It may be so acute that in rare cases the fingernail is lost.

Treatment

Application of moist heat, like soaking the finger in hot water; protection from further trauma (injury) by a bandage; and finally, when it comes to a head, incision and drainage to allow the pus to escape. After cutting into the pus pocket some antibiotic ointment should be applied, and the hot soaks continued.

GLOSSARY

Abrasion   rubbed or scraped wound
Acute   short duration
Chronic   long duration
Hangnail   strip of skin loose at base of fingernail
Incision   a cut

FURUNCLE

(Boil)

Cause and Nature

This acute infection of the skin is caused by staphylococcus, and usually starts in a hair follicle. The same person may have many boils, one right after the other. This is called furunculosis.

Signs and Symptoms

Red, tender, swollen, firm area begins around a hair follicle, gets larger and be-

comes more painful. Finally it comes to a head, pus is seen under the center of the lesion, and it will either burst by itself or be incised to allow pus and blood to drain out. After being opened, there is usually a core of white material which has to be removed.

Treatment

The skin around a lesion should be kept clean to prevent the spread of infectious material which might cause other boils. Hot, moist heat should be applied to speed up the pointing, or coming to a head. A small incision over the yellow spot will allow the pus to drain out, and the core to be removed.

If a person has repeated boils, he should be investigated for diabetes or anemia.

One should never squeeze a boil, especially if it is located in or around the nose. Lesions around the nose, face, and ear should be treated with great care, as they are dangerous.

GLOSSARY

Follicles   depressions or sacs
Incision   a cut
Infection   invasion of body tissues by foreign organisms
Infectious   liable to be communicated by contact
Lesion   wound or sore
Staphylococcus   substance causing infection

CARBUNCLE

Cause and Nature

This is larger than a boil, may extend deeper into the tissues, and is characterized by having many openings, or draining places, while a boil has only one. The staphylococcus causes the infection, and it starts in a hair follicle. Carbuncles are usually seen on the back, back of the neck, the hairy backs of the hands or fingers. These regions have fatty columns under the skin which allow the infection to go deeper and to spread. The principal identifying mark of a carbuncle is that it points (comes to a head) in several places.

Signs and Symptoms

Red, hard, swollen areas which are much more painful than a boil, and point in several places, are usually carbuncles. There are severe systemic reactions at times, such as fever and prostration. These lesions may go into serious complications, and may, if not properly treated, result in death.

Treatment

Underlying conditions, such as diabetes or anemia, should be investigated. Hot, moist applications should be made several times a day. The patient should have injections of penicillin, and when pus has formed the lesion should be incised, and the pus drained out. Local application of penicillin often helps after incision, and the dressing should be changed several times a day. Adhesive tape should not be used on the skin immediately surrounding the carbuncle, as this may irritate the skin and cause further infections. Never squeeze.

GLOSSARY

Anemia   deficiency of red corpuscles in blood
Staphylococcus   cause of infection
Systemic   the body as a whole

INFECTION OF SWEAT GLANDS UNDER THE ARMS

Cause and Nature

This is an infection of the sweat glands by staphylococcus which appears as tender, hard lumps under the arm. These become red and painful, and finally they become soft, after the formation of pus has occurred.

Signs and Symptoms

Multiple or single painful lumps under the arm which become soft and finally drain.

Treatment

Application of moist heat, and after the lumps become soft, they should be incised and drained.

Avoidance of rough clothing and the application of deodorants should be observed. Sometimes the use of a fat free diet, and small doses of thyroid by mouth will help.

GLOSSARY

Deodorant   something which destroys odors
Follicle   depression from which hair grows
Incised   cut into
Infection   invasion of body tissues by foreign organisms
Staphylococcus   cause of infection

SEBACEOUS CYST

(Wen)

Cause and Nature

A slow growing cystic tumor that is benign, not tender, firm and movable, it is caused by the stopping up of a sebaceous gland duct. Thus the oily, sebaceous material is prevented from escaping. It is forced to back up, and forms a cyst.

Signs and Symptoms

These non-tender, firm lumps usually are found in back of the ears, on the scalp, on the back, the face, or the scrotum.

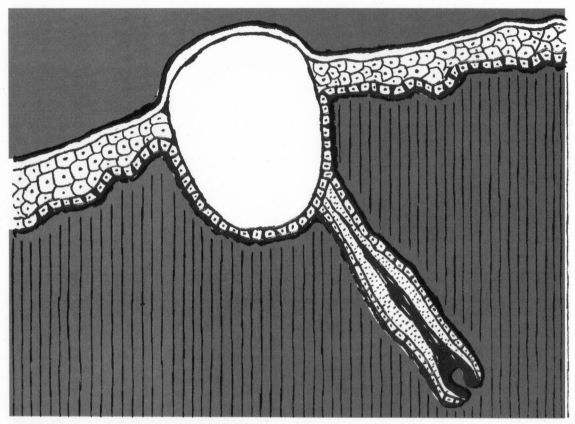

Sebaceous Cyst: Creamy material produced by gland at bottom cannot escape because skin outlet is plugged. The cyst is surrounded by membrane.

Fatty tumors, or lipomas, are usually not so well rounded and have a soft feeling rather than a firm one.

Treatment

Surgical excision of the entire cyst, getting all of the capsule or wall of the cyst. It is necessary to remove these tumors and thus prevent their recurrence.

GLOSSARY

Benign   not malignant
Capsule   a fibrous or membranous envelope
Cystic   pertaining to a cyst or sac
Duct   a tube
Excision   cutting away; taking out
Lipomas   fatty tumors
Tumor   swelling or abnormal mass of tissues

WARTS

(Verrucae)

Cause and Nature

This small, circumscribed epithelial tumor is caused by a filterable virus, and it is common for more than one wart to appear on a person, as the warts inoculate themselves into the surrounding skin. They are contagious—that is, they may be passed on from person to person. They usually appear on the hands, less frequently on the soles of the feet (plantar warts). They may occur on other parts of the body, including the genitals. When they appear on moist surfaces, such as the genitals, they may be in groups. These are called venereal warts. They are not caused by venereal disease, but by other warts.

Warts may disappear by themselves in weeks or months. Sometimes they persist for years. Those on the soles of the feet (plantar warts) are the least likely to disappear spontaneously.

Signs and Symptoms

A circumscribed, cauliflower-like lesion, that usually is raised above the skin. When seen on the soles of the feet, they may be depressed below the surface and covered with callus.

Treatment

If left untreated, warts may disappear spontaneously. This is why the simplest form of treatment often seems successful. Because they do often heal themselves, excision is not wise since it often leaves large scars. Superficial electrodesiccation by a doctor is often successful. Ten percent salicylic acid in collodion applied daily may give good results. Plantar warts, or those on the soles of the feet, are the most painful and the most difficult to treat. They should be treated by a doctor. Sometimes the simple injection of novocaine beneath a plantar wart will cause it to disappear.

GLOSSARY

Callus hard, thickened skin
Circumscribed within limits
Electrodesiccation removal by burning with electric needle
Excision cutting away; taking out
Epithelial covering of skin and mucous membrane
Filterable that which can pass through a filter
Genitals reproductive organs
Inoculate to implant
Lesion wound, local sore or growth
Virus a living cause of disease

HERPES SIMPLEX

(Fever Blister, Cold Sore, Herpes Labialis)

Cause and Nature

This lesion is caused by a virus. It may occur following any systemic disease, such as a common cold (in the form of a cold sore), or may follow an emotional disturbance such as the menstrual period. The lesion usually appears on the lips, but may be on the skin or on the conjunctiva of the eye. When these blisters occur in the mouth, they appear as small, punched-out ulcers, and are called canker sores.

Although called "fever blisters" they may occur without fever.

Signs and Symptoms

The onset may occur with burning and itching. Small, painful swelling occurs. This develops rapidly into a blister with a red, inflammatory base. The lesions are usually dry and form a crust. They will disappear spontaneously in five or ten days. Recurrence is common.

Treatment

Symptomatic relief and prevention of secondary infection should be attempted, as there is no specific treatment. Skin or lip lesions can be treated with spirits of camphor. Hydro-cortisone ointment may hasten the healing. Eye lesions should be treated by an eye specialist. If repeated lesions occur, they are sometimes stopped by vaccinating the patient for smallpox from four to eight times, at weekly intervals. If the original smallpox vaccination takes, it need not be repeated.

Cold sores caused by exposure to the sun may be prevented by the use of one of the sunburn lotions.

Conjunctiva   delicate membrane lining the eyelids and covering the front of the eyeball
Inflammation   condition characterized by pain, heat, redness, and swelling
Lesion   wound or local sore
Secondary   second in appearance
Vaccination   protection against
Virus   living cause of disease

HERPES ZOSTER

(Shingles)

Cause and Nature

The cause is a virus similar to that which causes chickenpox, but not the same virus. It is more common in males than in females, and practically never occurs before the age of fifty. It is an infection of the nerves, having visible skin manifestations.

This is exemplified in the most common form of shingles around one side of the chest, following the course of the intercostal nerve that runs between the ribs. This rash always coincides with the course of the nerve, and will not go beyond the mid-line, in the case of infection of the intercostal nerve.

One attack seems to confer immunity for the rest of one's life.

Signs and Symptoms

The patient may have chills and fever, burning pain over the area, or just "feel bad" all over for three or four days before the rash occurs. There is first a crop of blisters which soon dry and scab. The rash is always along the course of the affected nerve, and there may also be a deep burning or nerve pain. Neuralgia or pain may persist for months to years after the rash disappears. This is most common in older people.

Treatment

Treatment should be started early in the disease, and if this is done the course of the disease may be shortened, but there is nothing available now as a specific cure.

Large doses of vitamin B_1—100 milligrams twice a day should be started at once, with aureomycin, 250 milligrams three times a day, to be given also. Dusting powder or surfacain ointment may be used on the rash. If these are not available, tincture of benzoin compound may be used. This is to prevent scarring and to help control secondary infection.

Aspirin in adequate doses or aspirin and codeine should be given to control pain, and the lesions should be protected.

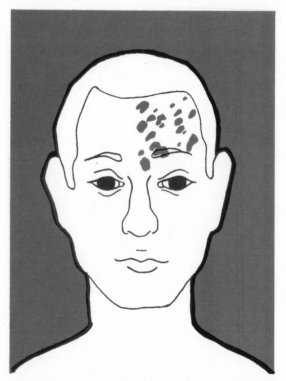

Shingles of the supra-orbital nerve. Note that the skin lesions follow the course of the nerve and do not cross the midline.

DANDRUFF

(Seborrheic Dermatitis)

Cause and Nature

The cause of dandruff is not clearly understood. It occurs on those areas most generously supplied by the sebaceous glands, such as the scalp, face, and ears. The lesion is usually subacute or chronic, characterized by ill-defined red patches covered by greasy scales.

Signs and Symptoms

The most common sign is the flaky scales from the scalp or other involved areas.

Treatment

This depends upon the stage and location of the condition. Dandruff of the scalp usually responds to selsun, applied locally. Seborrhea in other localities may respond to ointments containing hydrocortisone.

The hair should be washed daily, and selsun applied before washing for three days. Then do not use selsun again until dandruff reappears.

FUNGUS INFECTIONS

Cause and Nature

Superficial fungus infections of the skin are caused by many different types of fungi. The various parts of the body which are involved usually determine the name by which the infection is known. For example: ringworm of the scalp (tinea capitis); ringworm of the body (tinea circinata); ringworm of the groin is known as jockey strap itch (tinea cruris); ringworm of the feet is called athlete's foot, and is one of the most common forms of fungus infection; fungus infection around the finger nails or toe nails is known as tinea unguium.

While these infections may be caused by different fungi, and may need different

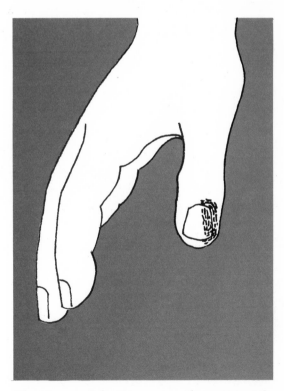

The Fungus infection commonly seen as Athletes Foot may also occur under the finger nails. This is difficult to cure.

kinds of treatment, they have a few important things in common. For instance, a primary fungus infection of the feet (athlete's foot) can cause antigenic substances which spread through the body and may cause secondary eruptions on the hands or other parts of the body. No amount of treatment to the hands will cure them unless the primary infection of the feet is cleared up first. This is important—always look for athlete's foot if an eruption appears on the hands which seems to be a fungus infection.

Second, strong medications, such as full strength iodine, used on the primary infection will set up the same reaction causing eruptions to appear on other parts of the body. Sometimes the disability from too vigorous treatment is greater than that caused by the disease.

Almost all fungus infections may become secondarily infected by bacteria, and thus two forms of treatment—one for fungus, and one for bacteria, may be needed.

These various fungus infections will be taken up separately, since different treatments are used for each.

GLOSSARY

Antigenic   having the ability to cause the production of antibodies
Bacteria   organisms causing infection
Fungus   a low class of vegetable organism
Infection   invasion of body tissues by foreign organisms

RINGWORM OF THE SCALP

(Tinea Capitis)

Cause and Nature

Various fungi are responsible. Sometimes these fungi may come from animals, such as cats and dogs.

Signs and Symptoms

Ringworm of the scalp usually occurs in children. It is highly contagious and often becomes epidemic in schools. One or more small, round, raised, grayish, scaly patches on any portion of the hairy scalp is the first lesion noted. The hair may become broken, dry, brittle, and lusterless in the affected areas; the hair usually is lost, causing round, bald areas. These may spread over the entire scalp.

There are few symptoms, except a slight itching. In spite of local treatment, the disease may persist for a long time—sometimes for years; but it usually disappears at puberty.

Treatment

A determination of the fungus causing the disease should be made by a doctor. Some forms are mild, curing themselves when the hair falls out. Others require extensive treatment. In resistant cases, X ray may be the treatment of choice. An antibiotic, griseofulvin, taken by mouth, has been found to be effective. This must be prescribed by a doctor.

The infected hairs can be detected by a fluorescent test (with a black light). These hairs should be removed with tweezers by hand, if possible. Three percent ammoniated mercury ointment is applied daily, and a linen cap worn about eighteen days. Then the scalp is washed daily, using a soft brush to remove the loosened hair. Warmed adhesive tape placed over the affected part and then removed quickly will sometimes help in removing the affected hairs. Pulling the hairs out with forceps or tweezers twice a week, and wearing adhesive tape over the infected areas between these times of hair pulling will often help. Three percent ammoniated mercury ointment applied daily to the entire scalp will sometimes prevent the spread to other areas.

Home Care

The patient is restricted from attending school or summer camp. Indoor play with children is prohibited, but outdoor play is allowed if there is no contact with other children, and the patient wears a cap at all times. Other children should not use the same comb and brush, hat or cap of the patient, nor should they sleep in the same bed.

Schwartze's formula, an ointment, is applied to the scalp nightly. Pets, such as dogs and cats, are examined with ultraviolet light to see if they are infected.

Children going to schools, camps, etc., should be examined (by black light) to determine infected cases because the condition is spread by contact. Barbers should use sterilized instruments, and the backs of seats in moving picture houses should be examined in the dark with fluorescent light to detect the fungus, as scalp ringworm is often spread in this way. Children returning from the barber shop should have their scalps washed.

If local measures are not successful then the hair should be removed or treated by X ray. This should be done by someone who knows his work, because an overdosage might cause permanent baldness.

After the scalp is apparently cleared, it should be examined several times (by black light) to detect fluorescent hairs which might still be infected.

GLOSSARY

Contagious communicable; catching
Epidemic when a disease affects many people in a community at one time
Fungus a growth
Lesion wound or sore
Puberty age when reproductive organs become functionally operative

RINGWORM OF THE BODY

(Tinea Circinata)

Cause and Nature

This classical ringworm is found on the extremities and body, and sometimes on the face. It is caused by a fungus, and is characterized by a clearing center with active margins, causing ring-shaped, round, discrete lesions—in other words, lesions which do not blend.

Signs and Symptoms

These ring-shaped lesions are usually scaly, and sometimes itch.

Treatment

Ringworm of the body is more easily cured than "ringworm" of the scalp. The

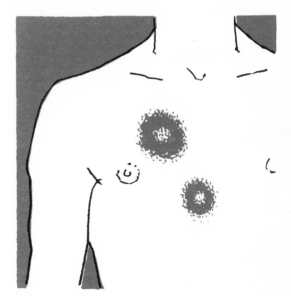

Ring worm of the body. Lesions are usually numerous and may be on any part of the body.

application, twice a day, of ointment such as Desenex or Timafax will usually clear them up in ten to twenty days. Iodine diluted half and half with glycerin and applied locally is also effective.

GLOSSARY

Fungus   an organism

RINGWORM OF THE GROIN

(Jockey Strap Itch—Tinea Cruris)

Cause and Nature

A fungus is the cause. The lesions, located in the region of the groin, may be dry and scaly or, if secondarily infected, will be red and weepy. Because of the sensitivity of this region, treatment should be mild.

Signs and Symptoms

There may be slight itching or burning in secondarily infected cases.

Treatment

Ointment, such as Desenex or Timafax, applied at night, and powder applied during the day, is usually effective.

If secondary bacterial infection is present, one of the antibiotic ointments, such as bacitracin ointment, will often help.

GLOSSARY

Fungus   low class organism
Secondarily   second in appearance
Sensitivity   being capable of responding to a sensation

ATHLETE'S FOOT

(Fungus Infection of the Feet)

Cause and Nature

This very common infection usually occurs between the toes. It is caused by a fungus, and is usually secondarily infected by

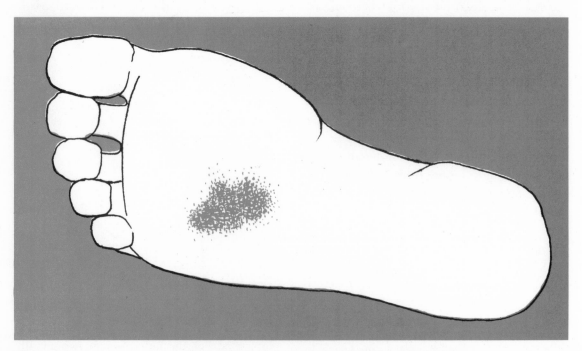

The appearance and common site of Athletes Foot—also seen between the toes.

bacteria. This disease is not caused by walking barefoot in shower rooms or gymnasiums, and swimming pools are not important in spreading the disease. The important causes of the disease are the presence of a fungus, poor foot hygiene, dampness of the feet from perspiration, not exposing the feet to air enough, and lack of immunity on the part of the individual.

Signs and Symptoms

The characteristic lesions are round, scaly patches or blisters found on the soles of the feet, palms of the hands, and between the toes or fingers.

Treatment

The use of strong drugs, such as iodine, for quick results, causes more trouble than a longer use of milder remedies. Never use full-strength iodine on the feet or hands. Desenex or timafax ointment, applied at night, and desenex or timafax powder applied during the day will usually take care of the fungus infection.

Keep the feet dry, expose them to the air, and if bacterial or secondary infection is present, use bacitracin or some other antibiotic ointment, after the fungicides have been used.

Four to six weeks may be necessary to clear the ordinary case, and the condition may recur.

GLOSSARY

Bacteria organisms causing infection
Foot Hygiene clean, healthy feet
Fungicides agents destroying fungus
Fungus a growth
Immunity power to resist disease or infection
Infection invasion of body tissues by foreign organisms
Lesions sores or abnormal spots
Secondary second in appearance

LICE OR LOUSINESS

(Pediculosis)

There are three varieties of lice that may infest man. The three areas involved are the head, the body, and the pubic areas. Transmission occurs through personal contact, hats, brushes, or clothing.

HEAD LICE

(Pediculosis Capitis)

Cause and Nature

Infestation of the scalp by lice. Most commonly found on people with long hair.

Signs and Symptoms

The lice can be seen, or their nits (ova or eggs) may be noted on the hair. The nits are fixed to the hair shafts, and can be moved up and down. There is sometimes itching, and occasionally infected excoriation of the scalp which is caused by scratching.

Treatment

All hats, combs, brushes, etc., should be thoroughly disinfected. Applications of DDT, in the form of powder or lotion, will usually destroy the lice.

LICE ON THE SKIN OR IN THE CLOTHING

(Pediculosis Corporis)

Cause and Nature

This is caused by lice which live in the seams of the clothing, and feed on the skin. This is a disease of poor hygiene, and occurs in crowded conditions, such as found during wartime housing.

Signs and Symptoms

Intense itching is the main symptom. The lice are found in the seams of the clothing, and the nits, or eggs, may be discovered on the body or in the hair.

Treatment

Boil the clothing for fifteen minutes. Bathe and scrub the body, applying DDT lotion to hairy areas.

CRABS OR CRAB LICE

(*Pediculosis Pubis*)

Cause and Nature

This is caused by a particular louse which usually infests the hair of the genital regions. It can be acquired through personal contact, from toilet seats, or from wearing unsterilized clothing previously worn by infected individuals.

Signs and Symptoms

The parasites in the genital regions are hard to find. Their nits, or eggs, may be found near the base of the hair. Intense itching may be present, and dangerous secondary infection may result from scratching irritated areas.

Treatment

Boil the clothing, disinfect the toilet seat, apply DDT lotion or powder to the affected parts, after bathing and drying. If secondary infection is present, use antibiotics, such as bacitracin or penicillin ointment.

GLOSSARY

Excoriation chafing or breaking of the skin
Genitals reproductive organs

Hygiene cleanliness; sanitary habits and conditions
Infestation invasion
Lousiness infestation by lice
Parasites organisms which live upon or within another organism

THE ITCH

(*Scabies*)

Cause and Nature

This condition is caused by the itch mite. The female mite burrows into the skin and deposits her eggs along the tunnel. Within four to eight hours the mites are hatched, and they make their way into the hair follicles. The condition is highly contagious through personal contact, and may involve an entire household. It is characterized by intense itching, which is worse at night.

Signs and Symptoms

The parasites are active at night and itching is most intense then. The burrow, or tunnel, appears as a fine, short, wavy, dark line, and an eruption may be present in the form of pimples, pustules, or scratch marks. These are found most frequently on the webs between the fingers, on the wrists, the forearms, the axillary folds, the breasts of women, the buttocks of children, and the genital regions. The lesions hardly ever appear above the neck.

Treatment

1. Hot packs, scrubbing thoroughly with soft brush especially where the burrows are apt to be found—the hands, arms, axillary regions, and genital regions.
2. Apply gamisco cream, kwell ointment, sulphur ointment, or benzyl benzoate. Any of the above are effective. The latter is perhaps the easiest to apply with a brush, but

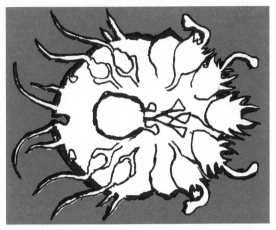

Itch Mite: Female burrows under skin, lays eggs which hatch and cause severe itching.

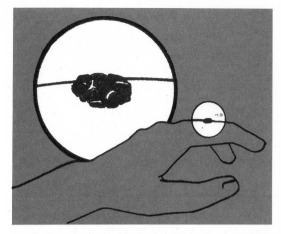

Senile Keratosis are harmless lesions caused by a piling up of scales on the skin.

may irritate the skin. Apply over entire body except head and face.

3. Next morning, apply ointment over body again. Omit bath.

4. Next night, repeat application of the ointment, but omit bath.

5. Second morning: take bath; put on all clean clothes; change and disinfect all bedclothes by boiling and airing.

If secondary or bacterial infection is present, antibiotic ointments such as bacitracin or neomycin ointment should be used. If first treatment is not successful, repeat in a week.

GLOSSARY

Axillary   the arm pit
Follicles   depressions or sacs
Pustules   small elevations of skin containing pus

SENILE KERATOSIS

(Warts of Old Age)

Cause and Nature

These are scaly, hard, slightly raised lesions seen on the face or hands, that is the exposed surfaces, of elderly people. They are seen more on people who have blue eyes and fair skin which has caused them to have freckles when they were younger. They are caused by exposure to the sun or at least aggravated by this exposure.

Signs and Symptoms

The scales usually form over a freckle and can be felt. They may be pulled off or fall off, only to build up again. If they are not treated, they may become larger, and in some cases may degenerate into an ulcer.

Treatment

The best treatment is prophylaxis, that is to try to prevent these lesions from forming. People with fair skin and freckles should try not to be over-exposed to the sun as they grow older. A bland ointment should be applied to the skin once a day to protect it from the rays of the sun.

When these raised, flaky lesions first appear they may be treated by a doctor who will scrape them off and touch the base with some acid; this will prevent a recurrence of that lesion, but others are likely to appear and should be treated promptly.

PSORIASIS

Cause and Nature

The cause is not known although this is a quite common skin disease and has been studied for a long time.

It is a chronic inflammatory disease and is seen in more men than women. The ages usually affected are between fifteen and forty-five.

The lesions are scaly, red papules which run together and usually appear in patches on the scalp, elbows, or knees, fingers, and back—although the lesions may appear anywhere. This condition sometimes tends to clear up spontaneously, but usually recurs again.

Signs and Symptoms

Psoriasis usually is painless and very seldom does it cause itching. The lesions are dull, red, and scaly; the scales are silver in color.

Treatment

A low fat diet is nearly always prescribed and foci of infection are sought and cleared up. Local treatment should be under the direction of a doctor who also may prescribe medicines to be taken internally.

LICHEN PLANUS

Cause and Nature

The cause has not been definitely determined but there is some evidence that virus infection may be the causative agent.

The lesions are raised, flat topped and may have a dimple in the center; they may be single or may run together, and are usually found on the inner surfaces of the thigh, the lower back, or the wrist, and flexor surface of the forearm.

Signs and Symptoms

The lesions as described may have a slightly violet color, and usually itching is severe.

Treatment

The treatment of this condition has not been uniformly satisfactory, and it may be best to consult a dermatologist (skin specialist). He may be able to at least relieve the severe itching.

ALOPECIA AREATA

(Bald Spots)

Cause and Nature

The cause of baldness or loss of hair is not known, although premature, partial baldness may be inherited and may be influenced by dandruff.

In alopecia areata, the hair falls out suddenly, leaving bald spots on the scalp. The skin is white and does not seem to be inflamed. These bald spots may increase in number until the entire head is bald. Indeed, the hair may disappear from the entire body. This is known as alopecia universalis. The hair may reappear spontaneously, and the younger the person the more likely the hair is to return.

Signs and Symptoms

A sudden falling out of the hair in patches over the scalp is the first sign. There are no symptoms.

Treatment

There is no satisfactory treatment for alopecia. The foci of infection should be sought out and cleared up. Any emotional strain or stress should be relieved, and the endocrine glands should be investigated. Mildly stimulating substances may be applied to the scalp, but this usually does no good. A skin specialist should be consulted in all cases of this distressing condition.

GLOSSARY

Dandruff   scales formed on scalp
Foci   points; sites
Pigment   coloring matter of the body
Premature   earlier than normally expected

VITILIGO

(White Patches on the Skin)

Cause and Nature

The cause of this condition is not known. Vitiligo is characterized by a sudden loss of pigment in different areas of the skin. The resulting spots are white in contrast to the surrounding skin, which has pigment. Indeed, by comparison, the surrounding skin may seem to have more pigment than ever and look browner, thereby making the white spots stand out.

Signs and Symptoms

There are no symptoms.

Treatment

The patient should avoid exposure to sunlight, so the surrounding skin will not seem so brown.

A skin specialist (dermatologist) should be consulted and he may be able to aid in the return of pigment. There is sometimes a spontaneous return of the pigment.

Various medications have been used, both internally and locally, to help in restoring normal pigmentation, and in some cases have been successful. At least there is enough hope that the condition may be corrected to make it advisable for the patient to consult a doctor.

MOLLUSCUM CONTAGIOSUM

Cause and Nature

The lesions are caused by a virus. They are globular tumors which come in groups and may appear on any part of the body. They are slightly raised and skin colored. There may be a small dimple in the center of each small tumor.

Signs and Symptoms

These tumors are unsightly and at times become secondarily infected; then they become red and tender. Usually there is no pain or itching.

Treatment

A skin specialist may remove them by cauterizing them with an acid, or by curettement. When there are numerous such globular tumors, they have been treated successfully by taking sulfadiazine internally.

LEUKOPLAKIA

(White Patches)

Cause and Nature

These are flat, slightly raised white patches which appear on the tongue or mucous membrane of the mouth. The lesion is usually seen in heavy smokers, and may be

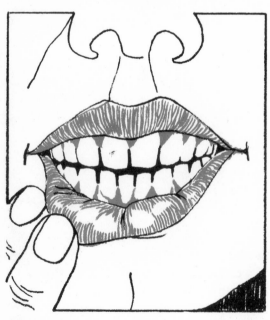

Oral Leukoplakia: White patches on the tongue, gums or mucus membrane of the mouth may be a forerunner of cancer.

connected with dental hygiene. If treated early, the lesions may clear up; but if allowed to go too long they become thick and rough and will eventually develop into cancer.

Signs and Symptoms

These lesions or white patches are not painful, and can only be detected by looking at the tongue or the mucous membrane of the mouth.

Treatment

The patient must stop smoking and never resume the habit, for to smoke may endanger his life. Good dental hygiene should be practiced and a dentist should be seen. If the lesions do not clear up in a short time the patient should see a skin specialist.

PAGET'S DISEASE OF THE BREAST

Cause and Nature

The cause is unknown. This is a cancer of the breast whose first symptom is an eczematous lesion around the nipple, starting out first with redness. This may begin to weep and crusts may form. If this lesion does not clear up promptly with the application of milk ointments, cancer of the underlying mammary ducts should be suspected. A skin specialist should be seen at once. If the diagnosis can be made before a lump appears the chances for cure are improved. Many other cancers of the breast are first detected by feeling a lump, but most of them do not have the eczema around the nipple.

Signs and Symptoms

A weeping, crusty skin lesion around the nipple should always be investigated if it does not clear up promptly under mild treatment. Eczema clears up with the use of proper mild ointments. Paget's disease of the breast does not clear up.

Treatment

Once the diagnosis has been made, the only treatment is prompt removal of the breast. This should be done before the lump or mass appears.

GLOSSARY

Eczema   skin disease
Lesion   wound or local sore
Mammary ducts   glands of the breasts
Weeping   exuding pus or moisture

PITYRIASIS ROSEA

Cause and Nature

The cause is not definitely known but it is suspected that some kind of an infection may be involved. Young people usually have the condition more often than older persons.

The diagnosis must be made by a doctor.

Signs and Symptoms

In this particular skin disease there is always a sign which is important and helps in the diagnosis—the so-called "herald patch." This single lesion appears on the body several days before the other widespread lesions appear, mostly on the trunk, very seldom on the limbs. The lesions are oval shaped, reddish, and have fine scales around the edges. Sometimes the itching is very mild, but at other times it may be much more severe.

Treatment

This condition usually clears up without treatment, within four to seven weeks.

Mild mentholated creams may be applied to control minor itching. If the itching is more severe, antihistamines may be taken by mouth, for symptomatic relief.

Pyribenzamine, fifty milligrams, is often a helpful treatment in relieving itching. One tablet of this preparation may be taken about every four hours.

GLOSSARY

Lesion   wound or local sore
Symptomatic   of the nature of a symptom or aimed at relieving symptoms

SKIN CANCER

(Malignant Skin Lesion—"Junction Nevus")

Cause and Nature

This lesion should be detected early because it can be very dangerous and may change into a melanoma, which is one of the most malignant tumors known to man.

This lesion may be present at birth or may appear at any time thereafter.

Signs and Symptoms

The junction nevus may resemble an ordinary mole but it has certain characteristics which should be watched for.

It is smooth and may be blue-black or slate-blue in color; it never has hair on it.

Treatment

Any lesion suspected of being a junction nevus should be seen immediately by a skin specialist who will remove it by surgery.

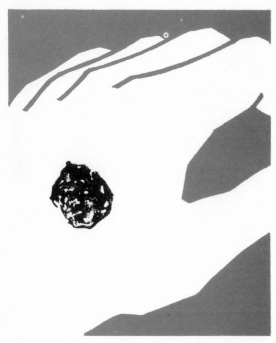

Melanoma: a smooth, dark, deadly mole with no hairs, may occur any place on the body.

MELANOMA

Cause and Nature

This is a deadly lesion which usually arises from a junction nevus or blue-black mole. When the melanoma has started to degenerate and spread throughout the body, death usually follows. Because of the widespread black color throughout the body where the melanoma has metastasized or spread, it has been called the "black death."

Signs and Symptoms

The melanoma makes itself noticed when a dark smooth mole begins to enlarge or break down.

Treatment

Because it is so deadly the melanoma should be thoroughly cut out or excised as soon as it is detected. Once the spread has started, excisions will not save the life of the patient. The spread of melanoma rarely starts before puberty, so for safety, all moles which are suspicious should be seen by a skin specialist and removed totally by surgery before the patient reaches the age of puberty. This is a very worthwhile safety measure.

GLOSSARY

Puberty age when reproductive organs are ready to function
Excise to cut out

BASAL CELL EPITHELIOMA

(Skin Cancer)

Cause and Nature

This lesion is the least dangerous of all the skin cancers, but nevertheless should be treated promptly.

The ordinary basal cell carcinoma does not metastasize or spread, and all the damage it does is through local destruction of tissue. The cause is not known, but it is most often seen in people who are at least middle-aged, usually older people, and the lesion is usually on the face.

Signs and Symptoms

Any lesion or sore on the face or ear that does not heal and remains for six months or longer should be seen by a doctor.

The color of the lesion is that of the skin, and the borders are often spoken of as being "waxy" in appearance. The small, firm, raised lesion usually is ulcerated in the center, and the borders slightly raised and rounded. The scab may be removed and local medication applied, but still the sore does not heal.

Treatment

This lesion should be seen by a dermatologist or skin specialist, who will remove it, usually by electrocautery or by radiation.

GLOSSARY

Electrocautery   electric apparatus for cauterizing tissue
Lesion   wound or local sore
Metastasize   spread to other parts of the body
Radiation   treatment with X-ray, radium, or other radioactive material

SQUAMOUS CELL EPITHELIOMA

(Skin Cancer)

Cause and Nature

The cause is unknown. This lesion is much more dangerous than the basal cell epithelioma as it can extend locally and spread to the other organs of the body. It can occur at any place on the skin but it is often seen on the mucous membrane of the lower lip. It is also seen, at times, on the tongue or other places on the mucous membrane of the mouth. Lesions in the mouth are especially dangerous.

Signs and Symptoms

This cancer usually comes on suddenly and grows rapidly. Any lesion with these characteristics should be examined by a skin specialist early. There is usually no sore or ulceration until the lesion becomes larger. It may spread into the skin and nearby tissues or may go to different parts of the body, causing death.

Treatment

A skin specialist (dermatologist) should be seen as soon as possible after the lesion is noticed. He can determine the type of lesion and extent of spread. Usually the growth can be stopped and the lesion destroyed by radiation, but sometimes surgery is required.

MOLES

Cause and Nature

Nearly everyone has one or more moles on the body and these are nearly always harmless. They are due to an overgrowth of some of the skin layers, and are usually light brown to dark brown in color. They may have hairs growing out of them. The kind with hairs growing from them are always harmless or benign. Moles may appear in any place on the body's skin.

Signs and Symptoms

These lesions are without symptoms unless they happen to be in a place where they are constantly irritated. In this case, they become tender or sore. Usually, the reason for wanting to get rid of a mole is because of its unsightliness, especially if it is on the face.

Treatment

Any mole that starts growing or becomes irritated should be seen by a doctor with the idea of having it removed by surgery.

There is one mole, blue-black or slate-blue in color, which may be present at birth or develop at any time after birth. It has a smooth surface and no hair. It may either be raised or level with the skin. This is called a "junction nevus" and is very dangerous for it may be the forerunner of melanoma, a highly malignant tumor. This kind of a lesion should be seen by a doctor who may refer the patient to a dermatologist, or skin specialist, to identify the mole and to remove it properly.

BIRTHMARKS

(Vascular Nevi)

Cause and Nature

These red or bluish lesions are usually present at birth, and are caused by an overgrowth of small blood vessels in a particular place. If the vessels involved are small superficial ones the lesions will not be raised, but will be flat. This has been called a "wine mark." If the deeper vessels of the skin are involved, the lesion or birthmark may be raised, reddish in color, and sometimes may grow larger.

Signs and Symptoms

The flat lesions are no trouble if they are not located on the face. The raised lesions sometimes cause trouble, even if they are not on the face, because they may become irritated or even be ruptured by repeated blows.

Treatment

The flat lesions should be left alone, as sometimes the treatment will make them worse; they can at times be covered by powder or some kind of cosmetic lotion. Sometimes they disappear spontaneously or fade out, as the person grows older.

A skin specialist, or dermatologist, should be consulted about the raised lesions, although these sometimes go away without any treatment. There are various methods which a skin specialist may use if he thinks the lesion should be removed. These methods are:

1. Surgical removal
2. Carbon dioxide snow
3. Radium

KELOIDS

(Enlarged or Ridgelike Scars)

Cause and Nature

A keloid is a raised or overgrown scar. Some people have a tendency to form these large scars, and the reason or cause is not known.

Any incision, such as an appendectomy scar or a cut on the arm from a barbed wire fence, may cause a raised red, hard scar called a keloid.

Signs and Symptoms

If these scars are on parts of the body where they can be seen, they are unsightly. There is seldom any pain or discomfort connected with them.

Treatment

This must be taken care of by a skin specialist, as just the simple excision or cutting out of such a scar will only cause a larger scar to form. The skin specialist will treat them before removal. The sooner he has a chance to work on these keloids, the more likely he is to be successful. Hence, if a scar has been enlarged for two or three months, it should be treated. After it has been present for a year or more, it is harder to remove.

CONTACT DERMATITIS

Cause and Nature

Contact dermatitis is an inflammation of the skin which may resemble eczema. It can be caused by exposure of the skin to irritating substances such as iodine, solvents, or lye. These irritants would cause inflammation of anyone's skin, and in industry it is important to rule out the chemicals which may cause dermatitis so that proper precautions can be taken.

A second type of contact dermatitis is caused by an allergic reaction of the skin in certain individuals who have been previously sensitized by exposure to this substance. The first exposure may not cause a dermatitis, but if the cells of the skin become sensitized, the person is said to be allergic to this substance and whenever exposed to it in the future will suffer an inflammation of the skin.

The chemicals which may cause contact dermatitis must be able to penetrate the unbroken skin and such chemicals are numerous. A few of them are named here.

Plants such as poison oak and poison ivy produce an oily substance to which many people are sensitized, and exposure to this substance causes dermatitis. Topical applications of some medicines such as sulfonilamide ointment or penicillin ointment will cause rashes on some people. Cosmetics and fingernail polishes are frequent causes of contact dermatitis. Certain metals such as mercury and nickel and the salts of these metals are known to cause dermatitis in some people because of a sensitivity to them. Dyes used in cloth, leather, and furs can cause an allergic reaction, as will industrial chemicals, such as used by photographers, metal workers, and beauticians.

The skin first becomes red and inflamed, then swollen; scratch marks produce a raw surface which sometimes oozes as in the case of poison oak. In most cases there may be seen the formation of blebs or blisters which are easily broken and cause the surface to weep.

Signs and Symptoms

Redness and swelling of the skin may become apparent within twenty-four hours of the exposure. Sometime later, this goes on to blister formation. When a person scratches, he may spread the irritating substances to other parts of the body where the dermatitis will start all over again.

Sometimes a swelling of the skin is the most important sign, and usually itching or burning are the most noticeable symptoms.

Other forms of dermatitis, such as seborrheic dermatitis, differ from contact dermatitis in that the rash is dry and scaly; in fungus infections the redness usually comes in between the skin folds such as between the toes. Eczema in a baby, the so-called atopic dermatitis, will occur on both sides of the body at the same time on such places as the elbows or the back of the knees. There is no blister formation. The baby usually inherits it from its parents.

Treatment

The first and most important step is to find the substance that is causing the dermatitis and withdraw the person from all contact with it. For instance, if a woman is sensitive to nail polish and suffers a dermatitis of the eyelids, the offending nail polish must be withdrawn before the eyelids can be treated properly. Mild cases may heal by themselves as soon as contact with the irritant has been discontinued.

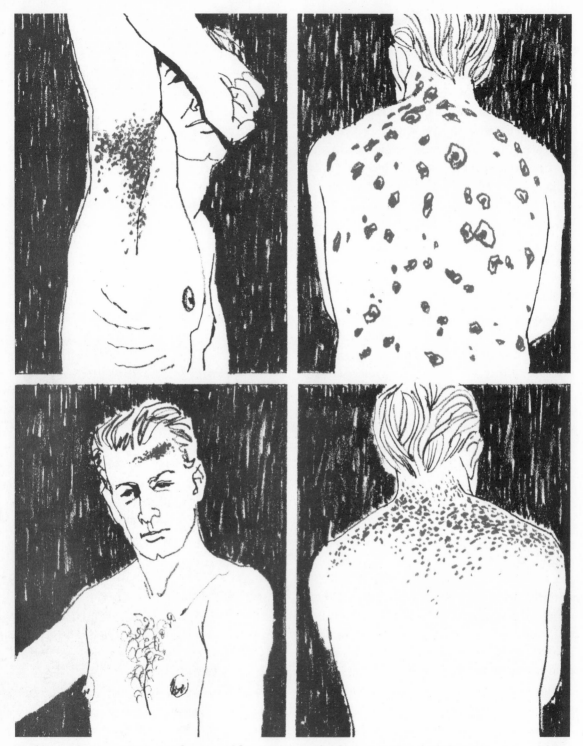

Rashes or skin eruptions may be caused by a variety of substances. Some of them are shown here: contact dermatitis from deoderant (*upper left*) and leather hat band (*lower left*), drug reactions from aspirin (*upper right*) and arsenic (*lower right*).

Local treatment depends upon the stage of the lesion. In acute, red weeping lesions, mild wet compresses of such substances as five percent aluminum acetate may be used, followed by calomine lotion with phenol to dry up the lesion and stop the itching. Prevention of secondary infection which may be caused by scratching is important. Some of the cortisone-type medicines used by local application tend to stop the spread of inflammation. People who have frequent attacks of dermatitis caused by something like poison oak can be partially protected by taking drugs or shots to desensitize them. Washing with soap and water after exposure will often lessen the severity of the attack or, if all of the offending substance is washed off before it penetrates the skin, the attack may be prevented.

GLOSSARY

Allergic   over sensitive
Desensitize   to make not sensitive
Eczema   skin disease
Inflammation   condition characterized by pain, heat, redness, and swelling
Lesion   wound, open sore, or degeneration

SUNBURN

Cause and Nature

Sunburn is caused by exposure of the skin to certain ultraviolet rays in sunshine. This type of reaction is usually seen only in the late spring and summer. In northern countries these particular rays are not present in the sunshine, but in southern countries, and especially in the summer time, they are present and harmful.

Many people think it is stylish and healthful to acquire a nice sun tan. On the contrary, overexposure to strong sunlight exerts a damaging influence on the skin, causing it to age early. This can be seen in the wrinkled skin on the faces and hands of people, such as farmers and sailors, who are exposed to sunlight a great deal. The exposed parts of their skin have aged prematurely.

In certain people there exists a very definite allergy or sensitivity to sunlight and these persons, after prolonged periods of exposure to the sun, may develop skin rashes which are difficult to treat. Such individuals are also more likely to develop skin cancers and keratosis—the so-called moles seen on the faces of older people. These are nearly always seen on areas which have been exposed to the sun and it is probably because these people are sensitive to sunlight.

Signs and Symptoms

Sunburn is like any other first and second degree burn. It causes redness and a burning sensation of the skin, and in severe cases there is a generalized feeling of malaise with fever.

It has been determined that people who are taking large doses of the so-called miracle drugs or antibiotics, may become sensitive to sunlight, and if exposed for any length of time while taking these drugs, may become ill from exposure to sunlight. This is not true of all antibiotics, only with some of them when taken in large doses.

Many skin conditions are aggravated by exposure to sunlight in spite of the general belief that warm sunshine is a cure-all. Two skin conditions only are known for sure to be helped by sunlight, and these are acne and psoriasis.

Treatment

If a person finds that he is sensitive to sunlight, he should avoid overexposure.

Certain suntan lotions will help protect the skin by cutting out some of the sunlight, especially the ultraviolet rays which cause sunburn.

In case of sunburn, a soothing lotion or ointment such as antipyrexol, or Kip, will help make the patient more comfortable. These are used to ease the pain in other first degree burns.

In cases of real illness caused by overexposure to the sun in people who have a definite sensitivity to sunlight, some of the steroids like triamcinolone are helpful in relieving the symptoms.

People who are definitely sensitive to sunlight may play golf or go fishing without suffering any harmful effects if they are taking one of the antimalarial drugs and at the same time try to prevent overexposure.

To sum up the subject of sunburn, no person should ever allow himself to become overexposed to the sun in order to get a suntan. Some people who are sensitive to sunlight should avoid exposure in order to prevent skin diseases and even generalized disease such as lupus erythematosus. People who are taking large doses of certain antibiotics—for instance, chlorpromazine—should avoid overexposure to sunlight while taking the drug. They may go ahead and play golf or fish after they stop taking the drug.

Use moderation and caution in acquiring a suntan.

GLOSSARY

Lupus erythematosus   a disease of the skin
Malaise   a feeling of discomfort
Ultraviolet   outside the visible spectrum

Chapter 19

Diseases Caused by Allergies

BEFORE DISCUSSING some of the allergic diseases, a general discussion of allergy may help in understanding the symptoms and treatment in these conditions.

Allergy is a term used to denote a hypersensitivity to some substance. This hypersensitivity is noted in different ways, according to which tissue of the body is sensitive to the substance. For instance:

1. If the tissue involved is the blood vessels of the skin, then we have reactions known as urticaria (hives), infantile dermatitis, and neurodermatitis

2. If the smooth muscles of the bronchioles (minute bronchial tubes) are affected we have asthma

3. If the tissue involved is the skin, we have contact dermatitis, such as poison oak

4. If it is the blood vessels of the subcutaneous tissue, we have angioneurotic edema

5. If the nasal mucous membrane is involved, we have hay fever

6. If the body as a whole is involved, we have anaphylactic shock

The exact cause of a person being sensitive to certain substances is not known, but it is thought that heredity may play a part.

The various substances to which a person may be sensitive may come from outside the body, such as pollens from trees, bushes, or grasses; dust from the air or animal emanations; contact with drugs, or certain drugs injected into the body—as with insect or snake bites, or serum injections by doctor.

It is also possible to take the offending substance into the body by eating. As we all know, some people develop hives after eating strawberries. A person may also become sensitive to some infection that he has harbored for a long time.

As mentioned above, heredity may play some part in sensitivity, but it is also felt that the sensitivity is affected by climate, nervous factors, and endocrine as well as metabolic influences.

The general principles which may be used in treating all allergies may be outlined below. This treatment should be in the hands of a doctor.

1. Determine the substance to which the person is sensitive

2. Avoid this substance

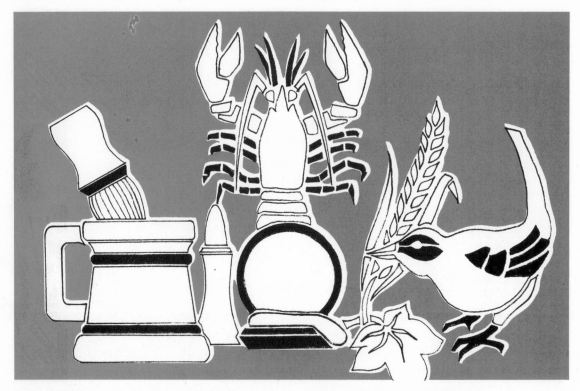

Allergies: A few of the substances which may cause allergies in susceptable persons.

3. Try to desensitize the individual to the substance by a series of injections of weak solutions which are gradually stepped up in strength
4. Give symptomatic relief with medicines such as antihistamine, adrenaline, and cortisone
5. Try to avoid the climate or contributing factors which may influence the sensitivity

GLOSSARY

Anaphylactic   severe reaction
Dermatitis   inflammation of the skin
Desensitize   to make not sensitive
Emanations   that which flows out of
Endocrine   secrete internally
Heredity   from one generation to another
Hypersensitivity   excessive sensitivity
Metabolic   chemical changes in the body
Pollens   fine dust from plants and trees
Sensitivity   susceptibility
Subcutaneous   under the skin

THE ALLERGIC DISEASES

Hay Fever

Cause and Nature

Hay fever is a form of nasal allergy in which the mucous membranes of the nasal passages react to some inhalant—dust, orris root powder, or pollens from trees, or weeds.

Running nose and sneezing which go with hay fever are often misdiagnosed as a cold.

Signs and Symptoms

Nasal blocking, running nose, sneezing, and sometimes conjunctivitis, or watery eyes. All of these symptoms occur when the person is exposed to the substance to which he is sensitive.

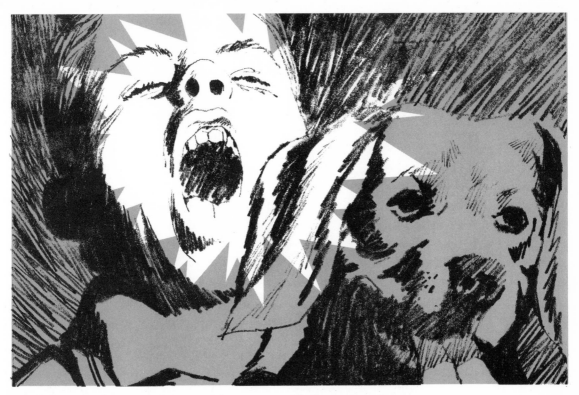

Hayfever and athsma may be caused by contact with dogs, cats or horses.

Sometimes the attacks occur only in certain seasons of the year, as when a person is sensitive to pollen from a tree.

Treatment

Tests should be done to identify the offending pollen or other substance. Then, when this is identified, an attempt is made to desensitize the patient by giving injections of a solution made to include the offending pollen in gradually increasing strengths. This treatment is often successful, but may have to be repeated each year just before the season of the pollen occurs.

The antihistaminic drugs give great relief in controlling the nose and eye symptoms.

GLOSSARY

Desensitize   to make not sensitive
Pollen   fine dust from plants and trees

Asthma

Cause and Nature

Asthma is a term applied to a group of symptoms which occur in recurrent paroxysms of shortness of breath, wheezing, a sense of constriction in the chest. Sometimes there is a cough. Allergic asthma is caused by a reaction of the bronchi to some agent to which the person is sensitive. The bronchi become constricted, and the mucous membrane of the bronchi swells, giving rise to a thick, tenacious mucous secretion.

Signs and Symptoms

Wheezing, shortness of breath, in which the difficulty is noted on breathing the air out rather than when breathing in. The patient may become slightly blue at times, and has difficulty trying to raise the thick sputum.

Allergic asthma must be differentiated from cardiac asthma, which is caused by a certain form of heart disease.

Treatment

The treatment should be started as early in the attack as possible. Drugs which relax the bronchi, such as adrenalin, give relief when injected. Similar drugs can be taken by inhalation or by mouth. Iodides, especially potassium iodide, may be given over long periods to loosen up the secretions and make it easier to raise the thick sputum.

GLOSSARY

Bronchi   small tubes leading to the lungs
Paroxysms   sudden, violent uncontrollable action
Tenacious   holding fast

SERUM SICKNESS

Cause and Nature

Serum sickness is a delayed allergic reaction caused by injecting some foreign serum. It usually takes from eight to twelve days for the symptom to appear.

One instance of injecting a foreign serum is when tetanus antitoxin is injected after an injury. This antitoxin is incorporated in horse serum, and a test should be performed by injecting a small amount of the antitoxin into the skin, and waiting five or ten minutes. If a large wheal, or welt, develops, the patient is sensitive to horse serum and the whole dose should not be given at once.

Signs and Symptoms

In about eight to twelve days the patient notices a fever, aching in his joints, swelling

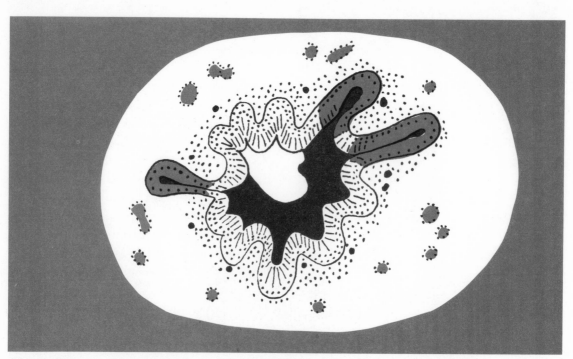

Cross section through a bronchial as seen in allergic asthma, showing red swollen mucus membrane and thick tenacious secretion.

of certain parts of the body, enlarged lymph glands, and skin eruptions.

Treatment

The patient should be given antihistaminic compounds, and should be given aspirin to keep him comfortable.

GLOSSARY

Allergic   oversensitive to some substance
Wheal   raised mark on skin

ANGIONEUROTIC EDEMA

Cause and Nature

Angioneurotic edema is often called giant hives. The swelling is below the skin rather than in the skin, as in urticaria, and is usually greater. It may be caused by eating or having injected some substance to which the patient is sensitive, by inhaling such substance, or from an insect bite. The swelling frequently involves the lips and eyelids. If the swelling is in the tongue, pharynx, larynx, or glottis, breathing may be obstructed.

Signs and Symptoms

The localized swelling may be transient and may or may not itch.

Treatment

Prompt treatment with antihistamine should be instituted. If breathing is embarrassed, adrenalin should be given and cortisone is often effective.

GLOSSARY

Glottis   opening between the vocal cords
Larynx   voice box
Pharynx   sac between the mouth and esophagus

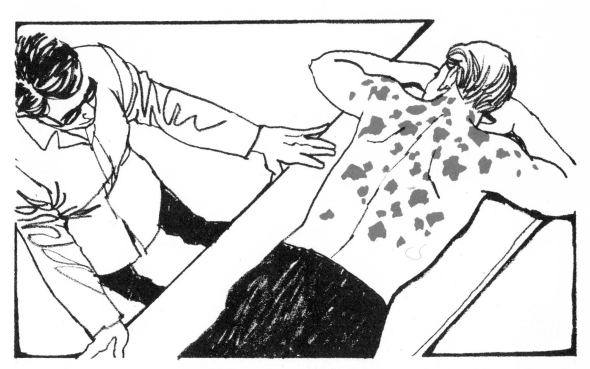

Giant Hives: A typical eruption which may be caused by eating strawberries, fish or other substances to which a person is sensitive.

ANAPHYLACTIC SHOCK

Cause and Nature

This severe shock-like reaction may follow very soon after injection of a foreign serum or protein into a person who may be very sensitive to the injected substance. Because injections are usually given in a doctor's office, this kind of a reaction most often occurs where a doctor is readily available. This is fortunate, for it is a very severe reaction which may cause death if not treated promptly.

Signs and Symptoms

Sudden onset of vomiting, fall in blood pressure, subnormal temperature, pallor, cyanosis, a thready pulse, diarrhea, and loss of consciousness, are the symptoms seen in anaphylactic shock.

Treatment

Tourniquet is applied to the extremity above the site of injection. Adrenalin is given by injection. The tourniquet is released from time to time. Patient should be kept warm.

GLOSSARY

Cyanosis   blueness of the skin
Pallor   absence of skin color
Onset   beginning
Tourniquet   a tight band used to stop bleeding

HIVES OR URTICARIA

Cause and Nature

The cause of hives in many chronic cases, or cases that tend to recur, may never be proven. However, there are many causes which are known. The most common cause of hives is sensitivity to some form of food. People who suffer acute cases of hives may give a history of having eaten fish or strawberries just before the attack. They are allergic to these foods. Some medicines will cause hives and in some cases, infestations by parasitic worms will cause the characteristic rash or breaking out. In some people, exposure to cold or heat or even the act of scratching may cause the wheals to appear, while in rare cases emotional factors may be the only cause. People who come from a family that has a history of allergy are more likely to have hives.

Signs and Symptoms

The lesion is a round or oval raised portion of the skin called a wheal. The wheal and skin around it may be red and will itch. One crop may disappear only to have another appear in twenty-four hours or less.

Sometimes hives or urticaria will resemble multiple insect bites, but a bite can usually be recognized by a small red spot in the center of the wheal. The itching in hives is usually quite severe, and this is aggravated by scratching. New wheals may be made to appear by scratching the skin.

Treatment

A doctor may relieve the acute symptoms by giving an injection of adrenalin. The prolonged relief which is also important may be obtained by taking some of the antihistamine drugs such as chlortrimeton or pyrobenzamine by mouth at regular intervals. Calamine lotion with phenol applied locally may help the itching, and, if the hives are caused by something a person has eaten, a dose of milk of magnesia may help remove the offending substance from the intestinal tract and thereby hasten recovery. In some severe cases doctors use the cortisone drugs with good results.

Chapter 20

The Collagen Diseases

THE TERM COLLAGEN DISEASES is applied to a group of diseases which show widespread involvement of the connective tissue. Among the collagen disorders are such diseases as rheumatoid arthritis, acute rheumatic fever, polyarteritis nodosa, disseminated lupus erythematosus, scleroderma, and dermatomyositis.

Since rheumatoid arthritis and acute rheumatic fever are discussed elsewhere they will not be taken up here, and because scleroderma, dermatomyositis, and polyarteritis nodosa are comparatively rare diseases, they will not be described.

Disseminated lupus erythematosus is not uncommon and will be described.

DISSEMINATED LUPUS ERYTHEMATOSUS

Cause and Nature

The cause is not known, but various conditions such as infections or sore throat with fever, overexposure to sunlight, and taking drugs for hypertension over a long period of time have been known to precede this con-

dition. The causative relation to it has not been established.

This condition is a chronic disease which may get better at times but is quite often progressive and usually fatal. It occurs predominantly in females. About eighty to eighty-five percent of the cases are seen in women. It may occur at any age but is most often seen between the ages of fifteen and forty years.

Signs and Symptoms

The symptoms of this disease are extremely varied. Most commonly seen early symptoms are fever, pain in the joints, pleuritic pains or pains in the chest, loss of weight, loss of appetite, weakness and shortness of breath.

The most characteristic sign is a rash that appears in a so-called butterfly distribution over the bridge of the nose. The cheeks on each side present a raised red, hard, and sharply outlined rash which has been likened to the wings of a butterfly.

Laboratory tests which confirm the diagnosis reveal an anemia, low white blood cell count, or leukopenia—from 2000 to 4000

299

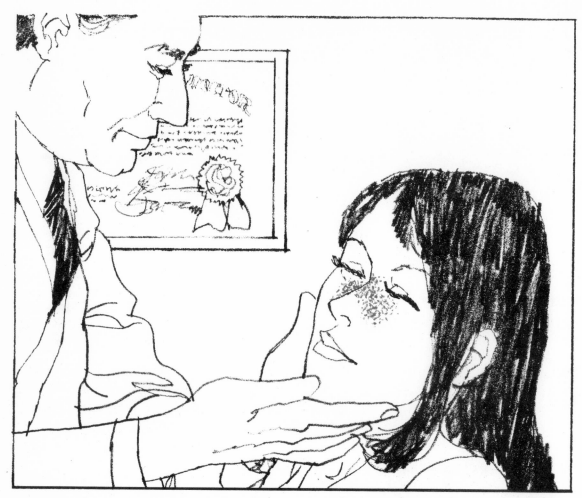

Butterfly rash as seen in disseminated lupus erythematosus is a serious condition.

white blood cells per cubic millimeter. The red blood cell sedimentation rate is markedly elevated.

In the urine there is usually found albumin and pus cells as well as red blood cells. The one laboratory test which is thought to establish the diagnosis in a suspected case is the demonstration in serum of so-called L. E. cells.

Treatment

The treatment of this condition must be in the hands of a doctor. The use of the steroids such as ACTH and cortisone has been of great value in relieving the symptoms. General supportive measures are important and the patient should avoid exposure to sunlight. Potassium chloride helps and a low salt diet is indicated.

GLOSSARY

Albumin   a clear thick protein substance found, among other places, in the blood
Anemia   deficient blood
Hypertension   high blood pressure
Pleuritic   pertaining to the pleura; painful respiration

Chapter 21

Cancer

NEXT TO HEART DISEASE, cancer is the second most common cause of death in the United States. Lung cancer became the leading cause of death from cancer in the United States in 1954, and continues to hold this position. It is estimated that approximately 52,000 persons in this country will die of the disease (42,000 men and 8,000 women) in 1967. When broken down, this amounts to 140 deaths a day. Since more than 75 percent of lung cancer is caused by cigarette smoking, the great majority of these deaths are preventable.

Cancer of the lung is also thought to be due to increased inhalation of irritants such as polluted air—so-called smog.

Cases of cancer of the uterus have decreased and this is perhaps due to early detection by wide-spread use of the "Pap" smear and early treatment.

Cause and Nature

The cause of cancer is not known; but millions of dollars are being spent every year in an attempt to determine this cause.

We know that cancer is a disorderly growth of body cells. In other words, a certain kind of tissue cell which has been growing and dividing normally for many years, will suddenly go wild and begin growing very rapidly. The cell will divide itself into two, then four, then eight, then sixteen cells, and so on, until it pushes away the normal cells around it. It also steals the food from the normal cells because it grows so rapidly. Sometimes a cancer will grow so fast that it cannot get enough food to maintain itself, and will break down. The result is an ulcer or sore.

Sooner or later some of these wild-growing cells will break off from the parent group and be carried through the blood stream or lymph channels to some other part of the body. Here they will start up another group of rapidly dividing cells. This migration of cancer from its original source to the other parts of the body is called metastasis.

Different types of cancer vary in their rapidity of growth. Some grow and metastasize very quickly, while others are slower. The slower the growth of the cancer, the better the chance a doctor has to find it and then remove it before it can be spread. It is

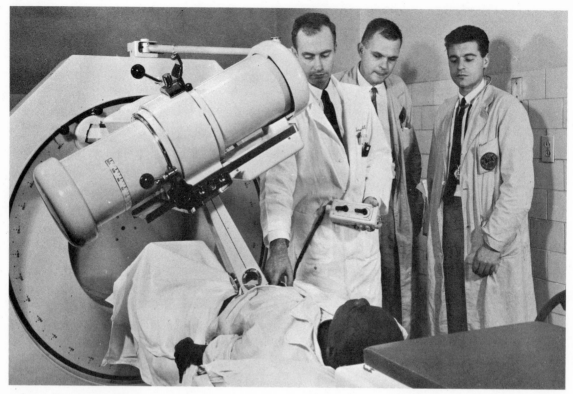

Illustration of patient receiving deep X ray therapy or treatment for cancer.

in this way that cancer is cured; and it *can* be cured if detected and treated in time.

If found early, cancer can be destroyed by radium or X ray, or removed by surgery, and the patient will be as healthy as ever. This is why it is so important for people, as they get older, to be on the lookout for cancer, and to have periodic examinations by their doctor.

Some types of cancer are more difficult to detect than others. However, it is known that sixty percent of cancers in women, and thirty percent of all cancers in men occur in areas of the body that can be easily examined.

It has been estimated that 150,000 Americans are being saved from cancer every year by early diagnosis and treatment; but we also know that 75,000 or more die who could have been saved if they had been treated early enough.

Statistics have been gathered to prove that the following types of cancer are now being cured, as compared to the number which could be cured if diagnosed and treated early:

Type of Cancer	Percentage Cured Seen Late	Percentage Cured Seen Early
Uterus	55	70
Breast	46	81
Rectum	25	77
Mouth	36	65
Skin	90	95
Lungs	4	34

Signs and Symptoms

How can you head off cancer in time?

If you will learn and pay attention to the following warning symptoms, you may be able to prevent or head off cancer. Look for:

1. Any unusual bleeding or discharge from the body openings, especially from the vagina
2. A lump or thickening in the breast or elsewhere. This applies to men as well as to women. Men do have cancer of the breast
3. A sore that does not heal
4. Persistent change in bowel or bladder habits
5. Persistent hoarseness or cough
6. Lasting indigestion, or difficulty in swallowing
7. Any change in a wart or mole on your body

The above seven points are cancer warnings which can be noted by you. There are other signs which can be detected by your family doctor. For this reason, every person over forty-five should be examined at least once a year by his or her family doctor.

Treatment

See your doctor immediately when any of the above signs are noted, for time is very important. The cancer can be cured if detected and treated before it spreads.

It has been estimated that cancer will occur in one out of every four persons in the United States. A yearly check-up by your doctor may save you, if you happen to be the one out of four.

In certain cancers, doctors have found that regional infusion and perfusion of cytotoxic drugs, (cell-killing or damaging drugs) have saved many cases. One of these drugs is called methotrexate. Many drugs used to cure cancer have undesirable side effects. Doctors have found that hypothermia, lowering of the body temperature, will prevent some of these side effects.

Millions of dollars and many millions of man hours are being used every month to find the causes and cures for cancer and it looks like we are coming closer to this goal.

Many new devices for detecting and treating cancer are being discovered continually. The chances of survival for five years or more after early diagnosis is better than ever (except for cancer of the lungs.)

RELATION OF CANCER TO CAUSES OF DEATH

Rank	Cause of Death	Percent of Total Deaths
	All Causes	100.0
1.	Diseases of Heart	38.8
2.	Cancer	16.2
3.	Cerebral Hemorrhage (Vascular Lesions)	11.1
4.	Accidents	5.9
	Motor-Vehicle Accidents	2.7
	All Other Accidents	3.2
5.	Influenza and Pneumonia	3.4
6.	Certain Diseases of Early Infancy	3.0
7.	Arteriosclerosis	2.1
8.	Diabetes	1.8
9.	Cirrhosis of Liver	1.3
10.	Suicide	1.2
11.	Congenital Malformations	1.1
12.	Nephritis	0.7
13.	Hypertension (without mention of Heart)	0.7
14.	Ulcer of Stomach and Duodenum	0.6
15.	Hernia and Intestinal Obstruction	0.5
	Other and Ill-Defined	11.6

NOTE: These figures are estimates by U.S. National Vital Statistics Division.

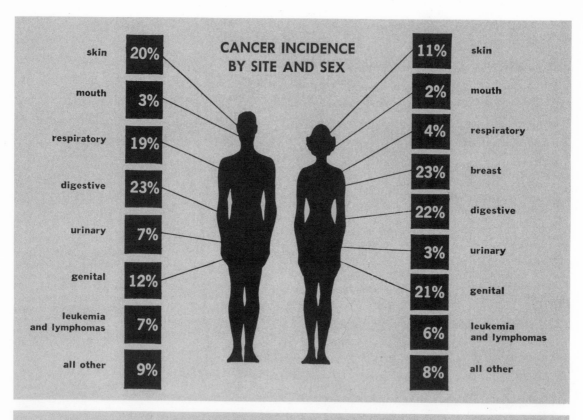

CANCER INCIDENCE BY SITE AND SEX

skin	20%
mouth	3%
respiratory	19%
digestive	23%
urinary	7%
genital	12%
leukemia and lymphomas	7%
all other	9%

11%	skin
2%	mouth
4%	respiratory
23%	breast
22%	digestive
3%	urinary
21%	genital
6%	leukemia and lymphomas
8%	all other

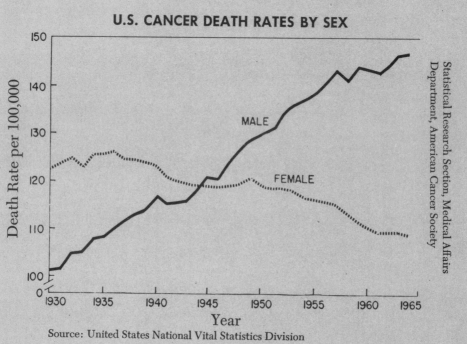

U.S. CANCER DEATH RATES BY SEX

MALE

FEMALE

Death Rate per 100,000

Year

Source: United States National Vital Statistics Division

Statistical Research Section, Medical Affairs Department, American Cancer Society

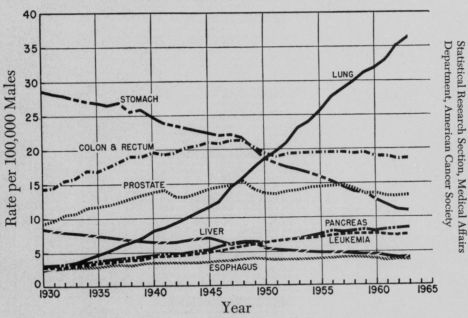

U.S. CANCER DEATH RATES BY SITE (MALE)

Rate per 100,000 Males

LUNG

STOMACH

COLON & RECTUM

PROSTATE

LIVER

PANCREAS

LEUKEMIA

ESOPHAGUS

Year

Source: National Vital Statistics Division and Bureau of the Census

Statistical Research Section, Medical Affairs Department, American Cancer Society

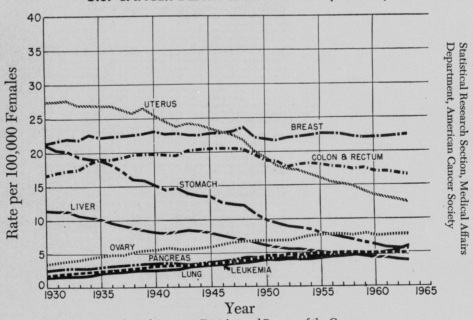

U.S. CANCER DEATH RATES BY SITE (FEMALE)

Rate per 100,000 Females

UTERUS

BREAST

COLON & RECTUM

STOMACH

LIVER

OVARY

PANCREAS

LUNG

LEUKEMIA

Year

Source: National Vital Statistics Division and Bureau of the Census

Statistical Research Section, Medical Affairs Department, American Cancer Society

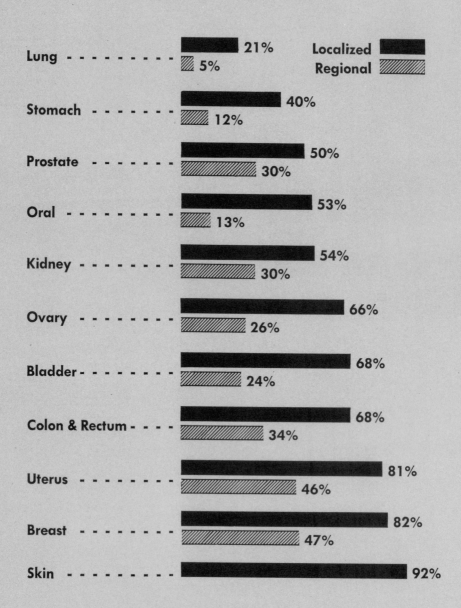

FIVE-YEAR SURVIVAL RATES
FOR SELECTED SITES OF CANCER

Lung — 21% Localized / 5% Regional

Stomach — 40% / 12%

Prostate — 50% / 30%

Oral — 53% / 13%

Kidney — 54% / 30%

Ovary — 66% / 26%

Bladder — 68% / 24%

Colon & Rectum — 68% / 34%

Uterus — 81% / 46%

Breast — 82% / 47%

Skin — 92%

Source: National Cancer Institute and Connecticut State Dept. of Health

LEADING CANCER SITES BY AGE AND SEX

Age	Sex	Five Leading Cancer Sites
Under 15	Male	Leukemia; Brain; Reticulo and Lymphosarcomas; Kidney; Bone
	Female	Leukemia; Brain; Kidney; Reticulo and Lymphosarcomas; Bone
15-34	Male	Leukemia; Hodgkin's Disease; Brain; Testis, etc.; Reticulo and Lymphosarcomas
	Female	Uterus; Breast; Leukemia; Hodgkin's Disease; Brain
35-54	Male	Lung; Colon-Rectum; Stomach; Brain; Pancreas
	Female	Breast; Uterus; Colon-Rectum; Ovary; Lung
55-74	Male	Lung; Colon-Rectum; Prostate; Stomach; Pancreas
	Female	Breast; Colon-Rectum; Uterus; Ovary; Stomach
75 and Over	Male	Prostate; Colon-Rectum; Lung; Stomach; Pancreas
	Female	Colon-Rectum; Breast; Stomach; Uterus; Pancreas

Source: Vital Statistics of the United States

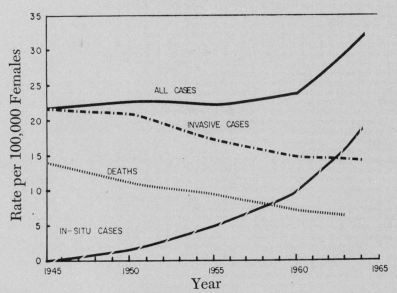

CANCER OF UTERINE CERVIX
INCIDENCE AND DEATH RATES

Source: New York State Dept. of Health (based on New York State except New York City)

APPLYING CANCER STATISTICS LOCALLY (ESTIMATES)

Size of City	Known Cancer Cases in 1967	Deaths from Cancer in 1967	New Cases of Cancer in 1967	No. Saved from Cancer in 1967	No. Who Will Eventually Develop Cancer	Deaths from Cancer (If Present Rates Continue)
1,000	4	1	3	1	250	150
2,000	9	3	6	2	500	300
3,000	13	4	8	3	750	450
4,000	18	6	11	4	1,000	600
5,000	21	7	14	5	1,250	750
10,000	43	15	28	9	2,500	1,500
25,000	107	37	70	23	6,250	3,750
50,000	215	75	140	47	12,500	7,500
100,000	430	150	280	93	25,000	15,000
200,000	860	300	560	186	50,000	30,000
500,000	2,150	750	1,400	465	125,000	75,000

PERCENTAGE INCREASE OF CANCER DEATHS FOR SELECTED COUNTRIES
(For men, ages 45-64, over an 8 year period*)

	Canada	England & Wales	France	Italy	Japan	Norway	U.S., White	U.S., Nonwhite
All Sites	+ 4%	+ 5%	+13%	+16%	+ 6%	− 2%	+ 5%	+12%
Esophagus	+ 8	− 5	+16	——	− 9	+39	+ 4	+24
Pancreas	+15	+ 9	n.a.	+30	+ 98	− 8	+11	+26
Lung/Bronchus	+38	+22	+56	+74	+139	+54	+34	+59
Prostate	− 2	−10	+36	+26	+ 50	− 2	−11	− 8
Leukemia	− 7	+10	+22	+30	+ 76	−23	+33	+51

*1952-53 to 1960-61   n.a.—data not available

Chapter 22

Arthritis

THERE ARE various types of arthritis and these may be classified into four groups as listed below:

1. Degenerative arthritis or osteoarthritis
2. Rheumatoid arthritis
3. Gouty arthritis (already described)
4. Arthritis due to specific infection

Of these, perhaps rheumatoid arthritis is the most commonly seen, and certainly is the most disabling. The term arthritis means inflammation of the joint, and various types of joint disorders will be described separately.

DEGENERATIVE, OSTEOARTHRITIS OR HYPERTROPHIC ARTHRITIS

Cause and Nature

This affliction is seen mostly in middle-aged and older people. Apparently it is caused by repeated use or trauma to the joint, and is not inflammatory.

Swelling, or hard knobs on the terminal or end joints of the fingers is one of the most common types of osteoarthritis. These are called Heberden's nodes and are usually not painful. X ray of the spine will often show spurs or overgrowth of bone, which is a manifestation of osteoarthritis. Indeed, the diagnosis is made most often by X ray examination, and the joints frequently affected are the weight-bearing ones, or the joints used most.

Signs and Symptoms

Swelling of the end joints of the fingers and pain or crepitation in the knee joints are common signs. There is seldom fluid on the joints and the joints rarely become fixed so they cannot be used. Osteoarthritis in the hip joints can be extremely painful. The feet, wrists, and elbows are seldom involved.

Treatment

This disease is seldom crippling and usually runs a mild course; but there is no way of reversing the damage which has been suffered in the joints. Heat to the joints and aspirin will relieve the pain. The patient should not become overweight, and should rest the joints as much as possible.

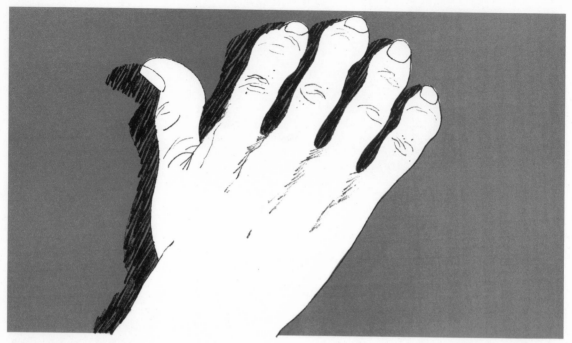

Osteoarthritis: Note that the swelling and distortion is in the distal or last finger joints nearest to the tips of the fingers.

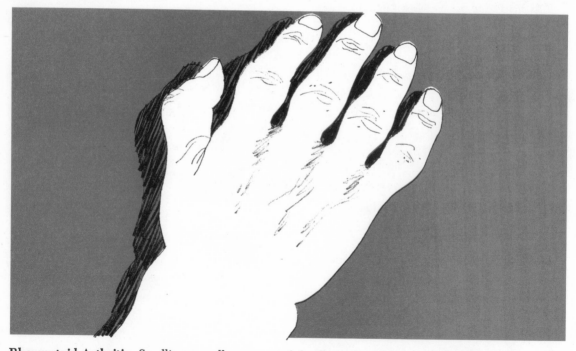

Rheumatoid Arthritis: Swelling, usually very painful, affects the middle and finger joints nearest to the hand.

RHEUMATOID ARTHRITIS
OR ATROPHIC ARTHRITIS

Cause and Nature

The cause is unknown but this disease can be one of the most disabling of all types of arthritis. It usually occurs in people between the ages of twenty and fifty, and is seen more often in women than in men.

Signs and Symptoms

The onset may be very slow, with mild pain in the extremities and slight fever, loss of weight, and easy fatigability. The hands, feet, and wrists are the most common sites, and then the knee, hip, elbow, ankle, and shoulder may be involved. Often the first sign is a spindle-shaped swelling of one of the first interphalangeal joints of a finger—that is, the finger joint, nearest the hand. This is an inflammatory reaction, and there is pain, swelling, and increased heat. On some occasions, it attacks the joints of the spine. This is known as rheumatoid spondylitis, and has a tendency to occur in young men. It may progress until the patient has an absolutely stiff, or poker, back.

The course of rheumatoid arthritis is very unpredictable. A few cases, about one out of four, get well. Another one out of the four will progress to absolute invalidism. The other two will be free of symptoms for a while, only to have them recur as bad as ever.

Treatment

Aspirin should be used to control pain. Rest is very important, but the affected joint should be used through its full range of motion every day, in order to keep it from becoming stiff. Cortisone and other steroids have been used to great advantage in help-

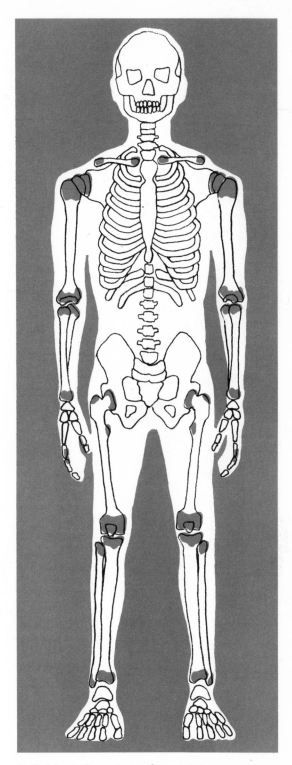

Arthritis—inflamation of a joint may occur where any two bones join each other.

ing the symptoms, but they do not seem to cure the disease. Physiotherapy should be used—that is, heat and massage to the part, and sometimes splinting for a part of the day at least, will help prevent deformity.

The gold salts, used intravenously, were considered at one time as one of the best treatments for this condition, but they should be used with extreme caution.

GLOSSARY

Fatigability   tiredness
Intravenously   into the vein
Onset   start
Spindle-shaped   swelling and pain in what is sometimes called the middle finger joint. This swelling tapers off at each end
Spondylitis   inflammation of the vertebrae
Steroids   medicine used in treatment of arthritis

INFECTIOUS ARTHRITIS

Cause and Nature

Infection of a joint caused by a specific organism usually is due to a gonococcus, pneumococcus, staphylococcus, or streptococcus.

The infection usually enters the joint through the blood stream, but it can on rare occasion be carried into the joint by a stab or penetrating wound.

Signs and Symptoms

The infection may attack several joints at one time or be confined to a single joint. The joint is swollen, red and painful, with increased warmth around the part.

Treatment

Rest in bed. Aspirin to control pain, and an antibiotic to attack the offending organism. Usually penicillin is found to be the most effective antibiotic.

PAINFUL SHOULDER SYNDROME

A very common condition and one which causes a great amount of suffering and disability is the painful shoulder. This painful shoulder syndrome may be classified in three separate groups as described below:

1. Calcified Tendonitis, Subacromial Bursitis, or Subdeltoid Bursitis

Cause and Nature

The cause is not precisely known, but injury and the aging process are suppose to play a major part in causing this condition.

There is a sudden acute onset of severe pain in one shoulder which prevents raising of the arm sideways and which, if untreated, will cause the patient great suffering and loss of sleep.

Several muscles are inserted or fastened to the humerus or upper arm bone just below the shoulder. These muscles are the supraspinatus, the infraspinatus, and the long head of the biceps. The muscles usually are attached to the bones in the form of tendons and inflammation of these tendons is called peritendonitis. Around the upper arm are small potential spaces between the muscles called bursa. Hence we sometimes call this condition subdeltoid bursitis when the inflammation is in the space or bursa underneath the deltoid muscle. After the inflammation has been present for some time, deposits of calcium appear and this is the reason for the term calcified tendonitis.

Signs and Symptoms

The onset of this disease is usually sudden. There is an acute pain in the shoulder region which is constant and prevents the person from raising the arm for such simple

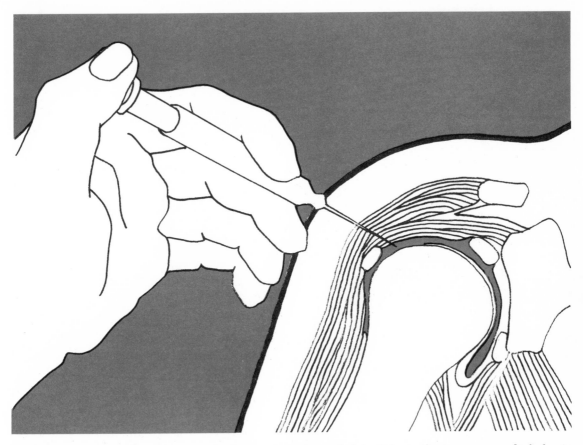

A doctor may inject novocaine or hydro-cortisone into subdeltoid bursa for temporary relief of pain in acute case of bursitis.

movements as combing the hair or shaving. There is no visible swelling or redness, but pressure on the muscles just below the shoulder will cause the pain to be increased.

X ray pictures of the shoulder will show a rounded smooth shadow which is a calcium deposit, and this will make the positive diagnosis of calcified tendonitis.

Treatment

The pain of calcified bursitis or tendonitis may be self limiting or may disappear without treatment, but this may take several weeks or months. The reason it stops hurting is that the small sac of calcium around the tendon ruptures into the bursa or small space between the muscles.

The pain is usually so intense that aspirin or aspirin and codeine must be used to make it bearable. X ray treatments to the shoulder have been known to lessen the pain, and injections of hydrocortisone or novocaine into the bursa will give temporary relief. These must be repeated many times before the condition clears up.

In some severe and persistent cases, an operation is needed to remove the calcium sac. In all cases the outlook is good, for the pain usually goes away and there is no disability or limitation of motion in the shoulder. Sometimes cortisone taken by mouth will relieve the pain.

2. Adhesive Bursitis

(Frozen Shoulder)

Cause and Nature

Frozen shoulder or adhesive bursitis is quite different from calcified bursitis. The onset of pain is gradual and less severe. The cause is not known but is thought to result from inflammation of the shoulder, caused by injury in some cases, which results in the formation of adhesions around the shoulder joint.

Other cases of frozen shoulder result from the immobilization of the shoulder over a long period as would happen if the shoulder were in a cast. A few cases of frozen shoulder are seen in people who have had heart attacks or coronary thrombosis, and sometimes a frozen shoulder will follow an acute attack of calcified bursitis.

Treatment

The treatment of this condition is not as satisfactory as it is in the case of calcified bursitis. Manipulation of the shoulder joint and a system of gradually increasing exercise of this joint must be employed in an effort to secure the return of function. Cortisone by mouth or injections of hydrocortisone do not help, and the use of X ray treatment is of very little benefit. Aspirin to reduce the pain while the exercises are being performed, hot packs, and massage are all helpful.

However, the most important treatment is active and passive exercise under the direction of a doctor.

3. The Shoulder-Hand Syndrome

Cause and Nature

The cause of the shoulder-hand syndrome is not clearly understood. It may follow a stroke, a heart attack, or may result from cervical arthritis. In some cases there is no apparent clear-cut cause. It is differentiated from other painful conditions of the shoulder by the fact that in addition to pain in the shoulder there is a swelling and pain in the hand on the same side. The onset as a rule is gradual and takes place over a considerable period of time.

Signs and Symptoms

A stiffness or slight pain in the shoulder may be the first sign. This may be followed by a swelling and discoloration of the hand on the same side.

The pain and limitation of motion in the shoulder may become quite marked, and if it were not for the swelling of the hand it would be difficult to tell the difference between this condition and subdeltoid bursitis.

As the condition progresses the swelling in the hand subsides and there is a shrinking of the tissues of the hand followed by a loss of use and finally by a contracture or clinching of the fist which cannot be opened up.

All cases do not go on to this deformity. Some get well either as a result of treatment or without any treatment. There is no calcium deposit in the subdeltoid bursa.

Treatment

The treatment in shoulder-hand syndrome is very unsatisfactory because the exact cause of this condition is not known. The use of heat, massage, and exercise does very little good, but the local injections of novocaine or hydrocortisone into the shoulder may give temporary relief from pain. This relief can sometimes be obtained from aspirin or aspirin and codeine. If injections are used they may have to be repeated many times. If cortisone or other steroids are given by mouth they may have to be used over a period of months and the usual precautions will have to be observed.

X ray treatment does not seem to help, but in some cases blocking of the nerve centers above the shoulder seems to give complete relief. Sometimes the nerve centers above the shoulder are completely removed by surgery and the results from this form of treatment are usually very satisfactory.

GLOSSARY

Adhesions union of surfaces normally separate
Cortisone a steroid
Deformity distortion of disfigurement
Immobilization immovable
Inflammation a diseased condition
Manipulation movement of a joint
Syndrome a set of symptoms which occur together

OLECRANON BURSITIS

(Swelling Around the Elbow)

Cause and Nature

Because of its exposed position at the point of the elbow the small bursa, or potential space known as the olecranon bursa, often fills with fluid. This has been called an engineer's elbow because of the frequency of the condition seen in locomotive engineers in the days of the steam engine. The position usually assumed by these men was bearing weight on the right elbow as they rested their right arm on the window while watching the track ahead.

Signs and Symptoms

This is a soft, painless swelling at the point of the elbow. It may be caused by any kind of trauma or injury to the elbow.

Treatment

The fluid from this type of bursitis can be aspirated by a syringe and needle. If a pressure dressing is applied it will seldom fill up again. If the swelling comes back it can be aspirated again. Moist heat may be applied and following that a pressure dressing. This treatment is nearly always successful in the hands of a doctor.

GLOSSARY

Bursa sac or sac-like cavity filled with fluid; found in places in tissue where friction might occur
Bursitis inflammation of one of these sacs
Trauma injury by bruising or wound

GANGLIONS

(Benign Tumors)

Cause and Nature

A ganglion is a cyst which arises within a tendon sheath or on the margin of a joint. This degenerative reaction is most commonly seen on the back of the wrist.

Signs and Symptoms

This enlargement or cyst is usually painless and the most important effect is a cosmetic one. Occasionally there is slight pain and if the lesion is tapped or aspirated by a needle and syringe it always recurs.

Treatment

Years ago the treatment was considered a sharp blow with a book or heavy object.

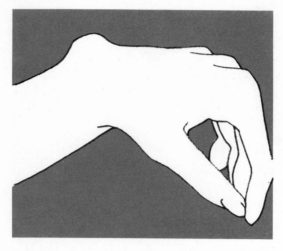

Ganglion: A cyst in a tendon sheath.

This would rupture the cyst, but it always was refilled with a thick gelatinous substance and came into existence again. The only real successful treatment should be removal by surgery and this must be in the hands of a doctor.

GLOSSARY

Aspirate   remove fluid with needle and syringe or special instrument

Cyst   sac containing fluid or partially solid material

Degenerative reaction   changing from normal functions or form to lesser functions. Becoming less useful

Ganglion   cyst within a tendon sheath

Gelatinous   jelly or gelatin like

Lesion   loss of function or break in tissue due to injury or disease

Rupture   break open through excessive pressure

Tendon   band of connective tissue attaching muscle ends to bone

HEEL SPURS

(Painful Heels)

Cause and Nature

Many people suffer from painful heels which are in some cases caused by new for-mation of bone on the heel bone. This is not always the reason however, for in some cases this pain is caused by an inflamed bursa or tendon. The tendon of Achilles is attached to the heel bone or the calcaneus bone. There are two bursa. There is one in front of, and one behind the attachment of this tendon. There is another bursa or small potential space just beneath the heel bone. When there is inflammation of the bursa, this causes pain just as a bursitis near the shoulder will cause pain. Often when the attachment of the tendons to the heel bone have been inflamed for some time, either by trauma or by infection, these tendons will become calcified at their attachments. This calcification or bone formation is called a spur on the heel.

Signs and Symptoms

Pain is the most consistent sign caused by these calcifications. In some instances the heel is extremely tender or painful when weight is borne upon it.

Treatment

The treatment of these painful heels should be conservative. Arch supports and a foam rubber pad cut out so the weight will be borne on other than the painful area will often help.

If the pain is on the back of the heel, then special shoes without a stiff portion behind the heel will reduce the tenderness.

Local injections of novacaine and hydrocortisone will temporarily relieve the inflammation, but they will not remove bone if any spurs are present.

Surgery should be used as the very last resort, because it is not always successful. New spurs may form after the old ones have been removed.

PART 3

Disorders of the Back

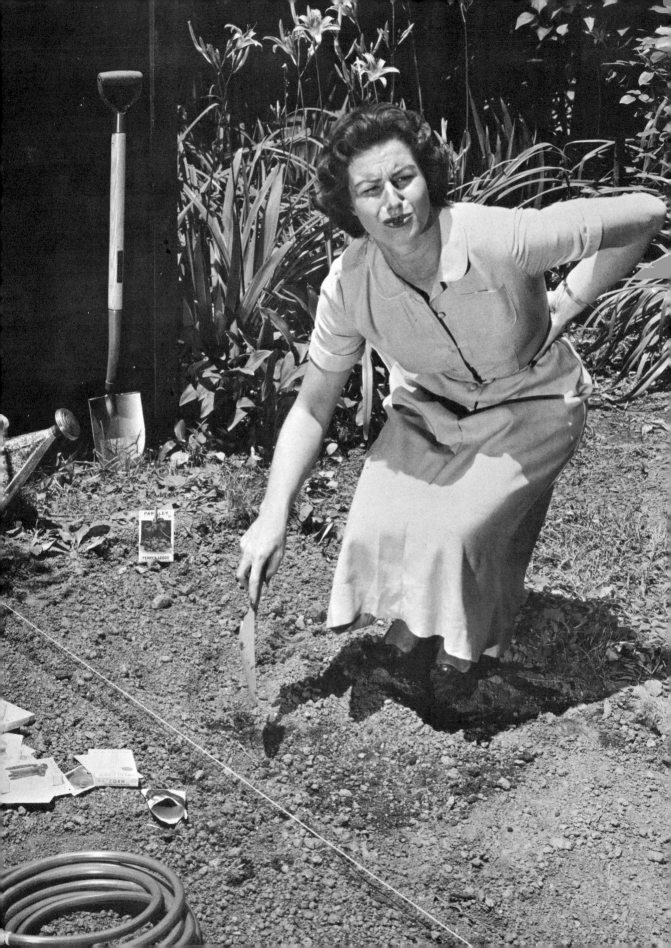

Chapter 23

Backache or
Pain in the Back

THERE IS perhaps no other symptom more commonly experienced than pain in the back. It is therefore important to have a basic understanding of the various conditions that can cause back pain. The following is a list of conditions which should be considered in looking for the cause of backache. These are listed in a sequence which shows the approximate frequency of various causes. For instance, the first listed cause, acute muscular and ligamentous strain, is by far the most common cause of back pain—and so on down the line. The last listed cause, visceral lesions, very rarely causes back pain.

CAUSES OF BACKACHE

1. Acute muscular or ligamentous strain
2. Fracture of the vertebra or vertebral processes
3. Postural defects
   a. dorsal hump-back
   b. lordosis
4. Intervertebral disc disturbances
5. Congenital abnormalities
6. Scoliosis (this is also poor posture)
7. Epiphysitis
8. Osteoarticular lesions (lesions in the vertebral joints)
   a. rheumatoid arthritis
   b. osteoarthritis
   c. vertebral lipping, or spurs
9. Infections
   a. typhoid
   b. tuberculosis
   c. blastomycosis
   d. pyogenic (pus-forming)
10. Neoplastic lesions (cancer, etc.)
    a. primary (arising from the spine)
    b. metastatic (coming to the spine from cancer of the breast or prostate)
11. Osteoporosis (decalcification of vertebra)
    a. senile
    b. post-menopausal
12. Painful coccyx
13. Herniated fat pad
14. Visceral lesions (gall bladder disease, etc.)

These afflictions are many in number, and we will try to describe most of them briefly, taking the back, or spinal cord, in sections and dealing with one section at a time. By beginning at the bottom of the spine we can first take the region that is most often involved in back pain.

319

GLOSSARY

Abnormalities   conditions that are not normal
Blastomycosis   disease caused by fungi
Coccyx   tail bone
Congenital   born with
Epiphysitis   inflammation of the ends of the bones
Herniated   protruding
Intervertebral   between the vertebra
Ligamentous   formed by ligaments
Lordosis   curvature of the spine
Osteo   of the bones
Scoliosis   lateral curvature of the spine
Senile   old
Tuberculosis   a disease
Vertebral   pertaining to the spine bones
Visceral   internal organs

PAIN IN THE LUMBAR AND LUMBOSACRAL SPINE

This may be described as the part of the spinal column that connects with the ilium, or hip bone. It extends upward to the point where the ribs come off the spine. In most cases pain is caused by muscle spasm, and this muscle spasm may result from a strain or injury to this part of the back which damages the muscles and ligaments found here. Sometimes it may be caused by a muscle spasm which is a protective mechanism. In other words, the muscles may stiffen up or go into spasm to protect a vertebra or a bone below, which has been damaged or dislocated. At other times there is some irritation or pressure on one of the nerves which leave the spinal column in the area, as in so-called sciatica.

The following conditions may cause low back pain, and are described separately below:

1. Intervertebral disc lesion (herniated disc); sometimes called discogenic disease

2. Postural lumbosacral strain
3. Acute muscle strains
4. Tumors, primary or secondary
5. Infection
6. Fracture
7. Rheumatoid arthritis
8. Herniated fat pad
9. Senile osteoporosis (decalcification of the bone in old age)
10. Osteoarthritis
11. Congenital anomalies
12. Coccygodynia (painful tailbone or coccyx)

DISCOGENIC DISEASE OF THE SPINE, HERNIATED DISC, AND HERNIATED NUCLEUS PULPOSUS

Cause and Nature

The intervertebral disc or nucleus pulposus is a ring of cartilage and fibrous tissue which lies between the vertebra. A degeneration of these discs is one of the most common causes of low back pain. The discs in the neck or cervical region often degenerate and press on the nerves arising in the spinal cord. This degeneration or herniation will cause pain over the shoulder blade and down the arm on the affected side.

The cause or reason for this degeneration is not known. When the disc degenerates it often herniates or is pushed out and causes pressure on the nerve roots which go out from the spinal column. Trauma such as lifting heavy weights is sometimes thought to be a causative factor.

When this condition is suspected X ray pictures of the vertebrae will show a narrowing of the space between the vertebrae where the disc has degenerated and herniated. Sometimes it is thought necessary to inject some opaque material and take X

ANTERIOR VIEW

1 Frontal Bone
2 Parietal Bones
3 Temporal Bone
4 Malar Bones
5 Bony Orbit
6 Superior Maxilla
7 Bony Cavity of Nose
8 Vomer
9 Teeth
10 Inferior Maxilla
11 5th Cervical Vertebra
12 6th Cervical Vertebra
13 7th Cervical Vertebra
14 1st Dorsal Vertebra
15 Manubrium, or Handle of
   Sternum
16 Body of the Sternum
17 Ensiform Process
18 Clavicle
19 Scapula
20 Coracoid Process of Scapula
21 1st ⎫
22 2nd │
23 3rd │
24 4th ⎬ True Ribs
25 5th │
26 6th │
27 7th ⎭
28 8th ⎫
29 9th │
30 10th ⎬ False Ribs
31 11th │
32 12th ⎭
33 Costal Cartilage
34 12th Dorsal Vertebra
35 1st Lumbar Vertebra
36 2nd Lumbar Vertebra
37 3rd Lumbar Vertebra
38 4th Lumbar Vertebra
39 5th Lumbar Vertebra
40 Sacrum
41 Ilium
42 Crest of Ilium
43 Crest of Pubis
44 Ischium
45 Thyroid or Obturator
   Foramen, round opening
   of Os-Innominatum
46 Humerus
47 Lower Head of Humerus
48 Ulna
49 Radius
50 Carpus
51 Metacarpus
52 Phalanges
53 Shaft of Femur
54 Upper Head of Femur
55 Neck of Femur
56 Great Trochanter of Femur
57 Lesser Trochanter of Femur
58 Outer Tuberosity
59 Inner Tuberosity
60 Patella
61 Tibia
62 Fibula
63 Inner Malleolus (of the Tibia)
64 Outer Malleolus (of the Fibula)
65 Tarsus
66 Metatarsus
67 Phalanges

Courtesy of Zimmer Manufacturing Company
Warsaw, Indiana

POSTERIOR VIEW

1   Occipital **Bone**
2   Parietal **Bones**
3   Sutures
4   Temporal Bones
5   Mastoid Process of
    Temporal Bones
6   Inferior Maxilla
7   1st ⎫
8   2nd ⎪
9   3rd ⎪
10 4th ⎬ Vertebrae of Neck
11 5th ⎪
12 6th ⎪
13 7th ⎭
14 1st Dorsal Vertebra
15 12th Dorsal Vertebra
16 1st Lumbar Vertebra
17 5th Lumbar Vertebra
18 Ribs
19 Clavicle
20 Scapula
21 Spine of Scapula
22 Acromion Process of Scapula
23 Coracoid Process of Scapula
24 Humerus
25 Great Tuberosity of Humerus
26 Ulna
27 Radius
28 Olecranon Process of Ulna
29 Carpus
30 Metacarpus
31 Phalanges
32 Sacrum
33 Coccyx
34 Ilium ⎫
35 Pubis ⎬ Of Hip-Bone
36 Ischium ⎭
37 Shaft of Femur
38 Head of Femur
39 Neck of Femur
40 Great Trochanta of Femur
41 Small Trochanta of Femur
42 Outer Tuberosity of Femur
43 Inner Tuberosity of Femur
44 Inter Condylar Notch of Femur
45 Tibia
46 Fibula
47 Os Calcis
48 Metatarsus
49 Phalanges

Courtesy of Zimmer Manufacturing Company
Warsaw, Indiana

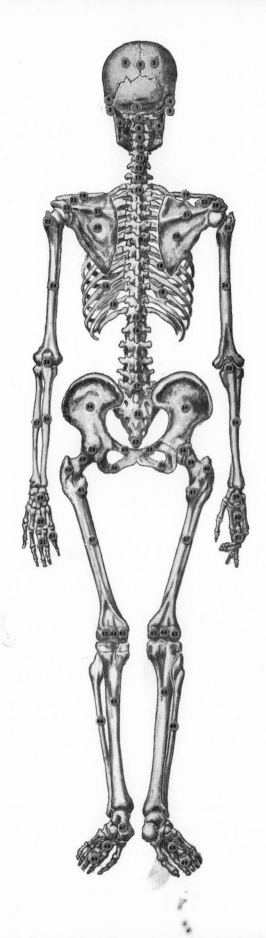

rays to try and determine the exact location of the herniated disc. This is called a myelogram and should be resorted to only when the diagnosis is not certain.

Signs and Symptoms

When the herniated disc is in the low spine or lumbar spine, there is pain in the low back and down the buttock on the affected side; this pain is often projected down the lateral side of the leg and foot. The motion of the back is limited because of pain and the patient tends to lean to the side opposite the pain as this may lessen the pressure on the nerve root. If the patient lies flat on his back he cannot raise the leg on the affected side and keep the knee straight without causing pain.

This condition was often diagnosed as sciatica before the real cause was discovered.

If the disc is in the neck the pain may be felt over the scapula or shoulder blade and it will radiate down the arm. Often the sensation down the arm will feel like needles and pins or an electric shock.

Treatment

The treatment should be conservative when this is possible and it will usually bring relief.

The patient with low back and leg pain should be placed flat on his back in bed. The bed should have boards underneath the mattress. Traction should be applied and moist heat will often help. Pain killers such as aspirin or aspirin and codeine should be used to relieve the pain. This treatment should be tried for two or three weeks.

The patient with a herniated cervical or neck disc should be placed in bed with trac-

tion applied to his head. When he is allowed up a high cervical collar should be worn until the pain is relieved. Analgesics such as aspirin or aspirin and codeine should be used.

If the pain in the low back is not relieved by the above treatment, traction, bed rest, and a back brace may help. As a last resort surgery should be attempted and the diseased or herniated disc removed. At times after removing the disc it is thought wise to ankylose or fuse the two vertebrae on each side of the herniated disc.

This surgery is not always successful and should be performed by an orthopedist and a neurosurgeon working together.

GLOSSARY

Cervical   pertaining to the neck
Herniated   protrusion of a loop, or knuckle, of an organ or tissue through an abnormal opening
Intervertebral   between the vertebrae
Opaque   substance light cannot pass through
Pulposus   any soft tissue
Sciatica   inflammation of sciatic nerve
Vertebra   anyone of the thirty-three bones of the spinal column

POSTURAL LUMBOSACRAL STRAIN

Cause and Nature

This backache occurs over long periods of time and is usually caused by poor posture; that is, a tilted pelvis which may result from one leg being slightly shorter than the other. In a woman it may be caused by wearing heels that are too high, and being overweight.

Signs and Symptoms

Careful measurement of the legs may reveal that one is shorter than the other. The pain is usually low-grade and constant, lasting over a long period of time. It is relieved by rest, and is aggravated by prolonged exercise.

Treatment

Correction of the difference in length of the legs by building up the heel on the short side may help. Bed rest with hot moist compresses will relieve the pain and cause the muscles to relax, but unless the cause is removed the pain will recur.

Women who are overweight and have prominent abdomens might reduce, and could perhaps relieve the discomfort by wearing low heels.

GLOSSARY

Aggravated   make worse

ACUTE MUSCLE STRAIN IN THE LOWER BACK

Cause and Nature

This severe pain may be brought on by a fall, by twisting the back suddenly, or by lifting a heavy object. The onset is sudden.

Signs and Symptoms

The muscles in the lower back are tight, and the pain is usually confined to the strained portion; that is, it does not radiate down the leg. This type of pain is usually severe and can be incapacitating.

Treatment

Rest on a hard bed for a few days, applying wet, hot compresses will usually relieve the pain. Aspirin or aspirin with codeine may be taken to lessen the discomfort. After the pain is completely gone, exercise to strengthen the back muscles may help prevent a recurrence.

BEND YOUR KNEES—DO NOT STRAIN YOUR BACK

Lifting heavy objects is one of the most important causes of pain in the back if the lifting is done in the wrong way.

The State Compensation Insurance Fund of California gives the following method as the proper way to lift in order to prevent injury:

1. Size up the load—make sure you can handle it easily yourself—if not, get help
2. Face the load squarely—get a firm footing and spread your feet about twelve inches apart
3. Bend your knees and get a firm grip on the load
4. Keep your back straight and lift by straightening your legs
5. Lift slowly and evenly without quick, jerky movements
6. Keep the load close to your body throughout the whole procedure
7. If it is necessary to turn, change the position of your feet—do not twist your body

FIBROSITIS

(Sore Muscles)

Cause and Nature

The term fibrositis is used by many doctors to identify a group of symptoms called a syndrome. There are so many types of this condition that it cannot be described as a single disease.

A comprehensive definition might state: Any condition causing pain, stiffness, limitation of motion, and soreness which is not located in the joints could be called fibrositis.

There have been many causes for this condition brought forward, but no one cause has been proven to be the single agent. For instance, it has been said to be caused by injury, by infection, by a faulty metabolism, and in some cases by a state of mind. It has not been proven to be a psychosomatic disease, but it is certainly seen most often in tense, keyed-up, or highly excitable persons.

One good explanation of the cause in some people has been tenseness which causes the muscles to tighten up and thereby cause poor circulation, which is followed by pain or soreness in the muscles.

Signs and Symptoms

The symptoms most often seen are pain or stiffness in the muscles. There may also be a soreness or tenderness of the muscles.

In some patients the doctor can find a real tender spot as if the muscle has a lump in it and this is sometimes called a "trigger point."

These symptoms may come on following mental or physical fatigue; they may come on gradually or the onset may be sudden.

Sometimes the pain is dull and aching and at other times it may be sharp or burning. It may be in the low back, the extremities, or in the chest. Often people with fibrositis in the anterior chest region think they have heart trouble and they should see their family doctor to rule this out.

One other characteristic of fibrositis which may serve to differentiate it from actual arthritis or injuries is that the person with fibrositis seems to feel better with exercise. The pain and soreness lessens when the affected part is used.

Treatment

If a person can be taught to relax, both mentally and physically, this will often relieve the pain. In many cases when they are reassured and told that they do not have arthritis or heart disease, they become better. A warm bath will often help the patient relax physically. A hot water bottle or heating pad applied to the painful area is often helpful. In cases where a "trigger point" can be found, a local injection of novocaine will cause the pain to dissappear.

People who suffer from this syndrome should be careful not to become too excited or tense. They should avoid sudden extreme changes in climate, and try to prevent getting wet and chilled by exposing themselves too much to unfavorable weather. They should also try and prevent either mental or physical fatigue.

GLOSSARY

Fibrositis   inflammed fibers
Psychosomatic   derived from the mind and the body
Syndrome   a group of symptoms

TUMORS, PRIMARY OR SECONDARY

Cause and Nature

The presence of a tumor known as a myeloma may cause pain in the back, and is known as a primary tumor. This usually appears in older people and is not very common.

A secondary tumor could result from metastasis, or spreading, of cancer from other parts of the body—such as cancer of the breast or cancer of the prostate.

Signs and Symptoms

X rays are needed to diagnose these tumors. The pain caused by them usually comes on slowly and is not helped much by heat.

Treatment

This is symptomatic and should be supervised by a doctor. Aspirin and codeine, and heat usually lessen the pain.

GLOSSARY

Symptomatic   treating the symptom

INFECTION

Cause and Nature

The cause may be infection of the vertebrae or intervertebral discs following typhoid, undulant fever, or blastomycosis. The pain follows infections of the entire body, and is not seen as often now that we have antibiotics.

Signs and Symptoms

There is usually a fever with chills preceding the pain in the back. In some cases the fever may go down, only to return time and time again.

Treatment

The treatment consists of treating the disease with antibiotics and should be under the supervision of a doctor.

GLOSSARY

Blastomycosis   an infection caused by fungus
Intervertebral   between vertebrae
Typhoid fever   a communicable disease
Undulant fever   a disease

FRACTURE

Cause and Nature

A fracture of one of the lower vertebrae is usually caused by a fall or other type of ac-

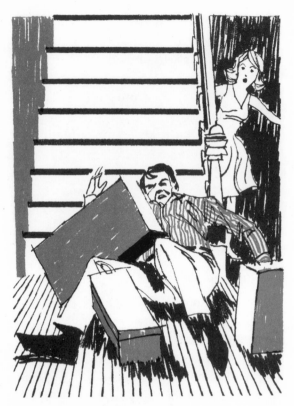

Don't move. Call Doctor.

cident, such as a car wreck. Sometimes we have a spontaneous fracture when the body of the vertebra is eaten away by a tumor.

Signs and Symptoms

The pain is sudden in onset following an accident, and X ray will usually reveal the trouble. As a rule, the pain and tenderness are pretty well confined to the site of injury.

Treatment

The patient should not be moved without using the greatest care to avoid increasing the fracture. In other words, the back should be kept perfectly straight when moving the patient. A doctor should be called at once and he will start the proper treatment. The object is to keep the spinal column from being pinched, and thus causing paralysis.

RHEUMATOID ARTHRITIS

Cause and Nature

The cause of rheumatoid arthritis is unknown. The onset or start of the pain is usually insidious and very slow, gradually building up. This usually occurs in younger people from twenty to forty years of age, and is seen more often in males than in females. Gradually it becomes a dull constant ache which seems worse in the morning, and is aggravated by exercise.

Signs and Symptoms

There are many tests a doctor may take to diagnose rheumatoid arthritis of the spine, and the disease may occur in any portion of the spine. X rays, blood counts, and sedimentation rates will usually help determine the diagnosis, along with the persistent gradually increasing pain, and a greater and greater limitation of motion in the back. In other words, the back becomes stiff—the so-called poker back.

Treatment

This condition requires long and careful treatment in order to prevent stiffening in a bad position, and to prevent suffering. A doctor should be in charge.

HERNIATED FAT PAD

Cause and Nature

The cause is a fat pad between the muscles, causing compression of the muscles in the back, and consequently pain.

Signs and Symptoms

The pain usually radiates down to the buttocks and up the affected muscle. A small tender mass can be palpated, or felt.

Treatment

Infiltration with procaine will give temporary relief, but surgical removal may be needed for permanent relief.

DECALCIFICATION OF THE VERTEBRAE IN OLD AGE

(Senile Osteoporosis)

Cause and Nature

Sometimes in old age the vertebrae become soft because of loss of calcium. This may cause a wedging of the vertebral bodies, or even a fracture from the slightest injury such as sitting down hard on the floor.

Signs and Symptoms

The curvature, or hump, in the back may become more prominent, and there will be pain at the point of injury.

Treatment

Rest in bed with the proper posture, moist compresses with heat, and aspirin for pain will often relieve the discomfort. Sometimes traction is needed, or even a brace may be necessary. X rays should be

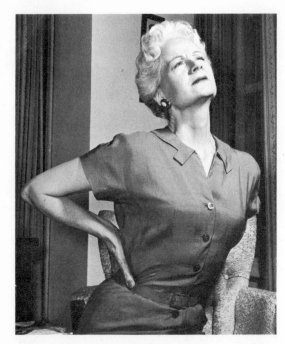

Women with Osteoporosis. Loss of calcium thins bones. Detected by X ray only.

taken under the supervision of a doctor.

The treatment of osteoporosis, has been improved upon by the discovery that if the disease is detected early enough, a simple thing such as taking "the pill" (contraceptive pill) every day will prevent the bones from becoming so brittle. Another form of treatment is called an anabolic or "building up" regime. This means taking thyroid, one-half gr., daily, taking "the pill" or some form of estrogen, by women, or androgen by men, every day; to this is added a strong vitamin such as Thex Forte three times a week.

OSTEOARTHRITIS OR VERTEBRAL LIPPING

Cause and Nature

In older people, sometimes a spur will form on the edge of a vertebra. This is called "lipping," and occurs in most old people.

Signs and Symptoms

This type of arthritis may be entirely painless and only detected by X ray. When there is pain it is usually aggravated by exercise, and relieved by a good night's rest in bed.

Treatment

Rest in bed with moist heat application and aspirin, ten grains, every three or four hours, will usually result in improvement.

The bed should be firm or it can be made firm by placing a board under the mattress. This prevents sagging of the back which puts a strain on the muscles which have been irritated by the arthritic spurs.

GLOSSARY

Spur   outgrowth from a tissue
Vertebrae   bones of the spine

CONGENITAL ANOMALIES

Cause and Nature

The cause of this is faulty development in the lower spine. Any part of the vertebra may fail to fuse, or may be absent, or may be in poor position, as in spondylolisthesis. These defects can be detected by X ray.

Signs and Symptoms

Usually the pain is mild and the abnormality may go unnoticed. Mild pain may be treated by conservative methods such as rest and heat.

Treatment

In large abnormalities causing severe pain, surgery may be needed to correct the defect. Sometimes it is possible to fuse the vertebrae together and get rid of the abnormal position, thereby correcting the pain.

GLOSSARY

Abnormality   not normal
Fuse   bring together
Vertebrae   bones of the spine

COCCYGODYNIA

Cause and Nature

The tailbone causes pain often after injury such as sitting down forcibly on a hard object. Sometimes there is arthritis in the joint between the coccyx and the sacrum.

Signs and Symptoms

This pain may be constant, and is not relieved by rest. It may be aggravated by sitting in a chair, especially a soft chair. X rays may show arthritis or a fracture.

Treatment

Conservative treatment, such as hot baths or sitting on an air-ring may help. Aspirin can be taken to relieve the pain. If all attempts at conservative treatment are not satisfactory, then removal of the coccyx by surgery should be considered.

GLOSSARY

Arthritis   disease of the joints
Coccyx   tail bone
Fracture   break
Sacrum   bone of pelvis

PAIN IN THE THORACIC SPINE

The thoracic region of the spine is that part which begins where the ribs begin, and extends up to the base of the neck. The causes of pain in this portion of the spine are very much the same as causes of pain in the lower, or lumbar spine, described before. The treatment is the same.

The one main difference in these two portions of the spine, as far as pain is concerned, is that often gall bladder disease will refer acute pain to the right thoracic spine or shoulder. The treatment of this condition, of course, consists of treatment of the gall bladder disease.

PAIN IN THE CERVICAL SPINE

The cervical spine is that portion of the spine known as the neck, and again the causes of pain in this region of the spine are similar to those in other parts of the back. One of the most frequent causes of pain in the neck is the so-called "whip-lash" injury which follows an unexpected snap of the neck following a rear-end auto collision. The pain may show up several days after the accident, and the pain and stiffness of the neck may be acute.

Bed rest, moist heat, traction and analgesics such as aspirin or aspirin with codeine, should relieve this condition in a few days. X rays should be taken to rule out fracture.

The ordinary stiff neck which is so often seen may be caused by any number of conditions, such as sore throat, a strain to the muscles of the neck, etc. This condition should be treated conservatively by placing the neck at rest and applying moist heat. Traction sometimes helps, and always take enough aspirin or other analgesics, because a comfortable patient will recover more quickly than one who does not get sufficient rest because of pain.

In summary, then, it may be said that most causes of neck pain are simple ones which cause muscle spasm, which in turn is painful. The most effective forms of treatment are:

1. Rest on a firm bed; always place a board under the mattress
2. Apply moist heat to the painful area several times a day
3. Take enough aspirin or other analgesic to keep comfortable
4. Traction is helpful in some cases, and this should be supervised by a doctor

If the above remedies do not bring relief, then X rays and a good examination by a doctor are in order.

When neck pain is caused by discogenic disease or herniated discs in the cervical spine the pain may be referred to the shoulder blade and down the arm on the side where the nerve is pinched. In these cases traction is the treatment of choice, and again this should be under the supervision of a doctor.

GLOSSARY

Analgesics   pain relievers
Fracture   break
Gall bladder   organ of body

PART 4

Disorders of Vision

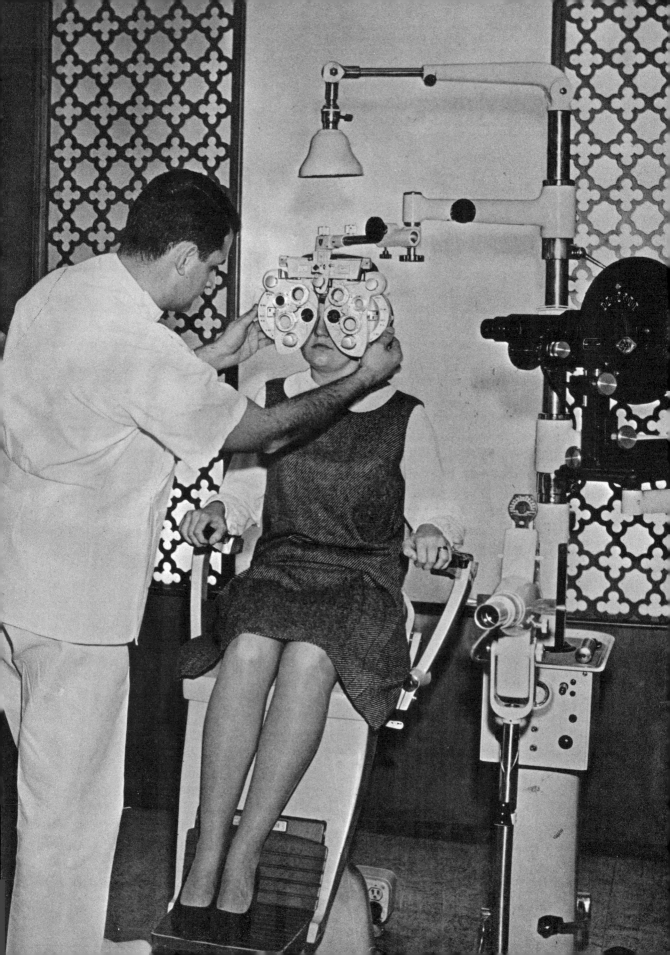

Chapter 24

Diseases of the Eyes

VISUAL DEFECTS are very common in the people of the United States. This fact was brought out by a recent survey. Vision tests performed on a large number of persons showed that only 43.5 percent of these people had normal vision. This brings out the unpleasant fact that over half the people in this country do not have normal vision. Almost one in every ten persons was found to have the use of only one eye, and about one out of two Americans wears glasses or contact lenses. There are 960,000 blind persons and an additional 2,064,000 people with serious visual impairments in our country. These facts would seem to indicate how important it is to detect visual imperfections early and correct them as well as possible, before they have a chance to become serious.

COMMON DEFECTS OF THE EYE

The most common defects of the eye are inherited and are caused by variations in the shape and size of the eyeball. These can usually be corrected by wearing the proper glasses. The process of correcting these defects is called correcting errors in refraction. These examinations are made by eye doctors. A few of these defects will be explained here.

First of all, we will take the normal eye. It can be considered as an optical instrument composed of different curvatures and different refractive materials or fluids, through which rays of light must pass. If the eyeball is perfect in shape, the rays of light in passing through the eye are bent so that they come to a point, or focus, on the retina in back of the eyeball, as in this diagram.

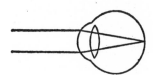

Diagram of Normal Eye

GLOSSARY

Impairments   diminishing in strength
Imperfections   defects
Inherited   from one generation to another
Retina   the back of the eye
Visual   pertaining to sight

333

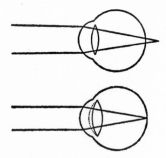

Diagram Showing Hyperopia
or Far Sightedness

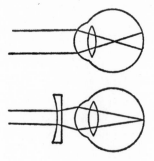

Diagram Showing Myopia
or Near Sightedness

HYPEROPIA

(Far-sightedness)

If the eyeball is too short from front to back, the rays of light will come to a focus behind the retina, and vision will be blurred. In slight degrees of far-sightedness the person is able to correct it by accommodating; that is, the eyeball is made longer, pushing the retina back, and the shape of the lens is changed, becoming fatter to bend the light rays more. This change is automatic, but if it goes on too much the person has symptoms, especially from reading or looking at nearby objects. These symptoms are a feeling of tiredness, fatigue, or headaches. This can be corrected by wearing proper glasses with a convex lens which bends the light rays, and causes them to focus at the proper spot.

MYOPIA

(Near-sightedness)

In this condition the eyeball is too long and the light rays are brought into focus ahead of the retina.

Since the eye has no mechanism for accommodating to this condition, the only way it can be corrected is by the proper concave lens which will cause the rays of light to be brought into focus further back on the retina. A near-sighted person does not have the headaches and eye strain which the far-sighted person experiences, because reading does not bother him. The only symptom he experiences is difficulty in seeing distant objects clearly. This can be corrected by proper glasses.

GLOSSARY

Focus   adjustment for vision
Retina   back part of the eye

ACCOMMODATION

If the object to be seen is close to the eye, the rays of light it sends are not parallel, but divergent. In order for these close objects to be seen clearly, the eyeball has to become longer, pushing the back of the eye, or the retina, further back so the rays will focus on the retina and not behind it. To help this out, the structure in the eye called the lens changes its shape, helping to bring the rays into focus at the proper place. These changes are called accommodation, and if it were not for this power, no normal individual would be able to see in detail any object closer to him than 20 feet away. This accommodation takes place automatically without our being aware of it. As a person gets older he loses this power of accommodation, and we see older people holding a paper out at arm's length in order to read small print.

GLOSSARY

Divergent   extend in different direction
Rays   small particles of light

ASTIGMATISM

This is a refractive error, which means having different curves in the same eye. It can be explained by saying that the normal eye has the curvature of the cornea like the inside of a bowl, but the eye with astigmatism has a cornea with curves like the inside of a spoon. Another comparison may be used—the normal cornea may have curves like a basketball, while the astigmatic cornea will have curves like a football. This condition must be corrected by using proper lenses.

In most cases, myopia or hyperopia may be mixed with astigmatism, and the lens in the glasses must contain cylindrical lens to correct the astigmatism as well as the lens for correction of the near-sightedness or far-sightedness. A person with a high degree of astigmatism must wear his glasses all the time.

GLOSSARY

Cornea   the transparent part of the coat of the eyeball which admits light

DISEASES OF THE EYES AND EYELIDS
Sty or Hordeolum

Cause and Nature

This is an acute inflammation of the eyelid, caused by a staphylococcus infection of one of the small glands in the eyelid.

Signs and Symptoms

The eyelid involved becomes quite red, swollen, and usually painful. The largest swelling appears at the root of one of the eyelashes.

Treatment

Hot compresses with just plain hot water applied to the lid for ten minutes at a time, three or four times during the day, will usually cause the infection to come to a head, or in other words, will bring about the formation of pus. This small pustule usually ruptures spontaneously, or it may be pricked by a sterile needle when it has become yellow. Once the pus is evacuated, the eyelid rapidly returns to normal. While the pus is draining out, the eyes should be washed out frequently with boric acid solution, in

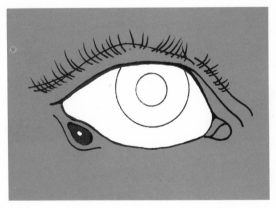

Stye: A painful infection of a small gland in the eyelid.

order to keep the infection from spreading. If the sty is large and quantities of pus drain out, it is well to use some antiseptic eye drops such as sulamyde ophthalmic solution.

Chronic Inflammation of Eyelid Margins

(*Blepharitis Marginalis*)

Cause and Nature

This chronic condition is caused by staphylococcus infection, or by Hemophilus duplex. Sometimes it is a result of seborrheic dermatitis. This condition is not caused by eye strain or improperly fitted glasses, but it may be aggravated by these things.

Signs and Symptoms

The lid margins assume a red scaliness and sometimes small ulcerations appear at the base of some of the eyelashes. There is very little pain.

Treatment

Seborrheic blepharitis should be treated by clearing up dandruff of the scalp or infections of the ears. Selsun may be used for curing dandruff of the scalp, but should never be allowed near the eyes. Penicillin ophthalmic ointment will usually clear up streptococcus blepharitis, or sulamyde ophthalmic ointment applied twice a day will act promptly.

Chalazion

Cause and Nature

A chalazion is a painless swelling that appears deep in an eyelid, not on the margin. It is a chronic condition which resembles a cyst in the eyelid. It is caused by an infection of one of the glands in the eyelid.

Signs and Symptoms

A painless swelling appears in the upper or lower lid. It may grow over a period of several weeks and then cease to grow. In some cases it may be absorbed and leave no trace.

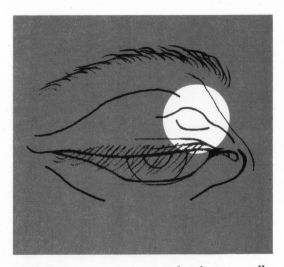

A Chalazion appears as a painless lump usually in the upper eyelid.

Treatment

If the chalazion or swelling in the eyelid does not disappear, it will have to be incised by a doctor who usually does this under local anesthetic, making a small cut over the lump on the inside of the eyelid, and expressing the contents.

GLOSSARY

Chronic   of long duration
Cyst   a sac
Expressing   taking out

Conjunctivitis

(Pink Eye)

Cause and Nature

Any infection of the conjunctiva is called conjunctivitis, and there are many bacteria which will cause these infections. The one described is called pink eye, and is common among children. It is caused by a specific bacillus called Koch-Weeks bacillus. It is highly contagious and is passed from one

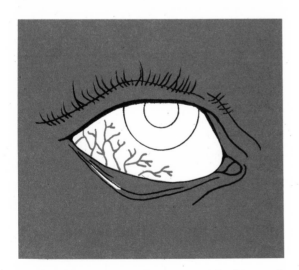

Conjunctivitis is an inflamation of the lining of the eye and eyelid.

person to another by using the same towel or wash cloth. Hence the person with pink eye should be isolated from other people to a certain extent.

Signs and Symptoms

The conjunctiva become pink. There is slight swelling but very little pain. Bright light aggravates the condition, so dark glasses should be worn in the sunlight. There may be itching or burning of the eyes.

Treatment

There are a great many ophthalmic solutions which will clear up this condition. Sodium sulamyde, ten percent, ophthalmic solution is one of the best. Drops of this should be placed in the eye three times a day. Again, let it be emphasized that one should use great care to avoid passing this condition on to someone else. After treating a person with pink eye the hands should always be washed.

GLOSSARY

Bacillus   organism that causes infection
Conjunctiva   the mucous membrane which lines the inner surface of the eyelid and covers the front of the eyeball
Isolated   separate; apart from
Ophthalmic   of or in the area of the eye

Trachoma

(Granulated Lids)

Cause and Nature

This disease of the conjunctiva is caused by a virus. It is one of the chief causes of blindness in some foreign countries but not in the United States. In this country it is commonly seen among Indians and in the

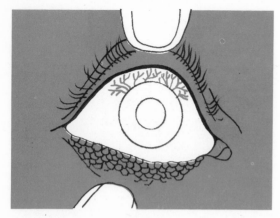

Trachoma or granulated lids: a chronic infection of the eyelids.

southern states. It is sometimes called "granulated lids" or "sore lids." If left untreated it may lead to blindness.

Signs and Symptoms

The onset of trachoma is usually acute, like catarrhal conjuntivitis, but after seven to ten days of red swollen lids, small follicles, or bumps appear on the inner surface of the lids. These gradually increase in number and size until after three or four weeks the diagnosis can be made. Secondary infection causes pus formation. There is itching and burning, and a feeling of having a foreign body in the eye. After about six weeks the under sides of the lids will have so many bumps on them that they will resemble a raspberry.

Treatment

The treatment of trachoma is difficult and should always be carried out by an eye specialist, if possible. The sulfa drugs and penicillin help, as does the use of copper. It takes a long time, and a doctor should be consulted during the early stages of the disease.

GLOSSARY

Catarrhal   pertaining to inflammation of any mucous membrane
Conjunctiva   mucous membrane lining the inner surface of the eyelid and covering the front of the eyeball
Granulated   rough or raw surface
Virus   cause of infection

ACUTE GLAUCOMA

Cause and Nature

There is a sudden rapid rise of the pressure within the eye, which is accompanied by severe pain in the eye and head.

Signs and Symptoms

There is sometimes a warning sign, such as seeing a halo around lights at night, sharp shooting pains in the eye, and a headache.

Treatment

This is a real emergency and should be seen by an eye doctor as soon as possible. If the patient is seen when the first warnings come, the treatment is much easier and is usually more effective. The doctor may be able to relax the pressure by the use of drops. If not, the patient should be seen within twenty-four hours by a competent ophthalmic surgeon who can relieve the pressure by surgery, and thereby save the vision.

SECONDARY GLAUCOMA

Cause and Nature

The cause is increased pressure within the eye, and the reason for this increase can be laid to something specific, such as an

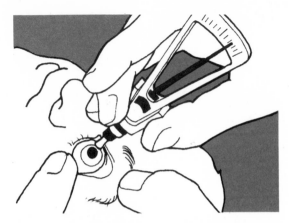

A Tonometer is used to measure tension in the eyeball for early detection of glaucoma.

acute infection of the eye with swelling of the parts, or by a tumor which may press on the drainage spaces.

Signs and Symptoms

There is pain in the eye and headache. The eyeball becomes hard and the doctor is able to read the increased intraocular pressure by an instrument called a tonometer.

Treatment

The treatment should be aimed at the cause of the glaucoma—the infection or tumor. The pressure can usually be kept down by using eye drops to dilate the pupils until the primary cause is removed. Very seldom is surgery needed in this type, although sometimes it becomes necessary.

PRIMARY SIMPLE GLAUCOMA

Cause and Nature

This is a disease of late middle life and does its damage because the increased pressure often is not noted in time to start effective treatment.

Signs and Symptoms

The early signs are:

1. A need for frequent changes of glasses
2. Difficulty in adjusting the eyes to new glasses and then having to change again
3. Blurred vision and seeing halos around lights
4. Sharp, shooting pains in the eyes
5. Headaches

The last two symptoms may not be present. Late signs are night blindness and reduction in vision.

Therefore, if you need to change your glasses often, see halos or rainbows around lights, or have spells of blurred vision, be sure you see a good ophthalmologist or eye specialist. Especially, if there is a history of glaucoma in your family, do not neglect to pay heed to these signs.

Treatment

The treatment of glaucoma should be in the hands of an eye specialist or ophthalmologist, and the sooner he begins treatment the better the outlook. Continuation of increased pressure will result in blindness if untreated. The ophthalmologist may be able to halt the progress by the use of eye drops and diuretics or other drugs. If this isn't possible, surgery is the only answer.

STRABISMUS, CROSSEYE OR SQUINT

This condition is usually called crossed eyes and it usually develops early—at birth or at least about the age of two.

Cause and Nature

There are many muscles which cause the eyes to move from one direction to the oth-

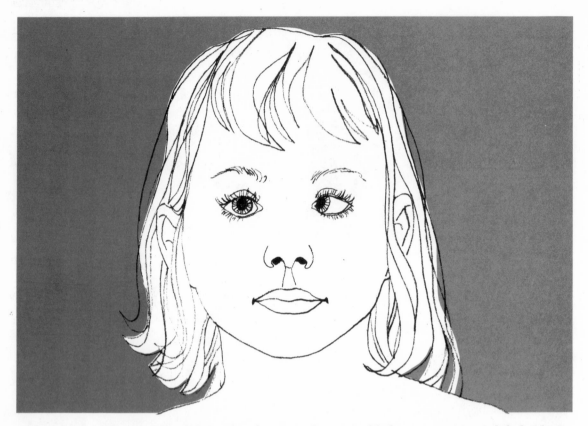

Crossed eye: Correction should be undertaken as early as possible by a competent ophthalmologist.

er, and the eyes usually move together. However, if a muscle or a set of muscles in one of the eyes is weak or paralytic, this eye rolls out or inward as the case may be. The squint may affect both eyes.

Signs and Symptoms

The crossed eye is easily detected in the young child, and if it is not corrected this may sometimes cause blindness in one eye. That is, if one eye moves normally, being supplied by adequate muscles, and the other eye rolls out, the child does not use the eye that is crossed, and does all the seeing with the one good eye. The bad or impaired eye becomes lazy with no work to do, and if this is allowed to continue, the child will become blind in one eye.

Treatment

The services of a good eye specialist should be sought as soon as the squint is detected. Sometimes the muscle imbalance can be corrected by glasses or by exercises. Other cases need surgery, and in some cases two or three operations are necessary. The condition can be corrected, and the sooner the better.

Often when one eye becomes lazy because of muscle weakness, the doctor will put a patch over the good eye and force the patient to use the weak eye. This strengthens the muscles of the weak eye. There are other exercises which may be used, but the services of a good eye doctor, an ophthalmologist, are imperative.

CATARACT

Cause and Nature

A cataract is a frosting or formation of opacity of the lens. It may occur in one or both eyes, and also may occur at any age, although nearly all cataracts occur after the age of fifty. There are many causes—infection, injury, diabetes, or just old age—which may contribute to the formation of the cataracts.

Signs and Symptoms

There is always one sure sign of cataract formation, and that is a gradually increasing blurring of the vision in one or both eyes, which cannot be corrected by glasses.

Treatment

This depends on whether the cataract involves one or both eyes, and also the extent of the loss of vision. There is no treatment for cataracts except surgery. This should be placed in the hands of a good eye specialist or ophthalmologist. The time of operation should be decided upon by the doctor. It is no longer considered necessary to wait until the cataract is ripe, or fully developed, before operating. Many things enter into this decision, such as the rate of growth of the cataract, the vision in the other eye, etc., but the doctor should decide this.

ACCIDENTS AND INJURIES TO THE EYES

Foreign Bodies in the Eyes

Cause and Nature

Any foreign body in the eye may cause a laceration or abrasion of the cornea, and since the foreign body may be covered with bacteria, infection may result and ulceration follow.

This ulceration could cause scar formation which could lead to loss of vision.

Signs and Symptoms

There is usually pain and watering of the eye when a foreign body is present.

Treatment

Never try to rub out a foreign body because this may scratch the eye. Try to wash the foreign body out with clean, plain water, or boric acid solution. If this treatment is unsuccessful, a doctor should be seen at once for expert assistance.

Contusions of the Eye

Cause and Nature

A blow from a blunt instrument, a fist, or a snowball may cause a contusion of the eyeball, and if severe enough this may cause hemorrhage within the eyeball.

Signs and Symptoms

There is usually pain, watering of the eye, and blurring of vision. The tissues around the eye may become considerably swollen and turn black and blue.

Treatment

The patient should stay in bed if possible, and cold applications or compresses should be applied every three hours for the first day. A doctor should be seen if the eye does not improve rapidly after the above treatment. If a perforation of the eyeball is present, a doctor should be consulted at once.

A drug which causes bruises, black eyes, etc., to clear up more rapidly is now on the market. It is called Varidase and should be taken only under doctor's supervision.

Chemical Injuries to the Eye

Cause and Nature

In modern industry, many chemicals are used; indeed chemicals may be present in fumes with which people come in contact every day. Hence, it is not uncommon for some of these chemicals to affect the eyes.

Signs and Symptoms

There is usually burning and watering of the eyes with some swelling and redness.

Treatment

This is one of the real emergencies which must be treated at once. The patient cannot wait until the doctor comes but must instantly begin to wash the eyes out with large amounts of cold water. Duck the head into a bucket of water with the eyes open. Then, if some bicarbonate of soda is handy, put some of that into the water. A small rubber bulb syringe can be used to irrigate the eyes under the eyelids, etc. Use large amounts of water. Then cold bandages or applications should be placed on the eyes, and a doctor consulted as soon as possible.

PART 5

Accidents and First Aid

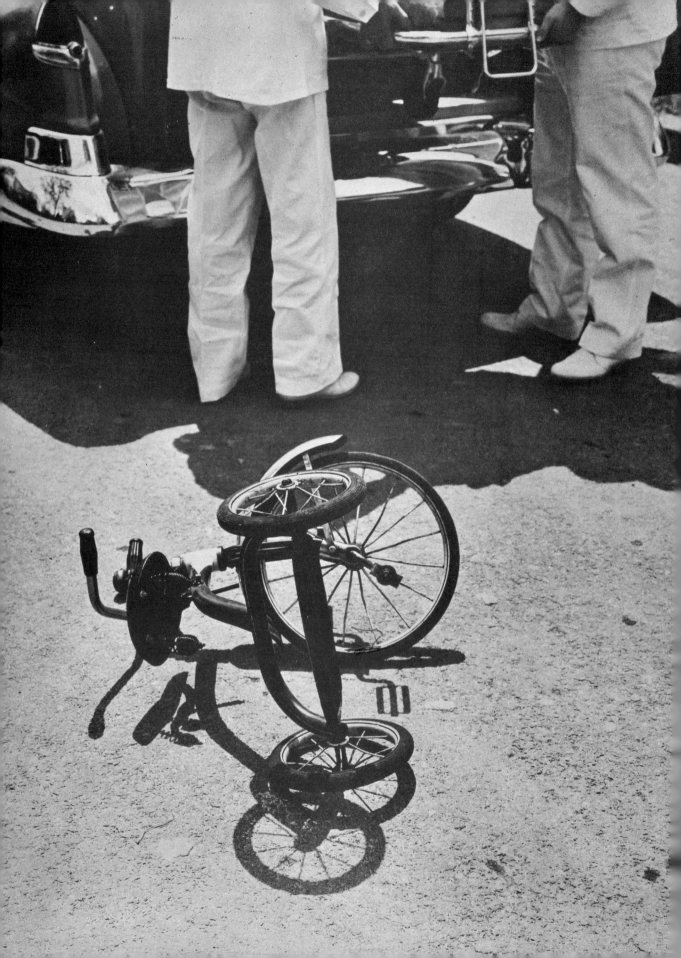

Chapter 25

Accidents: Their Cause and Prevention

THIS IS BY FAR the most important chapter in the entire book. It is important because if you read it and take the precautions which are recommended, you may save the life of one who is very dear to you.

Accidents are the greatest cause of death of children between one and nineteen years of age. Just as tuberculosis years ago, was called "The Captain of the Men of Death," today accidents have become the worst danger where children are concerned.

In order to prove the above statements and to impress upon the reader the impor-

tance of reading this chapter over and over again, a few statistics will be quoted. All of us worry about whether our children will catch diphtheria, whooping cough, lockjaw, smallpox, typhoid fever, influenza, and measles. The children can be immunized against all of these diseases, but they cannot be immunized against accidents by any injection the doctor may give them. They can only be protected against accidents by intelligent parents who know the causes of accidents and who, if they don't know them, are willing to study a chapter such as this and put into operation the things they learn. This can be done by protecting the child when he is too young to be taught facts, and by educating him as he grows old enough to learn.

All of us may worry at one time or another about the danger of our child becoming affected by pneumonia, cancer or leukemia, tuberculosis, poliomyelitis, stomach and intestinal infections such as appendicitis, kidney disease, or heart disease. Let us take a look at some reliable statistics on the causes of death for ages one through fourteen years.

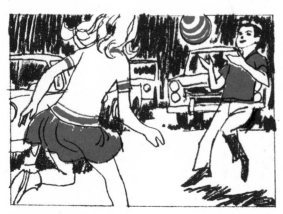

Playing in the street results in accidents.

345

DEATHS OF CHILDREN

The deaths caused by accidents outnumber the total of all the other dread diseases added together. The following statistics are from one year in the United States:

Deaths caused by accidents........ 10,313
Deaths caused by disease.......... 10,064
   Cancer and leukemia.......... 3,156
   Pneumonia 2,821
   Tuberculosis 1,263
   Polio 862
   Stomach and intestinal infections. 779
   Kidney disease 673
   Heart disease 510

Millions of dollars are being spent every year to find medicines and vaccines to fight these seven dreadful diseases, and it is only recently that money is being allocated to study the thing that causes more deaths than all of them put together. The results of this research is here for your use if you will only see fit to use it.

Before we proceed further with these gruesome statistics (and remember that every figure shown here is the absolute truth; most of the statistics were compiled by the National Safety Council), let us consider the other by-products of accidents, excluding death. Accidents cripple for life three or four times as many children as they kill. Forty thousand to fifty thousand children in the United States are crippled for life each year by accidents. Do you want this to happen to one of yours?

There are many things every parent can do to prevent injuries to his own children and the children of others. The hazards that cause accidents can be removed, and actions that lead to accidents can be avoided. Most important of all is the matter of cultivating the child's instinct of self-preservation by helping him to recognize dangerous situations and make a habit of avoiding them. Children can start to learn safe habits in babyhood, and thus prepare to minimize the chance of injury throughout life.

In trying to protect your child against accidents, it may be well to think of first things first; and it certainly would be wise to know just what accidents cause the most deaths during childhood. Listed below are the six most common causes of accidental death, divided into groups according to age.

First things first. We note from the chart below that motor accidents are more deadly

PRINCIPAL CAUSES OF ACCIDENTAL DEATHS

Numbers of deaths in one city during one year listed by age

	Under 1 year	1-2 years	2-3 years	3-4 years	4-5 years
Motor Vehicles	187	400	315	355	378
Conflagrations	185	185	160	140	130
Falls	135	90	55	25	20
Burns	150	210	150	160	130
Drowning	30	270	160	120	110
Poison	60	240	70	25	15

after one year of age, conflagrations hold about the same up to five years, with the greatest mortality between one and two. Falls are more dangerous up to one year of age. Therefore, be careful about your baby and see that he doesn't fall off the bed. Burns, drowning, and poisons seem to be more prevalent among the group from one to two years old, and all the other causes of accidents listed seem to be more deadly in this one to two year group. Therefore watch your child very closely between the ages of one and two, when he is first beginning to walk.

The baby at this age is very inquisitive. He will put anything into his mouth that will go into it, and will swallow what he can. He will put his hand or foot into an electric fan or any other machine he can find. He is not afraid of water, no matter how deep it is, and will walk into a deep pool if not watched. He is not afraid of automobiles or fire, and most important of all at this age, he will resent warnings if they are repeated too often in a nagging manner.

Then how will we protect the toddlers against all these dangers? First of all, if you are going to leave him alone, see that he is in a safe play pen from which he cannot escape. Be sure that the slots in the side of the play pen are not far enough apart so he can get his head caught between them. Keep all hot liquids, matches, etc., out of his reach. Do not allow the baby to wear highly inflammable clothing. Most important, keep medicines, poisons, kerosene, detergents, etc., under lock and key and definitely out of his reach. See that electric outlets have plastic plugs in them, or cover them with something so the baby cannot put his fingers into them; and see that all worn electric wires running from lamps, etc., are replaced by new ones, for he is just as likely as not to chew on a worn electric wire right in the place where the insulation is worn off. Be sure that when the young baby is first beginning to explore he is well supervised when he goes near roads, alleys, swimming pools, driveways, and especially near filled bathtubs. Never leave your baby in the bathtub while you go to answer the phone, and never leave a radio or any electric appliance in the bathroom for him to touch while he is in the water.

As the baby becomes a little older you can begin his education. For instance, when he starts to touch a hot radiator or stove, do not yell "No!" at him, but tell him "That is hot" or "It will burn"—then when he goes ahead and touches it the pain will convince him you were right, and he won't touch it again. You can teach him that not everything he sees that is liquid is fit to drink. For instance, if a bowl of vinegar is within his reach and he starts to take it, do not stop him—just say "You will not like that." After he tastes it he will get the idea more effectively than if you shout "No, No" or "Stop that!" This is all part of his education.

All children, and I repeat *all* children, should be taught how to swim at an early age. The two- or three-year old baby will walk into a deep pool without the slightest fear. He should be taught that water in the nose and eyes and mouth is not a pleasant thing, and he will respect water. Until he is old enough to be taught how to swim, even if you have taught him to respect water, he should never be allowed to go by himself near a deep pool or river, because he may just decide to walk right in. See that he is protected from all these hazards.

When he starts to climb, be sure he cannot climb high enough to hurt himself, but at the same time let him fall a short distance just to remind him there is a low point of gravity and that if he climbs and falls it may be painful.

Keep all sharp objects such as scissors, needles, etc., out of reach, and see that his toys, such as a teddy bear, do not have eyes which he can remove and swallow, or stuff into his nose or ears.

Above all, be sure that there are no guns within the reach of children. This applies to an even greater extent to children who are old enough to play "cops and robbers." Having seen so much of this on television they will not hesitate to point a gun at a playmate and pull the trigger. Any number of children are killed by being shot in this manner every day, and it is always the fault of the adult who allows a gun—loaded or empty—to remain in a place where a child can reach it. This is unforgivable. When a boy becomes older, fourteen or fifteen, he should be taught by his father or some other qualified person how to handle a gun safely, so that when he starts to hunt he will appreciate the danger involved and will never allow the barrel of any gun, either loaded or empty, to be pointed at himself or any other person. As a doctor, I have seen too many children die of accidental gunshot wounds which could have been prevented if the parents had afforded protection and education.

These are the two objectives—first of all, *protection* from these hazards when too young to be educated, and then *education* so they can protect themselves as they become older and can no longer be supervised at all times by an adult.

In one of our large cities there were 407 persons killed by accidents last year, and it may be of interest to see where most of these deaths occurred.

171 accidental deaths occurred in the home.
120 accidental deaths occurred in public places.
86 accidental deaths occurred on streets.
30 accidental deaths occurred at work.

From this we see that the most dangerous place in town is the home, and we know that with the proper care on the part of the homemaker these dangers could be greatly done away with. In this particular city, falls claimed the most lives—181, traffic accidents came second with 86, then came burns with 36, poisoning 27, and suffocation by food, 24. Again, we see that if we prevent falls in the home, fire and burning from hot liquids in the home, a great many deaths could be prevented. Is it any wonder that we ask you to read this chapter over and over again?

Nearly every day we read in the newspaper of the death of an infant or young child by asphyxiation caused by placing a plastic bag over his head. These plastic films have become very popular as bags in which to place vegetables. They are placed over your clothes by the cleaners and used in many forms, so that every home has to contend with them. The young child thinks it is fun to place these bags over his head because he can see through the bag. The film clings to the face and suffocates the child, causing death. There is only one way to prevent this, and that is to destroy all plastic or film coverings when they are removed from the object which they cover. Never allow a young child to play with them. Never use plastic as a waterproof cover for a baby's mattress. The baby may tear off a piece or

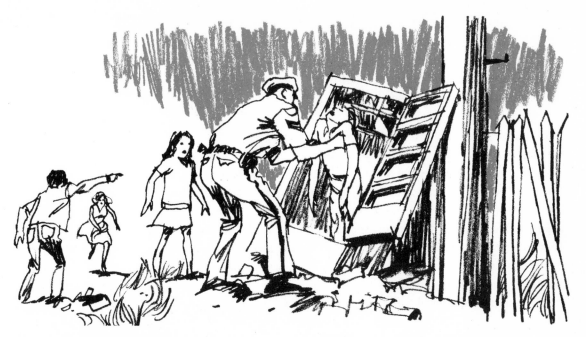

Every old refrigerator should be destroyed to prevent children from the danger of suffication.

pull it loose from the mattress, and place it over his face. Let me repeat, destroy immediately all plastic bags which are brought into your home as covering for food, laundry, clothes, or what not. Destroy them as soon as they are removed from the object they cover.

All of you have read of the tragic deaths caused by children locking themselves in old refrigerators which have been allowed to remain in the neighborhood after they are no longer in use. This is one case in which the remedy is easily found. Destroy all old ice boxes or refrigerators, or dispose of them by selling them. Do not allow them to remain around for children to play in, and perhaps to die in.

We have noted above that traffic accidents account for a great many deaths. In trying to protect your young child from such an accident always be sure the child is riding with a safe driver. In a city it is bet-

ter to send them in a taxi than to allow them to ride with a driver whom you do not know.

All cars should have safety belts, and some companies now manufacture them for children. Shoulder belts are more effective.

The seat next to the driver is the most dangerous. We know this because in traffic accidents resulting in death, the person sitting next to the driver is the one most often killed. If your car does not have seatbelts and your child is in the front seat with you, be sure he stands behind your shoulder.

Be sure the doors are locked by a safety device that cannot be unlocked by the child. Sometimes the tops of the little pushbuttons that lock the doors can be removed after the door is locked.

Never allow your child to go out at night dressed in dark clothing. He should always wear something white so the driver of a car who may be going at a rapid rate of speed can see him. Always teach your children to cross the street between the two white lines which mark the pedestrian crossing, and teach them to look both ways carefully before stepping out into a crosswalk.

Accidents are increasingly dangerous to adults as well as to children, and as a person becomes older he is more liable to suffer crippling accidents. Anyone who has been in an old folks' home or a county hospital and has seen the great number of older people with broken hips can vouch for this. A fractured hip caused by a fall can happen in an instant, but it takes six or eight months to heal, and sometimes the elderly person remains crippled for life.

We have learned that home is the place where most accidents occur, and that more dangerous accidents, those causing death or severe crippling to adults, are caused by falls. Now let us see what we can do in the home to prevent falls. We must first know what causes most falls in the home and then correct these conditions.

Listed below are some of the common causes for falls in the home:

1. Liquid on the kitchen floor
2. Light cords stretched across the floor
3. Throw rugs on a slippery floor
4. Highly polished hardwood floor or stairway
5. Darkness in rooms or on stairways
6. No rails to hold walking down stairs
7. No bars on wall in bathroom over the bath tub
8. No rubber mat in bath tub
9. Arising from bed suddenly and starting to walk while a little dizzy
10. Wearing bedroom slippers around the house
11. Getting up from a chair and starting to walk while one of your legs is "asleep"
12. Moving too suddenly over a slippery, highly polished floor.
13. Standing on unsteady chairs or stools to reach something on a high shelf
14. Small articles on the floor, such as spools of thread, books, or toys

If you can overcome these fourteen hazards, you can prevent many falls. Last but most important of all, if you feel yourself falling, turn quickly, if possible, and land on your back or your stomach.

In that way you may prevent a broken hip which is caused by landing heavily on your side.

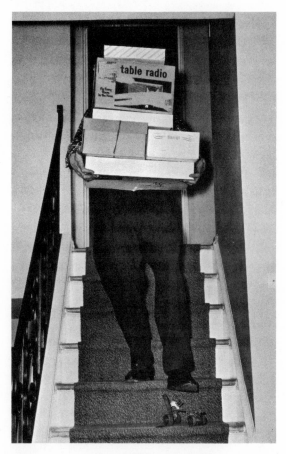

Stairways are one of the most common causes of accidents in the home. They should be kept clear of all objects.

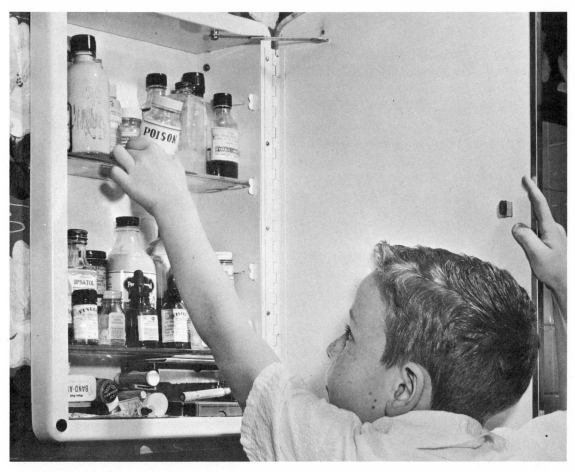

All drugs in the house should be locked to prevent children from eating them. The medicine chest should be locked since children can usually reach it.

Many fatal accidents and crippling ones too, may occur in the home and are not caused by a fall. For instance, the bathroom is a dangerous place, especially the medicine chest. The following rules may help prevent death or sickness.

1. Never take medicine without reading the label first. Never take a dose of medicine in the dark because you think you know the size of a pill or the place where the bottle you want has been left. Someone may have changed the bottles

2. Never keep poisons or cleaning fluids in the medicine chest

3. Always mark a big red "X" across the label of a bottle which contains a poisonous liquid, such as Oil of Wintergreen

4. If you keep pills beside your bed, never keep over one night's supply on the table beside you

5. When you pour liquid medicine from a bottle to a spoon, always pour from the side opposite the label so that the medicine will not run down over the label and obscure it

6. Always keep medicine in the box or bottle with the proper label. Never mix several kinds of pills in one box

7. Remember that even too much aspirin may be poisonous or fatal to some people

Even the kitchen, where a woman may spend most of her time, may be a very dangerous place. Here are some rules to use in order to prevent accidents in the kitchen.

1. If you are wearing loose clothing such as a bathrobe or nightgown, be especially careful, because these clothes are not close to your body, and if they catch fire you may not feel the fire soon enough to put it out

2. Have a flashlight ready when you open the oven door to prevent burned hands if oven lights are out of order

3. If you are using a wood or coal stove be very careful when adding fuel to the stove to prevent a spark from flying out and setting fire to your clothes

4. Use utensils with insulated handles when you can. This will help prevent burning your hands and help to keep pot holders from catching fire

5. Always turn the handle of a utensil containing hot liquid or food toward the back of the stove so it will not be accidentally pulled over by a child or knocked over by yourself. Do not place the handle over another burner.

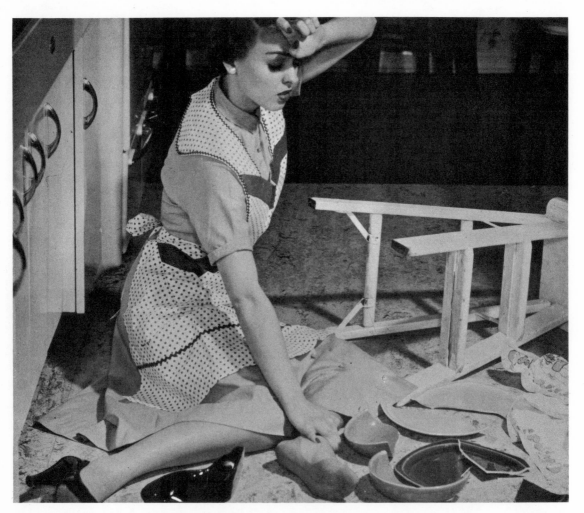

The housewife spends a great deal of time in the kitchen. Falls are common occurrences and should be guarded against. They may result in serious injury.

In the living room or bedroom, think of the following safety measures:

1. Always have a tight screen in front of the fireplace

2. If a room heater is used, either gas, electric, wood, or oil, it should be checked about once a year to see if it is still safe. In many places the Fire Department will do this checking for you, or the people who sell you your gas, oil, or electricity will be glad to check your heater for you

3. Always have a window opened a little, or a door opened into the next room, if a heater is on. You must have ventilation, and the automatic vent may be plugged up as it sometimes is during snowstorms

4. When you light a gas heater, always light the match before you turn on the gas

5. Never have oil, gasoline, or any other inflammable material near a heater

6. When you buy a heater second-hand, be sure it is checked first for safety

7. Never place a heater where it can be knocked over, and if you have a portable oil heater be sure it has a wide base so it cannot be knocked over easily

TRAFFIC DANGERS

As more and more automobiles crowd the highways and streets, and as the speed and power of cars is increasing, traffic accidents are becoming a leading cause of accidental death and crippling injuries.

1. As a pedestrian, always look both ways two times before crossing a street

2. Cross between the white lines of the crosswalk

3. Wear something white when out at night or at dusk

4. When walking on a highway, walk on the left side of the road so as to face all oncoming cars, and carry a flashlight with you at dusk or at night—in addition, wear something white. Step off the pavement when cars approach

As drivers or occupants of a car:

1. Never drive while drinking

2. Never ride with a driver who has been drinking. Taxicabs are much safer

3. Use common courtesy on the road

4. Look both ways two times before driving into an intersection

5. Be sure you have perfect control of the car at all times, and this means avoid excessive speed.

6. Keep your eyes on the highway at all times, for the slightest glance to one side or the other may mean your death, or the death of someone else

7. Be sure your brakes are working perfectly and that your tires are good, so that a blowout is not likely to occur

8. Safety belts should be installed in all cars, and should be used, for it has been proven beyond any doubt that many lives are saved daily by the use of safety belts

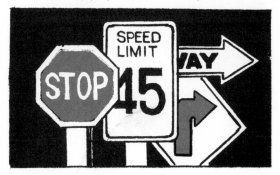

The above suggestions may seem trivial, and you may say "I do all of these things anyway," but remember that overlooking any one of them may cost you your life or health. A great deal of money and time are being put into the study of safety engineering, to improve the safety of the cars themselves; but the man who drives the car can learn by the mistakes of others, and these mistakes are too numerous to be listed. Be sure you are not guilty of such mistakes.

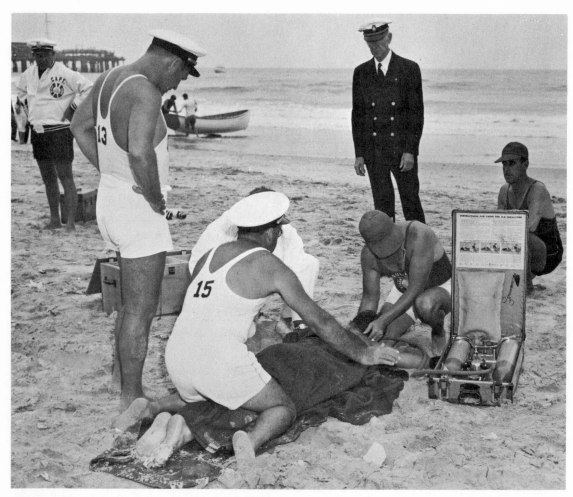

A pulmotor being used to resuscitate a drowning victim. If no pulmotor is available the use of mouth to mouth breathing and external cardiac massage should be employed after mouth is cleared.

DROWNING

Many lives are lost each year because of drowning, and some of these could be prevented if the following precautions were taken:

1. All swimming pools and fish ponds should be protected from small children by having high fences or other means of keeping young children away from them for their own safety

2. Every child should be taught to swim at an early age, and before that should be taught respect for deep water, and to know the dangers of it

3. Never leave a baby in the bathtub while you answer the door or the telephone

4. While out in a boat, use common sense, and do not stand up in the boat if it is a small one. By losing your balance you could turn the boat over

5. Treat all boats as dangerous

6. Never wear hip boots when fishing from a boat. They do no good, and if the boat should turn over, the hip boots may drag you to your death. This happens many times every year

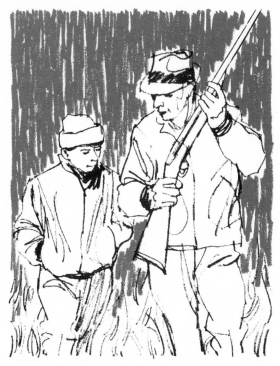

All young hunters should take hunters training courses. The gun is a deadly weapon.

HUNTING

Carelessness or ignorance while out hunting has caused far too many accidental deaths.

1. Teach all young people who are going to become hunters the proper way to use a gun safely
2. Never point a gun, loaded or unloaded, at anyone; and never allow your own gun to be pointed at yourself
3. Check the safety catch frequently to be sure it is on
4. In removing a gun from a car, never pull it out by the barrel, even though you might be sure it is not loaded
5. Never carry a loaded gun in the car
6. When hunting do not shoot into the brush because you see a movement there. Always see clearly and identify the object at which you are shooting. Every year during deer season a great number of hunters are killed because of failure to observe this rule
7. Never leave a loaded gun in the house even though there is no shell in the barrel, but there is one in the magazine. Children find these guns and play with them—quite often shooting and killing a playmate. This is not the fault of the child, but of the parent who left the gun where the child could find it

POISONING

Many commonly used household cleaning agents and other materials—even medicines—are poisonous.

1. Be sure these are locked away out of reach of children
2. Never place detergents or cleaning fluids in the kitchen under the sink where children can get them
3. Never leave rat poison or insecticides where the exploring child can find them
4. Always clearly mark the poisonous material so that adults will not be fooled and take them by mistake

Now we have said that accidents are the greatest cause of death and crippling in children. We know that accidents rate high in the ten leading causes of death among adults. Why don't we do something about this? We have cancer societies, poliomyelitis foundations, rheumatism societies, and each year millions of dollars are spent in trying to find ways and means to prevent death by these diseases. We are now beginning to spend money to find out the causes and preventions of accidents; but that money is only a drop in the bucket when we realize how many deaths are caused by accidents in comparison to these other diseases.

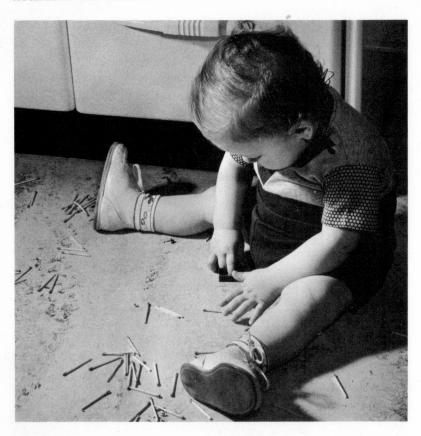

Matches should be kept away from children. There is danger of eating them (poison), burning clothes or house. Many forest fires are also caused by children playing with matches.

It is to be hoped that every one who reads this will try to do what he can to help in the study of ways and means to prevent accidents. As a final test, we have here a check list. Please go over it and to find out if whether you are guilty of practices which may lead to fatal accidents. If you are guilty, correct these things, and save the life of someone dear to you.

DO YOU EVER?

If you can answer all of these "Do you ever?" questions with a resounding "No," probably you and your family have good safety habits. This is a checklist of things *not* to do.

1. Keep a radio in the bathroom?
2. Place containers of hot fluids on the floor or in places where a child can reach them?
3. When cooking, allow the handles of pots or pans to be turned out toward the edge of the stove where a child could tip them over?
4. Have worn electric cords in your house?
5. Keep any medicine, cleaning materials, poison, etc., in a place where a child can reach them?
6. Throw away old medicine boxes or bottles by placing them in cans in the yard where children can reach them?
7. Fail to read the labels on medicines before taking them or giving them to someone else?
8. Leave matches or cigarette lighters in places where children can reach them?

9. Dress your child in flimsy inflammable materials?

10. Allow a fire to burn in the fireplace without placing a good screen in front of it?

11. Forget to teach your children never to stand close to something flaming or smoldering in the fire—where bottles or caps can explode and burn or cut them?

12. Fail to open a door or window in a room where gas heaters are used?

13. Keep firearms or guns in a place where children can get them?

14. Allow young children to eat meats, popcorn, or carrot sticks?

15. Allow babies to play with toys which have small parts that may be removed, such as eyes on a teddy bear?

16. Allow babies to play with sharp-pointed objects, such as scissors or knives?

17. Use a crib which has been painted with lead-base paint? Children chew on cribs.

18. Forget to destroy plastic bags in which suits are brought home from the cleaners, or in which food has been packed?

19. Leave a small baby in the bathtub for a second while you answer the telephone or front door? It takes only a second for a small one to drown or be scalded.

20. Forget to keep all windows on upper floors locked?

21. Forget to place gate at top and bottom of stairways when babies are around?

22. Forget to raise the sides of the crib when you leave the baby in it?

23. Use a crib or play pen with bars far enough apart so the baby can get his head caught between them?

24. Leave appliances such as lawn mowers where children have access to them?

25. Forget to teach children not to play in dangerous places such as streets or highways?

26. Forget to instruct your child never to run into the street without looking both ways?

27. Forget to instruct your child never to run into the street from behind a parked car?

28. Fail to keep a good fence around the yard so your child cannot wander into the neighbor's swimming pool or fish pond?

29. Have a pond or pool of your own when your children cannot swim?

30. Neglect to teach your children how to swim at an early age?

31. Forget to look behind your car carefully when you are backing out of the garage?

32. Forget to delegate some certain person to watch the children when a group of children and adults are together?

33. Allow your son or daughter to wear hip boots when fishing from a boat?

34. Leave a child alone in the bathtub?

35. Try to remove wax from the ears with a foreign object?

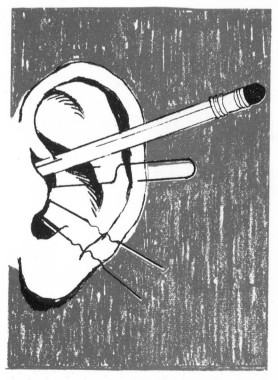

Do not remove ear wax with objects such as these. They may cause serious injury.

We have seen how people, especially children, may be killed or crippled for life by accidents which could be prevented. How are we to prevent them? There are three ways in which we can help in the prevention of accidents.

1. Education—teach children and adults safety habits
2. Engineering—encourage the manufacturers of cars, toys, etc., which have safety devices
3. Enforcement—not only tell your child to practice good safety habits, but see to it that he does. Apply this rule to yourself

GREEN LIGHT: GO FOR ROAD SAFETY

Nine out of ten road accidents are the driver's own fault and only one in ten is due to defects in the car or the road. This frequently heard statement may serve to awaken drivers to their responsibilities, but it is of little help to anybody making a serious study of traffic problems and traffic risks. Carried to its logical conclusion, indeed, it would mean that 100 percent of all road accidents should be blamed on the driver, since nothing happens on the road which he did not, in some way, start.

The truth is, of course, much less simple. Any traffic accident depends on three main factors—the driver, his vehicle, and the road—although the degree to which any one of these is involved may vary. There are certain subsidiary factors too, some constant and some not, which may be difficult to assess but which must nevertheless be taken into account.

The part played by speed, for instance, has long been greatly oversimplified. There is evidence that, taken over a driver's total mileage, most of his accidents on modern highways occur at the lower operating speeds. The proportion of accidents per driver drops with increasing speed, reaching its lowest value at about sixty-five m.p.h., but rises sharply again at higher speeds. It is true that accidents at high speeds are far more serious. However, the number of injuries on a miles-travelled basis, is at its minimum between forty-five and seventy m.p.h. The fact that moderately high speeds are associated with lowest accident rates on highways should lead to the setting of more realistic speed limits.

Not all discoveries made in this field are quite so unexpected, and many of them confirm everyday experience. It has long been known that in all countries twice as many accidents occur at night as during the day, and that dawn is the most dangerous time of all. The holiday peaks in road accidents are recognized facts, but no one has yet discovered the real reason for them. Investigations have shown only that the average number of accidents at holiday periods is twenty-five percent greater than at other times, *even if all other traffic conditions are the same*.

It is also known that there are now fewer road accidents involving pedestrians than there were twenty-five years ago, and a number of reasons may be advanced for this.

People walk less nowadays and many pedestrians are drivers as well and are more aware of the dangers; road signals are also better; both in towns and on the open road.

What Road Accidents Cost

The cost of accidents has been assessed from every angle. In the United States the

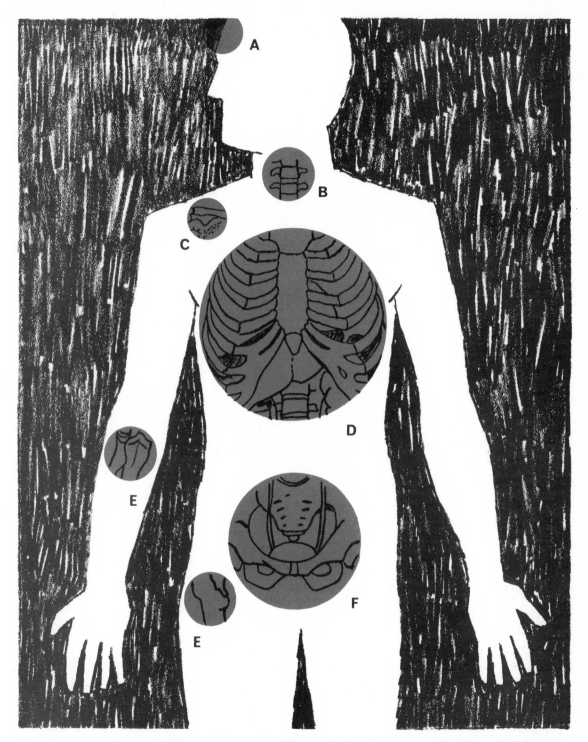

Injuries commonly seen following an automobile crash: (A) Laceration of scalp or skull fracture. (B) Broken neck. (C) Fractured collar bone. (D) Chest injuries caused by steering wheel. (E) Fractured arms or legs. (F) Ruptured bladder of fractured pelvis.

press has given wide publicity to the loss to the American economy from road accidents.

But how can we assess the economic loss due to the premature death of young drivers who are at the beginning of their most productive period, and who are the primary victims of traffic accidents? Some seventy-five percent of fatal accidents involve men; what are the effects on a family of the death of its breadwinner?

There is both a simpler and a better way of looking at the human factor. As an expert of the Harvard School of Public Health has put it, "People drive as they live."

According to another expert, marital status has a definite influence on accident-proneness. Married persons are less liable to accidental death than widowers, who are in turn safer on the roads than divorcees. The only exceptions to this rule are people under twenty years of age; they have a higher percentage of accidents when married than if they are single.

Over-indulgence in alcohol, fatigue, and sheer lack of attention are, obviously, responsible for a very large number of accidents, but little systematic study has been made of the causes underlying these factors, whether physiological, psychological, or social.

Until a clearer light can be thrown on these obscure matters, more limited but more immediately realizable goals may still be pursued.

When all possible information has been obtained, it may at last be possible for effective prevention to be undertaken and for the green light of safety to shine on the roads of the world.

Meanwhile each of us can do his part by knowing and scrupulously observing the traffic laws, following the rules of courtesy and safety on the road, and taking advantage of every mechanical means of protection, such as safety belts for both passenger and driver and careful attention to the tires, brakes, and operating efficiency of the car.

ACCIDENTS IN FARM AND JUNGLE

At home and at work peasants or farmers are more exposed to accident risks than perhaps any other occupational group. The farmer's home is also his work place and combines the dangers of both. When he works on the land, the experience of his kind is often insufficient to guard him against all its hidden dangers.

The family character of many farms, the comparatively isolated existence, poorer schooling than in the town, and fewer opportunities for obtaining the knowledge he needs, less support from social services, all these factors make the farmer into a kind of poor cousin in the modern world.

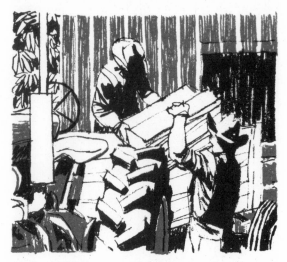

Farm machinery must be operated with caution.

The answers to these questions are still not known, but a good deal of basic research is being carried out in most countries of the world.

What About the Driver?

Finally there is that great unknown, the human factor. If the psychologist is to put forward anything better than mere theories, he must work closely with the engineer, the policeman, and the doctor.

Some not very successful attempts have been made to draw up a composite picture of the man who is "accident-prone" on the roads, as has been done for other types of accidents. It has not been possible to establish any certain link between accident-proneness and physical or psychophysiological failing. One series will show that quick reactions lead to accidents, while another demonstrates that quick reactions and slow reactions cause about the same number of accidents. One medical report will state that it is dangerous for people with high blood pressure to drive; another that persons with low blood pressure are liable to accidents.

The one conclusion to be drawn from these few examples is that interpretations of tests of psychomotor ability seem peculiarly liable to error.

The United States may be considered one of the countries where agriculture has made most progress in the last hundred years or so. Yet a study of the frequency and type of agricultural accidents on seven thousand Indiana farms has shown 28.6 percent of them to be due to light agricultural equipment, hand tools, fire, hot liquids, drowning, poison, and domestic animals. A further 29.6 percent were due to

falls, the majority and the most severe being falls from ladders. This figure bears a striking similarity to that for deaths from falls in Ceylon. Of a total of 2,799 deaths from all accidents in one year in Ceylon, 554, or over one tenth, were caused by falls; and in 349 cases the men who fell were tapping palm trees or picking coconuts or fruit. Despite the dissimilarity of their occupations, one is forced to the conclusion that the Indiana farmer and the Ceylonese peasant run just about the same risk of a fall; and there is not much to choose between falling from a tree and falling from a ladder.

Agricultural accidents—like accidents in the home, the workshop, or the factory—are to a large extent linked to traditional forms of activity, and by and large they are the same the world over.

Advice That Gets Ignored

Rural schools should be provided with textbooks describing and warning against the risks encountered on farms, and rural councils might well promote adult education along similar lines. However, there is no hiding the fact that such basic education is the most difficult of all, since it deals with a subject which everyone thinks he knows all about already.

The peasant trusts his instinct and the pragmatic knowledge handed down through his father or the village elders—he is naturally suspicious of the city "expert." No agricultural safety campaign can afford to overlook this vital factor. To be effective, such a campaign should be entrusted to a man of the soil, for good advice that otherwise would be ignored, will be listened to if it comes from a respected elder or a young farmer whose good crops bear witness to his ability.

"... Never hold a sharp instrument pointed toward yourself. Don't leave your pitchfork lying about. Test your axe-handle before use. Never leave a scythe standing in such a way that it can fall blade upward. Be careful with storm lanterns in hay barns. Never leave a harrow with its points in the air. Don't try to mend your ladder with a couple of nails or a piece of twine. Never climb over a fence with a load on your back ... "

Adages like these should, from earliest youth, have impressed on land workers' minds the need for elementary precautions, but they seem often to breed overconfidence.

Trusting, consciously or not, to his own cleverness or physical strength, the peasant or farmer, like the housewife in her kitchen or the workman at his bench, all too often forgets the risks with which he is overfamiliar. This may result in serious accidents.

Getting Used to Machines

The introduction of mechanized farming brings new dangers. Although they free the agricultural worker from his most arduous tasks and increase his productivity, the new machines require of him a much greater degree of care and vigilance.

The study carried out recently in Indiana showed that only about fifteen percent of accidents were due to agricultural machinery, but those accidents were by and large the most serious. A sort of "sixth sense" of self-protection which guards the worker more or less against the usual kind of accidents, gives little protection against threshers or mechanical harvesters. Although he

may be careless about it, the farmer knows very well that his horse may kick out at him; but when he gets his first brand new tractor, he usually has no idea that this machine he is so proud of has a treacherous and often fatal habit of capsizing at the least expected moment.

There are several ways of countering these new risks. One is to require the manufacturer of agricultural machinery to fix clear, legible, and indelible safety warnings on his products. Certain countries have even considered introducing agricultural driving licenses, which would provide an opportunity to give agricultural workers the safety training they so badly need.

THE FACTORY'S BEST PRODUCT IS ITS SAFETY

In the United States, out of a total of 91,-000 accidental deaths from all causes, 14,-000 are due to industrial accidents. In the same country, two million workers annually have occupational accidents resulting in incapacity for work. The number of work days lost in this way was estimated at 230 million in one year, and the corresponding economic loss at $4,200 million.

An analysis of all types of industrial accidents shows that only one in eight is caused by machines. Vehicles, electricity, sources of heat, and similar causes account for one quarter of the total. More than half are made up of what a British expert, W. T. McCullough, Chief Inspector of Factories, has called the Big Five: (1) falls from a height; (2) falls on the level; (3) handling of materials, etc.; (4) falling objects; (5) hand tools. One technician has even claimed that today there are fewer risks in manufacturing nitroglycerine than in transporting a heavy crate.

Making Accidents Impossible

Two different tendencies have developed in efforts to improve industrial safety. One is toward more and more detailed legislation and measures to improve the physical conditions of work. An English safety engineer recently said: "It is my job to see that even the clumsiest and least intelligent of our factory hands runs no risk of an accident."

The other tendency is to lay stress on the importance of education. According to partisans of "Education first," the evidence shows that a "human factor" is involved in more than eighty percent of occupational accidents, and that therefore preventive measures should be directed toward the worker. Moreover, they say, when legislation and inspection procedures become too complex and cumbersome, they are no longer respected.

These two approaches are of course complementary. No accident is entirely due either to an outside cause or to a human failing. Most experts on the question agree today that industrial accidents, like all other accidents, have multiple causes.

The "Fatal Action"

For an accident to cease to be potential and become actual, there must be a conjunction between the victim and the material cause, which supposes a precipitating factor. This factor which determines or precipitates an accident may be independent of the victim, as for instance in the case of a falling stone or other object, a plank that gives way, or a machine that breaks down. But in a large number of cases, this factor is simply a movement or act of the victim himself. For this, Professor Victor Raymond of France has coined the phrase "le geste néfaste"—the fatal action.

Most frequently, this fatal action is an uncorrected conditional reflex. By their very repetition, many work movements become stereotyped. The man becomes a kind of robot, slave of the machines and objects he works with. His work movements become mechanical, and always follow the same pattern. Now suppose that the machine or the objects the worker is concerned with suddenly present some departure from the usual pattern. Unless the worker's conditioned reflex is quickly corrected, the "fatal action" will be made.

Fortunately for him, the human being possesses protective mechanisms against these "fatal actions." First there are the primary reflexes which produce an "instinctive" withdrawal from a danger usually perceived through the sense of touch. Conditioned reflexes can also produce similar protective reactions. "Once bitten, twice shy" says the proverb—reaction to fire is the classical example.

A child who actually touches a burning object will withdraw his hand by a primary reflex action. An association between the sight of fire and the sensation of burning is established, and a conditioned reflex is created which lasts throughout his life. Whenever he sees a burning object getting too close, he withdraws.

Such protective reflexes can be developed by creating associations between a danger and certain sights and sounds—warning by sirens or bells, and, very important, notices and labels.

Finally the instinct of self preservation that everyone possesses can be strengthened and trained so that it corrects, checks, or coordinates habitual actions and prevents them from becoming "fatal actions."

Built-in Safety

Unfortunately this instinct of self preservation cannot be relied on absolutely—there will always be occasional lapses. Much can be done, however, to limit their effects by technical and mechanical safety measures. To be effective such measures should protect all workers alike and should require no effort or cooperation from the individual.

They are based on the elimination of all risk. An example is the prohibition of the use of white lead in paint, which has automatically prevented white lead poisoning among the people working with paint.

If safety devices are built into machines, fewer precautions are needed when using them. Of course the workers know about these safety devices and their role, and it sometimes happens that they resent them because, they say, such devices complicate their work. Therefore they sometimes remove them or put them out of action, temporarily or permanently.

Machines should always be provided with an automatic stop that operates whenever its safety devices are not working. The less such a device interferes with the worker's habits, the more easily it will be accepted and used by him.

These safety measures are collective in nature and do not require the cooperation of the individual worker. There are others which do require his more or less active participation. As we have seen, this is often problematical and such measures, even though necessary, are therefore less reliable.

Vague Uninformed Fears

It is difficult enough to obtain even the worker's passive cooperation, for instance, in following certain rules, or going for a medical check-up. If he is asked to take more active precautions, like wearing gloves, special glasses or a mask, experience shows that the results are usually unsatisfactory.

It is of the first importance that each worker should know and understand the risks to which he is exposed. Instructions must be complete, detailed, and precise in order not to create simply a vague, uniformed fear of accidents. For example, everyone knows vaguely that electricity is dangerous, but what is important is to know how dangerous and in what way. It is not enough for someone to know the dangers of lightning, or of high tension currents, if he does not realize the dangers of the common 110 volt or 220 volt household electricity supply.

Again, it is not enough just to tell people about such risks—they must really understand their nature. It is for this reason that dependence cannot be placed on rules, warnings, "forbidden" notices, etc. They become so familiar that after a while they have no further effect in preventing the "fatal action."

None of these "individual" safety measures can be really effective unless the person they are intended to protect is made to feel a partner in the scheme, and this will depend largely on the attitude of the works manager. He must set the pace. If he is genuinely concerned about safety measures, the engineers and foreman will follow suit, and the accident rate will soon reflect the success of their combined efforts.

EDUCATION,
THE ONLY VACCINE AGAINST
ACCIDENTS

Dangers surround a child from the moment it draws its first breath. The whole of human life is indeed, in a sense, an unceasing struggle against danger.

Most accidents are the result of unnecessary risks taken either because of faulty judgment, or, what is worse, through lack of physical fitness or simple ignorance. Education, both physical and mental, is certainly the best vaccine against this murderous affliction that we call accident.

During his first year, a child is incapable of judgment. Unable to move or to do anything for himself, he depends entirely on his mother. At first then it is the mother who has to think and act for him, and protect him against all the dangers to which he is exposed.

There is one particular danger against which the mother must be constantly on guard—suffocation. The first precaution is to make sure that within the baby's reach there is nothing that might interfere with his breathing. Eiderdown pillows should never be tolerated. In recent years, a new danger has appeared in the shape of plastic curtains, trimmings, etc. Static electricity may cause this filmy substance to cling tightly to the face of a new born child, blocking its nose and mouth and suffocating it rapidly. In the United States, plastic bags bear a notice drawing attention to this

danger and warning parents to keep them out of baby's reach.

Food is the second great cause of suffocation. Even an overworked mother should realize that she is running a terrible risk if she leaves her baby alone to suck his bottle. Third, far too many mothers appear not to know how easy it is to stifle a baby sleeping in the same bed with them.

While a mother should always protect her child against danger during the first months of his life, it is very important for her to let him start to fend for himself when he is about one year old. Little by little she should lose the habit of doing things for him, of fussing over him. A mother who is over-worried and over-careful is perhaps the child's greatest danger; for the moment he escapes her supervision—as of course he will sooner or later—he is likely to assert his freedom by doing some forbidden and perhaps fatal action.

One precaution against this instinct for self-assertion is to make the child's environment as safe as possible. A French doctor, Philippe Gravel, stresses in this context that psychological as well as physical factors need to be taken into account.

For example, a fall on a staircase may be due to the pattern and color of the carpet, failing to provide sufficient contrast between one step and the next so that it is difficult to see where each begins and ends.

Learning to Know Danger

But passive protection is not enough: it is necessary for the child to learn to understand the risks he runs. Adults frequently make one of two mistakes: either they credit the child with more intelligence than he possesses, or they assume he is quite unable to think for himself. In both cases they fail to understand that they are dealing with a mind and a body in constant development.

Between twelve and fifteen months the child is absorbed in examining the world around him. He will explore the house. He will try to touch everything he comes across, particularly if it is on a level with his eyes. He will try to put almost everything in his mouth. Around two, he becomes capable of opening a door. He likes to lift up a lid and empty a box, only to fill it up again afterwards. He has little idea of distance and tries to climb here, there, and everywhere. To play with water becomes a favorite pastime. At about three, he is surer of his movements and likes to go walking. He learns to distinguish right and left. He enjoys feeling responsible and making himself useful. At the age of four, he thinks of nothing but running about and playing ball. He can ride a tricycle and climb trees. He can concentrate mentally for longer periods.

Should all this exploration and these increasingly dangerous activities be prohibited? "No," says Monsieur Robert Sallé, head of the teaching and publicity section of the French *Institut National de Sécurité*. "You cannot base accident prevention on the principle of taking no risks. In life you get nowhere if you don't take risks."

Safety education should accordingly be pursued along two lines:

(1) Teach the child to distinguish between the risks he may take and those he had better avoid.

(2) Teach him the best way of dealing with the dangers that cannot be avoided.

If parents are to provide their children with a judicious blend of advice, reprimand, and prohibition, they must learn to know their children better. They should, for instance, admit once and for all that, as the statistics show, boys are more liable to have accidents than girls. Knowledge of possible accidents should not be an excuse for resignation or inaction, but rather a guide to where preventive efforts should be concentrated.

Critical Moments

An important factor in accidents is the time of day. A survey carried out recently in Stockholm by the pediatricians of the Swedish Committee for the Prevention of Accidents in Childhood showed that a large number of accidents occurred between ten a.m. and eight p.m., with a slight increase from eleven a.m. to midday, and a very marked increase between three p.m. and six p.m.

In Stockholm, these are the hours immediately preceding the midday and evening meals, and are probably also those during which children are less well supervised. Hunger and fatigue, particularly toward evening, make the children more accident prone.

The time of year also plays a part. According to Dr. Barbara J. van den Berg, summer is the season in which most of the accidents among children between the ages of one and fourteen occur in the Netherlands.

A pilot study carried out at Columbia University on children who repeatedly suffered accidents revealed a number of psychological factors. It was found that hostility to the environment, a conflict with the parents, or simply a state of tension within the family may create a predisposition to accidents. Also that a child who strains his powers in order to gain acceptance by a group of older children may take dangerous risks.

In different regions or countries, children are exposed to different dangers. In Scandinavia and in the Netherlands, drowning is the most frequent cause of accidental death among children of preschool age. Among home accidents in Great Britain, burns are second only to suffocation. In all countries where motor traffic is intense, it is responsible, perhaps not for the most frequent, but certainly for the most serious accidents.

It has often been said that the education of the children starts with the education of the parents. This is especially true in matters of safety. "If I had only known . . ." says the mother in despair after her child has been crippled or killed in a traffic accident. Why did she not know that a child under five should never be allowed to venture alone on the road?

"But," she says, "my little boy was playing quietly on the footpath and all of a sudden he rushed into the middle of the road after a ball . . ."

She should have known that there are a number of simple things a four-year-old can be taught, including the rule, "Stay out of the street."

Learning Road Safety at School

Once a child goes to school, there are more opportunities for safety education. But instead of relying exclusively on the teacher, parents should increasingly take part in this aspect of their child's upbringing. It has been quite clearly shown that in a factory where the manager is not interested in safety there is a high accident rate, despite the observance of rules, the good will of workers, and the devotion of engineers. The same applies in a family where the parents are not sufficiently concerned with their children's safety.

Safety education must therefore be considered part of general education and should certainly be included in the school curriculum. It is also an essential part of that "savoir vivre" that the child acquires mainly from its parents.

The motorist or the cyclist driving in town traffic must have his eyes everywhere, right, left, in front, and, with the help of his mirrors, even behind. This *diffuse* kind of attention is exactly that of an animal, or a man for that matter, moving through a probably hostile forest. Schooling, on the other hand, tends to develop *concentrated* attention. A strong case can be made out for training this *diffuse* kind of attention and one of the best ways of doing so is probably through team games and sports.

Sport indulged in reasonably may help young people to avoid traffic accidents, not only because it sharpens reflexes, but because it accustoms them to the observance of rules, and encourages a well-balanced way of life, health, food habits, and moderation in drinking.

There is no doubt, moreover, that the best way of substantially reducing the number of drowning accidents is to teach swimming at school.

Practicing How to Fall

Regarding falls, an analysis of industrial and home accidents shows the usefulness of distinguishing two kinds: falls on the level and falls from a height. The large number of falls in all human activities and the statistical predominance of falls on the level suggest that one remedy might be to give young people the right kind of physical training—perhaps including elementary Japanese wrestling (judo) and simple acrobatic exercises on the ground.

Falls from a height are less frequent but often more serious. A French school for building workers has developed special methods for teaching apprentices to fall even from a height of two stories without injury.

There is no doubt that accidents are fewer following efforts to make children realize the risks they are running and to teach them how to meet the dangers they encounter. Education offers the only hope of, little by little, overcoming this great malady of our times without sacrificing other human values.

THE WHY AND HOW OF ACCIDENTS

Take two apparently quite different accidents. In one, a man walking peaceably down the street has his head cut open by a flowerpot falling from a windowsill. In another, a man clearing undergrowth, severs his thumb with his billhook. The man in the first accident seems clearly the innocent victim of circumstances, while the other is in a sense "punished" for his carelessness. Yet the two accidents have something in common: each is the result of a series of events which contained the seeds of a potential accident.

In twenty years, the laborer had never cut himself with his billhook. Why, just this once, had he not taken his left hand out of the way quite fast enough? The reason was that he was tired after six solid hours of doing the same work. His fatigue increased the risk of injury with each repetition of the stereotyped action—the right hand making swift cutting movements with the billhook, the left moving more slowly. Then a moment came when coordination failed and the accident happened.

The man was not really the victim either of his own clumsiness or of bad luck; he was simply exposed to an unnecessary risk due to fatigue—a risk which could have been minimized if the work had been better planned.

What then of the unfortunate pedestrian hit by the flowerpot? Was he imprudent to walk along that pavement? Had he taken an unnecessary risk? Certainly not!

Yet two dangerous acts had been committed by others. The primary responsibility lay on the housewife who put the flowerpot on the sill. No doubt she knew that "accidents will happen," but failed to understand that they can also be avoided.

The second dangerous act was committed by her boy who actually knocked the pot over when he leaned out of the window to watch the people in the street below. There were, of course, other factors as well. The house could have been built in such a manner that the window did not give directly onto the roadway; or the housewife might have been stopped from breaking the city law which prohibits flowerpots on overhanging window ledges. There would have been no accident if any one of the dangerous acts which led to it had been prevented or if any one of the factors which rendered the flowerpot's fall possible had been eliminated. It is the same situation as for the woodcutter. Neither accident "had to happen"—both could have been prevented.

Big Risks and Little Risks

An accident can be considered in several ways. On the one hand there are the material circumstances that made it possible, on the other there is the human action that brought it about.

Then again there are the factors that influence our decision either to accept or to avoid the known risks which surround us in our daily lives.

Let us look at four typical risk situations:

A man who lights a cigarette runs a minute risk of burning himself and the possible consequences are of trifling importance —the risk is therefore easily accepted.

If the same man kisses his wife and she has a heavy cold, the risk of catching the cold is considerable, but the possible consequences are not very serious.

When he travels by air, the risk is extremely small but the potential accident involved is of the utmost gravity.

Finally, if this man were to handle high explosives in circumstances where the usual precautions could not be taken, the risk would be enormous, with correspondingly severe consequences. Fortunately, few of us, save in wartime, are exposed to such great danger; and should we be, society would generally offer us an equally exceptional reward.

Of all the ills that continually beset us, the accident is the most common, the most insidious, the most deadly, and perhaps the one about which we know least. Accidents take third place, after cancer and the cardiovascular diseases, among the principal causes of death in the world. They take first place at the time of man's youth and maturity—from one to forty-five years of age.

Yet this "plague" of the present age was not regarded as a public health matter until a few years ago.

Accidents Are Predictable

The first epidemiological studies soon showed the advantages of dealing with accidents in the same way as illness. Like diseases, they affect different age groups differently, and detailed studies have shown that they have an etiological history, just as do influenza or boils.

Accidents are never the result of pure chance. They generally occur in certain environments and in well-defined circumstances with a more or less predictable frequency.

Since accidents have been subjected to the methods used in medical research, three factors have become increasingly prominent: a "subject" susceptible to "infection," an environment favoring such "infection," and an "agent" which precipitates the accident.

When this analogy with illness was accepted, a number of other questions arose. If accidents are caused, and are not simply unpredictable pieces of bad luck, can they be systematically prevented? Can the "subject" be rendered less susceptible to "infection," the environment made less "infectious," and the "agent of infection" kept under control?

Modern methods of accident prevention are based on the assumption that the answer to these questions is "yes."

However, the variety and complexity among the causes of accidents is such that it is not easy fully to analyze and understand any given accident.

Technical experts must work on the environment, that is, the house, street, workshop, or office, and all the innumerable tools and machines which man has developed to serve him.

The epidemiologist goes beyond the particular problems involved in an individual accident, and, taking in the whole accident picture, develops general preventive measures covering the three main factors—subject, environment, and agent.

Last but not least, students of human behavior have recently made great contributions to the study of accidents.

Self-destructive Tendencies

An American psychologist, Dr. Lydia G. Gilberson, who is adviser to the Metropolitan Life Insurance Company, states unequivocally that ninety-five percent of all factors leading to accidents are of human origin. "Serious accidents can often be attributed to causes which are apparently quite unconnected with them," says Dr. Gilberson.

"There may be a link between the size of the grocer's bill and a broken leg which is undreamed of in the philosophy of the average man."

Dr. E. Eduardo Krapf, Chief of the World Health Organization Mental Health Section, considers that accidents may be directly caused by self-destructive tendencies, and quotes in support of this view, the case of a man who had already had forty surgical operations and asked for yet another on his brain, although it was not medically necessary. In his youth this patient had had four accidents and the only period of his life in which he had had neither accidents nor operations had been the very happy time when he was engaged to be married. Dr. Krapf believes there is no doubt that many persons who have accidents are unconsciously punishing themselves.

Certainly carelessness and lack of physical coordination are two human factors frequently involved in accidents, but the underlying psychological cause of these failings must be discovered and corrected before fully effective prevention can be undertaken.

Fundamental research of this kind has hardly begun. Fortunately, however, it is already possible to avoid much death and infirmity through accident prevention measures that were first developed by trial and error but have become increasingly scientific over the last fifty years.

What Is an Accident

There are still arguments about the definition of the term "accident." An advisory group convened by the World Health Organization considered it to be "an unpremeditated event resulting in a recognizable injury."

The American National Safety Council expands this definition: "An accident is that occurrence in a sequence of events which usually produces unintended injury, death, or property damage."

The Manual of the International Statistical Classification of Diseases, Injuries and Causes of Death prepared by the World Health Organization lists over 135 types of accidents* which more or less fit one or the other of these two classifications.

In statistical practice, however, physi-

---

*Not including complications due to non-therapeutic medical or surgical procedures, therapeutic misadventures and late complications of therapeutic procedures, or late effects of injury and poisoning.

cians and prevention specialists have grouped accidents into half a dozen major categories which vary only slightly from one country to another. For example, the classification of the American National Safety Council has six main headings: work, motor vehicles, public, farm, home, and school accidents. In the National Safety Council classification, drowning is considered a "public" accident; elsewhere it may be grouped, along with accidents caused by firearms, in the domestic accident category.

Accidents in the air or on railways, which are statistically insignificant, may be classed either as public or as transport accidents.

Poisoning is characteristically a "home" accident, while "school" accidents are very similar to home accidents except that they occur outside the home.

Earthquakes, Eruptions, and Floods

Imperfect as they may be, the various classifications do at least provide a basis for concrete preventive measures. One reason why they exclude natural catastrophes such as earthquakes, volcanic eruptions, and floods is that all these spectacular tragedies together take a far smaller toll in human lives than the unending succession of commonplace accidents.

One natural catastrophe which may be avoided by building homes on higher ground and away from streams is floods.

They must be fought as one of mankind's most serious enemies, these innumerable everyday accidents that happen all around us, at work and at play, in the home and at our doors, in the farmyard and in the city streets.

WHERE RISKS ARE GREATEST —AT HOME

The kitchen, the stairs, or the bedroom of a modern house hold more dangers than the fastest car or plane, the steepest mountain, or a ship in a storm.

Simple things such as a bottle of aspirin left lying on a table, a kettle of boiling water, a forgotten edge tool, will make more cripples and kill more children this year than will poliomyelitis and tuberculosis together.

Perhaps it is because the dangers are so commonplace that accidents in the home seem hard to avoid. Even the absent-minded or reckless will look before crossing a road; even the most prudent will unthinkingly run across a polished floor to answer the phone.

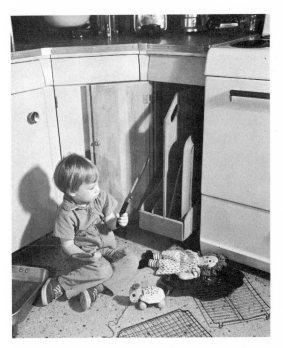

Caution: All children explore. A carelessly stored knife is dangerous.

Take Mrs. Ruth Galley, seventy-five years old, living alone in her room in Lewisham, England. She is in perfect health, yet every day for years she has risked a fatal accident. Like many English houses, hers has a coin-in-the-slot gas meter. For some mysterious reason, the meter is so fixed that she has to climb on a chair to put in the shilling. There she was one day when a health visitor called. (The National Health Service has seventeen health visitors for the 400,000 inhabitants of that part of outer London). A telephone call to the gas company, and the next day Mrs. Galley's meter was fixed where she could reach it easily. At the same time, the rubber pipe of her gas cooker, which was just as old and even more fragile than its owner, was replaced. All free of charge of course.

So her name will probably not be among the 4,500 or so persons over sixty-five who die every year in Great Britain as the result of a fall, or among the 1,500 persons who die as the result of poisoning by gas or other substance.

In the United States the number of home accidents in one recent year was estimated at 4,000,000, whereas the total of road and industrial accidents for the same period was reckoned to be only 3,350,000. If we take into consideration the 2,000,000 victims of accidents occurring outside their homes, but not at work or in automobiles, it would seem that twice as many people are hurt in the United States while engaged in activities that are supposed to be safe than are hurt at their jobs or in traffic. It is true that proportionally as well as in absolute numbers, there are more deaths in industrial and traffic accidents (50,000 in the United States in one year); yet there were no fewer than 43,500 deaths in accidents of other kinds, of which 26,000 occurred in homes.

In Great Britain, it is estimated that one accident in two occurred in or around the home and garden, or in playing grounds. The proportion may well be greater, since accurate figures are available only for accidents causing death or serious injury leading to hospitalization.

This seems probable, judging from the results of a survey undertaken recently in Stockholm by the Committee for the Prevention of Accidents in Childhood. It was found that of the Swedish capital's 227,000 children, 24,466 had had accidents of which twenty-nine were fatal; i.e., a proportion of one fatal accident to 840 less serious ones.

Previous estimates in Sweden were between 100 and 400 less serious accidents for every fatal accident. And Sweden has one of the world's lowest accident rates.

Care and Vigilance

Considering all the manifold dangers, what is surprising is that there are so comparatively few home accidents. Today, the safety of the home is a question of the least national dimensions. This is the point of view of the Royal Society for the Prevention of Accidents, whose home safety department extends its activities throughout the United Kingdom.

"Our great problem," says Barbara Naish, who directs this vital department, "is not to lose touch with everyday reality and to keep going with confidence even though we have no accurate way of measuring the results."

The people whom it is important to reach are those who are naturally careless. It is usually the very poor who need help most—those who do not go to safety meetings organized by the 135 local Home Safety Committees in Great Britain. They neither read the pamphlets, nor see the films, nor visit the expositions.

These potential victims of accidents must be sought out in their own homes. A neighborly visit by a member of the Local Home Safety Committee or an inspection of the gas and electricity installations will do more good than all the public lectures in the world.

Serious Burns

Door-to-door visiting is not always enough, however. Some problems require a more massive attack on old, ingrained habits. Recently, for example, the Royal Society for the Prevention of Accidents, with backing from the Home Office, launched a nationwide campaign to provide all open fireplaces with safety screens in order to bring down the number of serious burns, which over the years had been remaining fairly constant.

Similar campaigns could well have been launched in many other countries, for a bad burn is one of the most horrible accidents. The pain suffered by the victim, whether burnt by fire, acid, boiling water or steam, is only the first of his trials. Then comes treatment lasting on an average from one to three months, while subsequent operations and grafts are sometimes spread over several years.

Furthermore, any permanent infirmity or mutilation may lead to psychological consequences, the seriousness of which is only now beginning to be realized. Psychiatrists see these results everyday.

Every year, five to ten times as many children as adults suffer burns. In Great Britain, only 700 persons die of burns every year, but 550 hospital beds are permanently occupied by the victims of burns, and 126,-000 persons alive today have at some time been in a hospital with burns from the one single cause of clothes on fire.

The problem is even more severe in some of the rapidly developing countries because of the widespread use of gas and explosive substances (acetylene, butane, or propane lamps, fireworks, etc.).

Everywhere, boiling liquids claim innumerable victims.

Avoiding Burns

After the children, it is the elderly who most frequently suffer these terrible accidents which indeed cause more deaths among the old than among children. In Great Britain, victims of burns over the age of sixty-five are three or four times as numerous as those among young adults. Twice as many women as men suffer burns from clothing on fire; dresses, skirts, and nightgowns, particularly when made of cotton, are much more likely to catch fire than men's clothing.

In Great Britain today, a highly developed system of legislation and regulations provides some guarantee of safety. Every heating appliance—electric, gas, oil, or other—has to meet certain well-defined standards of safety, and it is against the law to expose a child to an insufficiently protected fire.

Dr. Leonard Colebrook, who is one of the pioneers in the prevention of burns in England, considers, however, that this is not enough. Speaking to a group of American colleagues several years ago, he expressed surprise that certain highly inflammable textiles were put on sale without the public being warned of their potential danger; for the quicker the material burns, the worse the damage.

"We have closed our eyes to the danger and, for that reason, have lost thousands of lives," says Dr. Colebrook. "If we want to fight effectively, we should, I think, put into practice a three point program:

1. Collect maximum information on the most inflammable textiles
2. Reach international agreement on ways of indicating the degree of inflammability of each textile and the rapidity with which it burns
3. Get the safest textiles used for children's and old people's clothing"

Guilty and Ashamed

Dr. Joan Woodward, a psychiatrist attached to the Burns Research Unit in Birmingham, England, considers that after the accident has happened no effort should be spared to soothe the anxiety and guilt feeling of the parents. She recently examined 200 children who had had severe burns two to five years previously. According to their mothers, eighty percent of the children still suffered emotionally from the effects. But during her survey, Dr. Woodward was to realize that many of the mothers suffered in this respect at least as much as their children.

"They all, without exception, feel guilty and ashamed," says Dr. Woodward. "Many of the mothers asked me bitterly why it had to happen to *their* child." This question indicates how deeply rooted is the sense of failure in a mother whose child has suffered a severe burn.

Many mothers read in the newspapers about accidents caused by fire. On television they may see propaganda films dealing with safety in the home. But they cannot believe that such a thing could happen in their own family.

All that can be done is to repeat: Watch that fire, careful with that boiling water. And an absolute rule for baby's bath: always put the cold water in first before the hot water. If possible, do not have children around the kitchen when the meal is being cooked. Do not have pots and pans on the stove with the handle pointing outward. Do young girls really have to wear nightdresses? A pair of pajamas, which catch fire much less easily, may mean the difference between life and death.

Spot removers, paraffin oil or gasoline should be kept in a safe place and in small quantities only. Such simple precautions can save life and prevent lives from being wrecked.

Poisoning Accidents

This is even more obvious when one comes to the third great class of home accidents: poisoning. Again, it is the children and, to a lesser degree, the old people who are the main victims. Unlike other home accidents, poisonings generally increase in number with a rise in the standard of living.

According to figures supplied recently by the American National Safety Council, 1,200 people die annually in the United States from poisoning and about 200,000 people become ill from the same cause. A study carried out by the New York Poison Control Center showed that half the victims of poisoning are under the age of twenty, and three-fourths of these are less than four years old, with children between the ages of one and two years leading the sad procession. This pattern, with slight modifications, applies the world over.

Enforcing strict regulations concerning the description and packing of poisonous substances is one obvious way of helping prevent poisonings in the home. But even here much remains to be done. International standards are urgently necessary in the description and labelling of poisons, whether they be medicines, cleaning fluids, insecticides, or any other dangerous chemicals. Paint used inside the house should be free of lead, as should all paints used on toys. This is already a law in a number of countries.

According to the health authorities, ninety-five percent of all poisonings can be prevented. But this requires watchful parents and the strict application of a certain number of rules.

The survey conducted by the New York Poison Control Center revealed that in ninety-three percent of child poisoning accidents an adult was present in the house at the time. In seventy-six percent of the cases it was the mother. Over fifty percent of the cases were caused by household products that were assumed to be harmless.

A country policeman in southern Sweden recently invented a special kind of latch for closing a cupboard. To release it, two separate movements are required. All the tests have shown that this is too difficult for a child under four. This device is quite inexpensive and has advantages over the key that so often gets lost, or that people sometimes, perhaps on the fatal occasion, forget to turn in the lock.

Working along similar lines, a young pediatrician has invented a stopper for a bottle that simply goes on turning round with a clickety-click noise when a child tries to open it, and an aspirin tube made of plastic which has to be squeezed slightly before a tablet will come out. These two inventions stood up very well in tests with children.

It is necessary to know which products to keep out of children's reach. Who would ever think of locking up cosmetics and perfumes? How many people realize that, in some countries, aspirin tablets are the principal cause of child poisoning? Barbiturates and the family pharmacy in general should be carefully put away where they are inaccessible to a child. The same is true of polish and cleaning products. On no account should toxic substances such as paraffin oil, gasoline, or acids be kept in containers originally intended for other purposes—lemonade bottles, jam jars, etc.

Falls, burns, and poisonings are not the only risks that must be guarded against. The greatest enemy of family safety, and one from which the others stem, is negligence, with its corollaries, untidiness and dirt. A badly lit room may cost much more than would a stronger lamp. A properly insulated electric plug, a step repaired in time, a safety bar or wire netting fixed in the window—it is on "details" such as these that the life of a child may depend.

To turn off the main switch before mending a fuse, to wipe up immediately a spot of grease fallen onto the kitchen floor, to leave the window ajar in a room where a gas or coal stove is alight—attention to these seeming trivialities will transform a house into a true home where a family can live in security instead of in constant danger.

With a little extra thinking and some small amount of extra work many tragedies could be avoided.

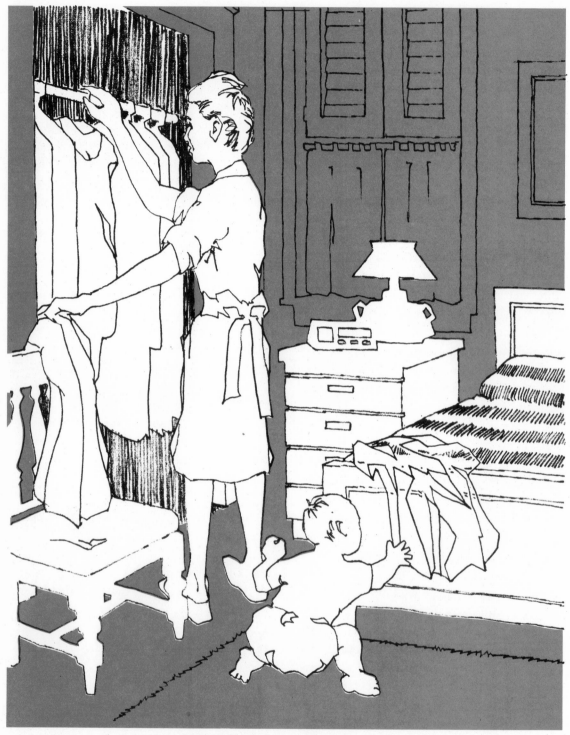

Many children die every year from suffocation caused by placing a plastic bag over their heads. Plastic bags are used by cleaners to cover dresses and suits. When they are removed they should be burned immediately. Never place within reach of a child.

ACCIDENTAL DEATH CAUSED BY PLASTIC BAGS

Since the advent of plastic bags there has been a great increase in the number of accidental deaths. These deaths usually occur in children ranging from a few months to two or three years of age.

In spite of the fact that the bags are usually labeled as dangerous and should be destroyed, they still continue to be one of the leading causes of accidental death in small babies.

These plastic bags are used for many different purposes; to cover clothes coming from the dry cleaner, to contain vegetables and fruits, and to contain bread. They should be destroyed immediately and not just thrown into the garbage can or waste paper basket.

A few cases of accidental death reported recently will help show just how dangerous these bags are.

1. A two-year old girl was found dead from suffocation with a plastic bag around her head. This bag had been used as a ukulele cover and had been removed by the baby while playing with it and placed it over her head.

2. A vegetable bag used as a diaper container and left on the dresser was found over the head of a one-year old baby who was dead from suffocation

3. A sweater bag, discarded into the trash can in the kitchen, was over the head of a two-year old child, found dead on the kitchen floor from suffocation

4. A nine-month old baby was found dead in his crib with a plastic bag over his head. This bag had been used to hold sea shells and had been left over the end of the crib. The baby found it and pulled it over his head

5. Dry cleaner's bag over garment in front seat of car. Five-months old baby dead with bag over head

6. A plastic bag was used to protect baby's bed. This five-weeks old baby was found dead with plastic wrapped around its head

7. A bag used to pack frozen turkeys was put into service as a diaper container and left on the bed. An eleven-month old baby was found dead of suffocation with the bag over its head

8. A dry cleaner's bag was used as a protection to keep the mattress dry. The eight-month old baby was found dead with the bag twisted around its head

9. A dry cleaner's bag had been left on the crib while the baby was sleeping. This five-months old boy was found dead with a portion of the bag over its face. Cause of death—suffocation

10. A dry cleaner's bag had been placed in the garbage can for burning. The two-year old sister had recovered it and placed it over her four-month old brother as a cover. The baby was found dead of suffocation

These are just a few actual cases reported in one state over a period of eight months.

The lessons to be learned from the above statistics are that the plastic material used in bags should be destroyed immediately. They should not be left in the garbage can but should be burned at once. And never should they be used as a covering for the baby's mattress.

Destroy immediately or lock up where children cannot reach them—ALL plastic bags.

GLOSSARY

Allocated   distributed

Ambiguity   not clearly understood; could have more than one meaning

Analogy   comparing similar aspects of two or more dissimilar things

Asphyxiation   suffocation

Cardiovascular disease   disease of the heart and blood vessels

Conflagration   a fire

Corollaries   results or consequences

Empirical   depending on experience or observation alone without regard to science

Epidemiological   the field of science dealing with factors that cause epidemics

Etiology   the study of the cause of disease

Etiological   pertaining to the cause of disease

Hazard   a danger

Immunized   given protection against a disease

Inflammable   capable of being easily set on fire (better word: flammable)

Luminous   shining; reflecting light

Mortality   death rate

Mutilate   to destroy part of; to cripple

Obscure   not easily understood

Pedestrian   pertaining to travel by walking; one who walks

Pragmatic   matter of fact

Precipitate   to cause to happen suddenly

Prevalent   widespread

Psychomotor   pertaining to a muscular action resulting from a mental process

Psychophysiological   the relation between the mental and physical process

Psychosocial   pertaining to the social aspects of mental life

Stereotyped   repeated without variation

Therapeutic   healing

Trivial   of minor importance

Chapter 26

First Aid: Used Only in Minor Injuries

NOSEBLEED

The patient with nosebleed should be kept quiet. The best position is to have him lie face down, so the blood will not run down his throat. Pressure should be applied from the outside, to both sides of the nose. This will usually stop the nosebleed in a short time.

If this fails, the nostril from which the blood is coming can be packed firmly with cotton, or with a narrow bandage. This will place pressure on the bleeding point, and control the hemorrhage. This packing should be left in place for about twenty-four hours.

If the above methods fail, the patient should be seen by a doctor.

SPRAINED ANKLE

This injury is usually caused by turning the ankle outward, and may be very painful. At times, there is considerable swelling, and the injured person is unable to bear weight on his sprained ankle. At other times, especially when the ankle puffs up immediately, there may be very little pain, and weight may be borne without difficulty.

The cases which swell up so rapidly with little pain are usually on the outer side of the ankle, and the swelling is probably caused by a broken blood-vessel.

When there is a great deal of pain, this usually means that the tendons on the outside of the ankle have been torn or stretched.

The treatment in both cases is the same. Immediately following the accident, cold should be applied to discourage swelling or hemorrhage. Then a pressure bandage, such as an ace bandage, should be applied firmly. The patient's leg should be elevated on a pillow—again to discourage swelling.

After keeping the leg elevated with an elastic bandage on it for maybe a day and night, and the swelling has decreased, the ankle should be taped. This is best done by using a so-called basket weave taping—that is, first placing a long piece of adhesive tape from the inner side of the leg around the heel, then up the outer side of the leg, keeping the foot at a right angle, and turned slightly outward on the ankle. The second piece of tape, about one inch in width, is placed in a circular manner around the ankle. This circular piece of tape should cross on itself in the front of the foot. Then the next piece of tape is placed down the leg, around the bottom of the foot, and up the side of the leg.

By alternating the tape—first up and down, and then around the ankle, the taping will soon firmly support the ankle and allow weight to be placed upon it without much pain.

After first applying cold water for a few hours to discourage swelling, the patient should always use heat thereafter to hasten healing of the torn ligaments. The heat may be applied in either the wet or dry form—that is, hot compresses or a heating pad.

Aspirin may be given to control the pain.

Remember to keep the ankle elevated, in case the pain is severe.

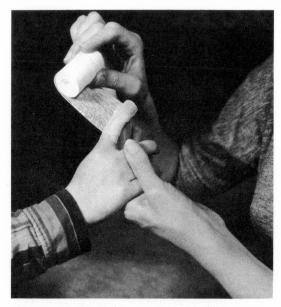

Thorough cleaning and dressing of wound promotes quick healing.

SCRATCHES AND CUTS

When a scratch is suffered on any part of the body, the first thought in the treatment should be to cleanse the wound. Ordinary soap and warm water can be used to wash the scratched surface until it is clean. Then some kind of a bland ointment may be applied.

There are many ointments sold in tubes now which contain antibiotics such as penicillin, aureomycin, etc. Some of these have, in combination, cortisone and other steroids.

After washing, drying, and applying the ointment, a dry dressing such as a Band-aid should be placed over the scratch to protect it from further injury until it can heal.

If no disinfectant, like an ointment, iodine, or merthiolate, is at hand, soap is just about as effective as any of these in preventing infection. Hence, to wash with soap

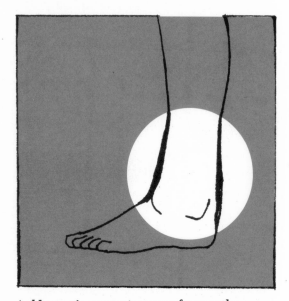

Ankle sprains or strains occur frequently.

and water, dry, and cover with a dry dressing is all that is absolutely essential.

In the case of cuts, the bleeding should be controlled by direct pressure over the bleeding spot. This is very important. When the bleeding has ceased, the cut should be cleansed with ordinary soap and water, and the edges of the cut should be drawn together. This may be done, in the case of a long cut, by stitches which must be placed by a doctor. In the case of a small cut, the edges may be held together by placing a piece of adhesive tape (sometimes a Band-aid will do) across the cut, pulling the edges together by placing the tape at right angles or across the line of the cut. Then the area should be covered by placing a clean bandage over the adhesive tape.

The most important points are control of bleeding by pressure, and cleansing the wound with soap and water.

BLISTERS

A blister on any part of the body should be treated as an open wound, and care taken to prevent infection. If the blister is intact, that is, the fluid is still present in it, there is no better dressing than the skin which is over the blister. So, if there is not enough fluid to cause discomfort, you may leave it alone.

If the fluid is abundant, sterilize a needle by holding it in a match flame, and stick the needle into the raised skin of the blister near the edge. Several holes may be made in this way, and the fluid will escape. Leave the skin over the blister, and apply a clean dressing, as the holes make it possible for bacteria to enter and cause infection.

If the skin over the blister has been bro-

ken in many places it is better to take some sterile scissors and cut it off, applying antiseptic ointments and a clean dressing.

BURNS

Burns are sometimes classified as to depth of tissue involved. Hence, a first degree burn causes redness of the skin only; a second degree burn causes blisters to be formed; and a third degree burn causes destruction of the entire thickness of the skin and of varying depths of underlying tissue, muscles, etc.

The first degree burns and small second degree burns may be treated at home, the main objective being to reduce pain and prevent infections.

By holding a burned area under cold water for a while, the pain may be reduced.

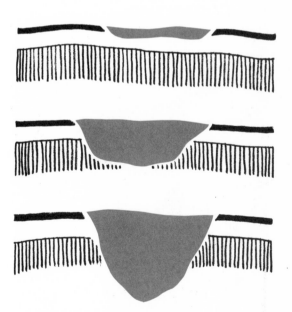

Classification of burns: 1st degree, only skin affected; 2nd Degree, blisters form; 3rd Degree, skin and underlying tissue affected.

The application of a bland ointment (antipyrexol, sold in tubes under the name of Kip) over the burned area, will protect it from the air, and reduce pain. The patient may also take aspirin to obtain relief.

Blisters which still contain fluid should not be opened, as this increases chances of infection.

Any burn greater than a first degree or small second degree, should be treated by a doctor.

ANIMAL BITES

The bite of any animal is dangerous, as it may be the means of introducing into the body the virus that causes rabies. No person has been known to recover from a case of rabies caused by the bite of a rabid dog. Therefore, dog bites or bites from other animals should be treated with respect.

If the dog is healthy, then the wound should be treated like any other wound—cleansed with soap and water, and after applying a good antiseptic ointment, such as erythromycin, polymyxin, bacitracin, etc., the wound should be dressed.

The dog should be observed for ten days, and if he does not develop symptoms of rabies in this time, the person who has been bitten is in no danger.

Do not kill the dog. If the dog is killed accidentally before the ten days is up, his brain should be sent to a laboratory to determine whether or not he had rabies.

If the dog was obviously mad or rabid, the prophylactic treatment against rabies should be started at once. The so-called Semple treatment has largely replaced the old Pasteur treatment, and it has saved many lives.

If the dog develops rabies within ten days, then the series of injections (Semple) should begin at once.

The treatment is sometimes helped by using antirabies hyperimmune serum, in addition to the Semple vaccine.

INSECT BITES

Most insect bites are not dangerous, and should be treated conservatively with the application of a mild antiseptic solution or ointment, such as Listerine or a Calomine lotion.

INSECT STING ANAPHYLAXIS

Cause and Nature

Every year there are reports of sudden death caused by the sting of certain insects. The most common of these insects are the honey bee, the yellow jacket, the wasp, and the hornet.

This form of anaphylactic reaction only occurs in people who are extremely sensitive to the poison injected by the insect when it stings them. This is the kind of reaction that occurs when sensitive people get injections of penicillin or tetanus antitoxin which has horse serum in it. Many people die each year from injections of penicillin. To suffer this kind of a reaction the person must be extremely allergic to, or sensitive to the substance injected.

Signs and Symptoms

The manifestations of an anaphylactic reation to an insect bite are seen a very short time after the bite—seldom longer than two minutes. The symptoms are weakness, nausea, shortness of breath, generalized burning pain, perspiration, swelling of the mucous membranes, chills, and dizziness. If death is going to occur it may come within thirty minutes after the bite.

Treatment

The treatment must start at once and the only effective treatment is the injection of .5 cc. of a one to 1000 solution of adrenalin. People who know that they are allergic to these stings should always carry a kit with adrenalin amphins that they can use to inject the adrenalin. This may be life-saving.

A tourniquet should be tied above the sting in all instances.

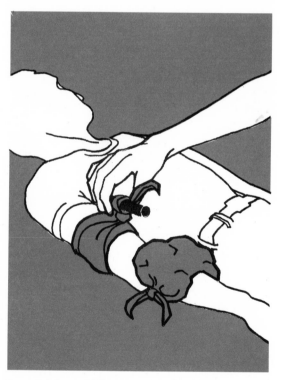

Insect stings: When a person is sensitive to insect bites, a tournequet should be tied lightly above the sting immediately, and ice packed around the bite.

Remove the stinger from the skin.

After the immediate emergency treatment it may be necessary to repeat the adrenalin injection.

In order to prevent a delayed reaction such as hives or urticaria, injections of antihistamines such as chlortrimeton or pyribenzamine should be given intramuscularly. Another useful tool used to prevent delayed reactions are injections of seroids such as cortisone.

Any person who knows that he is allergic to these insect stings should be desensitized by taking repeated injections of very weak solutions of the poisons over a long period of time. This desensitization will be performed by a doctor.

GLOSSARY

Anaphylaxis   a state of increased susceptibility to a drug or toxin

Toxin   any poisonous albumin or base of bacterial origin

BLACK WIDOW SPIDER BITE

The only dangerous spider in the United States is the black widow. This spider has been found in every state in the union except seven or eight.

The venom from the bite of a female black widow is said to be about fifteen times as potent as the venom from a rattlesnake. In spite of this, the death rate following a bite from a black widow is very low.

It is important to recognize the symptoms following the bite of a black widow spider and to start early treatment. This treatment must be in the hands of a doctor.

There is local pain, swelling, and redness at the site of the bite. In ten or fifteen minutes, a burning sensation spreads from the bite over the entire body. This may last for twenty or thirty minutes. Then there may be a sudden severe cramp-like pain in the abdomen, which may be mistaken for a surgical condition. The cramp-like pains may extend to the arms, legs, and back. There is extreme weakness, restlessness, and fear. Lastly, there is a burning of the soles of the feet. Children may have convulsions.

There are many drugs which can be used to cure this condition, and a doctor should be seen at once.

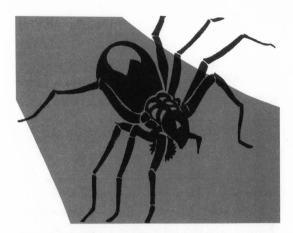

The bite of this small brown spider results in a local painful ulcer.

SPIDER BITE OR ARACHNOIDISM IN THE U.S.

Cause and Nature

While the black widow spider bite causes the most severe reactions, there are several other species of spiders found in the United States whose bites may or may not cause mild reactions. In foreign countries these poisonous bites are more common.

Since the spider is not an aggresive insect, it will seldom bite human beings, and because its fangs are not strong, they rarely puncture the skin. However, in the United States a great deal of investigation has been done on the effect of spider venom. Some cases of injurious effects have been reported when a spider other than a black widow has bitten a child or an adult.

The spider likes to hide in dark places and may be found in barns, old buildings, and even at times in clothes and bedclothes.

Signs and Symptoms

The effects of spider bites are divided into two classes: (1) That which has only a local effect or attacks the cells in different parts of the body, is called cyototoxic; (2) The venom which attacks the nervous system, as in the case of the black widow, is called neurotoxic.

The effects of the bite of a black widow spider (Latrodectus) have been described, but there is a species of spider known as Loxosceles found in the central and southern part of the United States which can cause a moderately severe local reaction. The bite of this small brown or tan spider will cause a sloughing or destruction of the skin which makes an ulcer that may require several weeks to heal. It is a good idea, therefore, to warn children to be careful of spiders when they are playing in dark places, such as, barns or old buildings.

The unreasoning fright which some people have when they see any kind of a spider is not called for.

Treatment

In most cases specific treatment is not required. However, if there is a severe general reaction as seen in children or older people, such as muscle spasms and shock, this should be treated by a doctor with muscle relaxants, perhaps a warm bath or other appropriate measures. Local treatment is aimed at the prevention of infection.

In cases of severe nerve reaction or neurotoxic reaction, there is specific treatment in the form of specific antivenom which must be administered by a doctor. This is much like the antivenom used in the case of a rattlesnake bite as it neutralizes the poison injected by the spider.

It should be emphasized, that ill effects from spider bites in the United States are extremely rare. An attitude of caution rather than one of fear should be maintained toward spiders.

GLOSSARY

Cytotoxic   a toxin or antibody which has a specific action upon cells of special organs

Neurotoxic   a toxin or antibody which has a toxic action on the nervous system

HICCUPS

There are many remedies for hiccups, and usually one of the following simple cures will work:

The patient should lie down and rest, if possible. Sometimes drinking a glass of cold water will terminate the attack.

If the person with hiccups can be made to think of something else, as in the case of a sudden surprise, hiccups often disappear.

One of the best ways to treat a case of hiccups is to get a paper bag and fit it closely around the mouth and nose. Breathing into this bag, the patient can breathe the same air over and over again. In this way, the carbon dioxide builds up, and helps to stop the hiccups.

In very persistant hiccups as seen in people who are ill or very weak, a few whiffs of

straight carbon dioxide will stop them. Remember this is a dangerous gas and should be used with caution, under the supervision of a doctor.

FAINTING

The sudden loss of consciousness is called fainting. While there are many causes for fainting, the most common is lack of blood at the level of the brain. This is usually caused by pooling of the blood in the lower part of the body. A common example of this is seen when a soldier faints after standing at attention for too long.

The treatment is to allow the person to remain in a lying position. If possible, the head should be lower than the rest of the

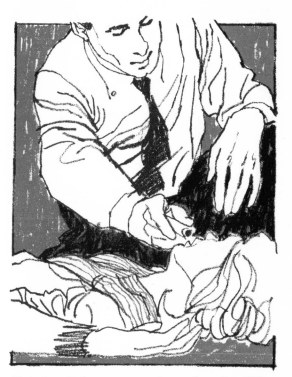

Fainting: When a person faints they should be placed with their head down or level. A whiff of smelling salts will help.

body. In this way, the blood is allowed to rush back to the brain.

The person who has fainted should be allowed to breathe plenty of fresh air, and the clothing around the neck and chest should be loosened. The use of cold water or stimulation by holding "smelling salts," that is, aromatic spirits of ammonia, under the nose to be breathed by the patient, will hasten the return of consciousness.

When a person feels a fainting attack coming on, he should immediately lie down.

SNEEZING

Sneezing is not a disease, but is a protective effort on the part of the body to expel or force out any irritating substance which tickles the mucous membranes of the nose. Hence, when we inhale black pepper, we sneeze violently. Therefore, one should not try to stop a sneeze as it really helps us by cleansing out unwanted substances in the nostrils. Once the nose is clear, the sneezing will stop.

CHARLEYHORSE

This is a term used to describe the rupture of a few small fibres of muscle, usually in the leg. This rupture of muscle fibres may result from a direct blow, or could be caused by excessive strain. There is usually a very tender swollen spot at the point of rupture, and walking becomes painful.

Application of heat to the spot, with gentle massage, will usually allow the fibres to heal in a few days. Rest of the injured limb is important in order that the healing may be more rapid.

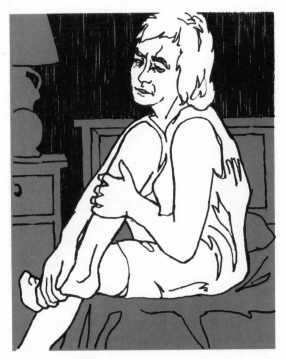

Painful muscle cramps usually occur during the night and interfere with sleep. They may be prevented by taking five grains of quinine at bedtime.

MUSCLE CRAMPS

All of us have experienced painful muscle cramps at one time or another, and upon feeling the painful area, a definite lump can be felt. This lump or cramp of the muscle can be relieved by massaging the area. Also, this condition is often helped by the application of heat, and by putting the part at rest.

If a person has repeated cramps, it is likely that a shortage of calcium exists. By taking dicalcium phosphate with viosterol, three capsules daily, for about two weeks, these recurrent cramps can often be prevented. The best treatment for curing or preventing muscle cramps is to take quinine sulfate, five grams, three times a day.

MOTION SICKNESS

(Car Sickness, Train Sickness, Sea Sickness, Air Sickness)

Many susceptible people exhibit a series of symptoms when they are subjected to motion for long periods, as in taking a long automobile drive over a very curvy, winding road.

The first feeling noticed is an uneasiness in the stomach. This is followed by muscular weakness, dizziness, turning pale, and sweating. The last symptom to appear is vomiting, and then the person may feel better for a while, only to have the same set of symptoms appear again, if he continues to ride.

The treatment is to eat and drink lightly before starting on a trip. There are many drugs, such as dramamine and bonamine, which if taken before and during a trip, will prevent motion sickness.

MASHED FINGER

(With Blood Under the Fingernail)

This painful condition occurs frequently following a blow on the end of the finger by some object such as a hammer. The pain is severe and throbbing in nature. The blood may be seen beneath the fingernail, where it cannot escape.

The treatment is to use a sharp-pointed knife, or some other sharp instrument, to bore a hole through the nail. This can be done by rotating the knife point over the same place on the nail, and applying a little pressure. When a hole is bored through the nail, the blood escapes and the pain ceases.

The hands and instrument should be washed well before the hole is bored.

BRUISES

A contusion or blow to any part of the body may result in a bruise, which becomes black and blue and swollen.

The treatment is to first apply cold, in order to prevent the swelling. A pressure bandage (ace bandage) should be applied, if possible, for the same purpose. The part should be treated in this manner for forty-eight hours. Then heat and massage should be used to hasten absorption of the blood, which has spilled out into the tissue.

INGROWN TOENAIL

This condition has two main causes:

1. Wearing shoes that are too tight
2. Improper cutting of the toenails

The toenail should not be cut in a rounded manner as the fingernails are cut, but

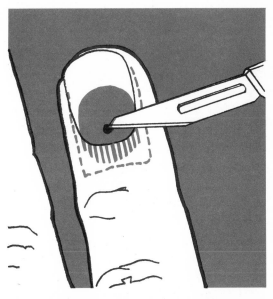

Boring a hole through a nail with blood under it will relieve throbbing pain.

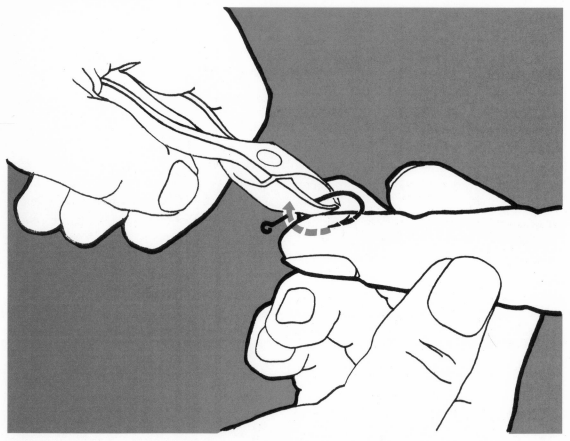

Removing fish hooks: 1) Push the hook on through the finger (red arrow above), 2) Cut off the shaft of the hook, 3) Pull the hook the rest of the way out with a pair of pliers.

should be cut squarely across, and not cut too short.

If an ingrown toenail or infected granulations start growing around the toenail, hot water soaks should be used. A small piece of cotton should be placed under the nail where the irritation exists, and large shoes should be worn. If conservative home methods do not cure the condition, a doctor should be consulted.

In addition to cutting the toenails squarely across, and not too short, it helps to cut a small V in the center of the nail. Most important of all—do not wear tight shoes.

SPLINTERS OR FOREIGN BODIES

Foreign bodies or splinters in the skin should be removed. First wash the part with soap and water. Then sterilize a needle or pin by holding it in the flame of a match. The skin over the splinter should be opened with the point of the needle, and then the needle should be placed at the deepest end of the splinter, and gentle pressure used to push the splinter out. When the end is free, the splinter or foreign body can be removed by using a small pair of tweezers or forceps. Simple antiseptic precautions should be observed.

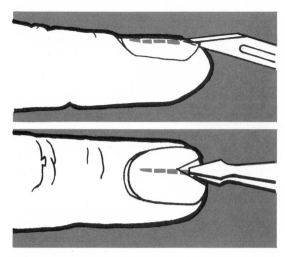

A **splinter** under a nail may be removed by cutting a V-shaped notch in nail and grasping the splinter with a pair of tweezers.

SPLINTER UNDER FINGERNAIL

If the splinter can be seen, the finger should be washed with soap and water and a sharp pair of scissors should be used to cut a V-shaped piece out of the nail down to the edge of the splinter. The splinter may then be grasped by a clean pair of tweezers, and pulled out.

INFECTED HANGNAIL

Any infection around the fingernail should be treated promptly. Moist heat should be applied; the part should be elevated and at rest; and finally, some antibiotic, such as penicillin, may be prescribed. If the infection comes to a head or pus is formed, then a small incision should be made next to the nail and the pus allowed to drain out.

GLOSSARY

Gangrene   decay of a part of a living person
Hemorrhage   bleeding

BUNION

(Hallux Valgus)

Cause and Nature

The bunion is caused by the great toe turning toward the outer side of the foot. The tendency to this condition may be inherited, but it is usually caused by wearing narrow, pointed shoes.

Signs and Symptoms

The base of the big toe which has pointed towards the outer side of the foot presses against the shoe, and the soft tissues are thickened and become very painful. Often there is an enlargement of the bone at the base of the toe and this increases the thickening and discomfort.

Treatment

Do not allow a child to wear narrow, pointed shoes. If there is a mild tendency towards turning outward of the big toe, sometimes this can be corrected by proper shoes and wearing a pad between the great toe and the next toe. If the condition has become permanent and painful, it should be corrected by surgery.

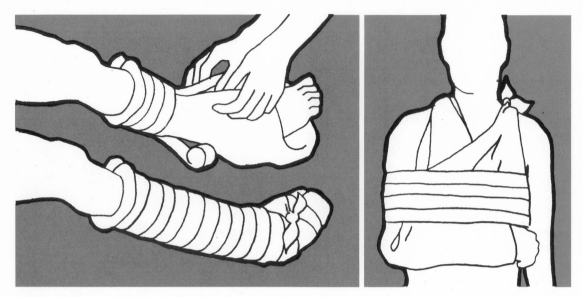

Fracture first aid: If it is necessary to move a person with a fracture in order to reach medical help, place the injured limb in a splint or sling. When a foot or ankle is fractured, a pillow splint may be used as shown on the left. Use a sling and bandage for a fractured collar bone as shown on the right. For a dislocated shoulder use only the sling. Whenever possible, do not move the injured person, instead bring medical help to him.

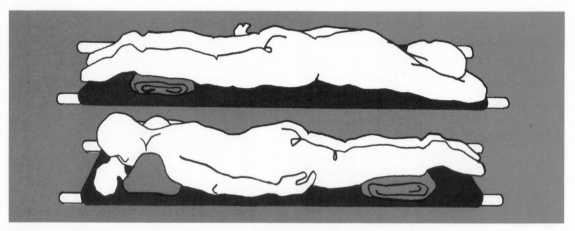

Back and neck injuries: Great care must be exercised when moving a person with a back or neck injury. Do not move the patient unless it is absolutely necessary.

Lower back injuries (thoracic or lumbar vertebra): Transport the patient face down. Do not allow the back to be bent forward or flexed. Place a blanket under the legs (see upper portion of drawing).

Upper back or neck injuries (cervical vertebra): Transport the patient face down. Do not allow the back to be bent forward or flexed. Place a blanket under the legs. Position the patient's arm and a sandbag under his head to prevent it from moving (see lower portion illustration). A slight traction on the head is desirable if practical.

Chapter 27

Emergency Treatment

FRACTURES

The basic techniques for handling injured persons with broken or fractured bones are illustrated and described briefly on the facing page.

FIVE POINTS IN TREATING ANY INFECTION

1. REST. The part should be put at rest to help the body fight the infection
2. HEAT. By applying heat to the part, more blood is brought to the area, and the blood contains elements which fight the infection
3. ELEVATION. The infected part should be placed higher than the other parts of the body to prevent swelling, which would delay the healing process
4. DRAINAGE. If pus is formed, it should always be drained out. It usually is best to get a doctor to make the necessary incisions
5. ANTIBIOTICS. By using one or more of the present-day antibiotics, such as penicillin, ilotycin, terramycin, or erythromycin, in addition to the first four measures, most infections can be cured

ARTIFICIAL RESPIRATION

(The Mouth-to-Mouth Method)

One of the most important first aid techniques is mouth-to-mouth resuscitation. This has largely replaced the old method of pressure on the chest which was used in artificial respiration. The old method can sometimes be used in connection with the new, although as a rule it is not necessary to use both of them.

When a person has ceased to breathe because of immersion in water, electric shock, or any other form of stress, his breathing should be restored as quickly as possible so that the tissues of his body, especially the brain, receive oxygen.

The pulse should be felt to see if the heart is still beating in spite of the fact that the person has stopped breathing.

If the heart is beating, this makes the task of successful resuscitation easier. This is the method.

The mouth of the patient is cleared quickly of water or any other foreign matter. The patient is placed on his back and the index finger is passed through his open

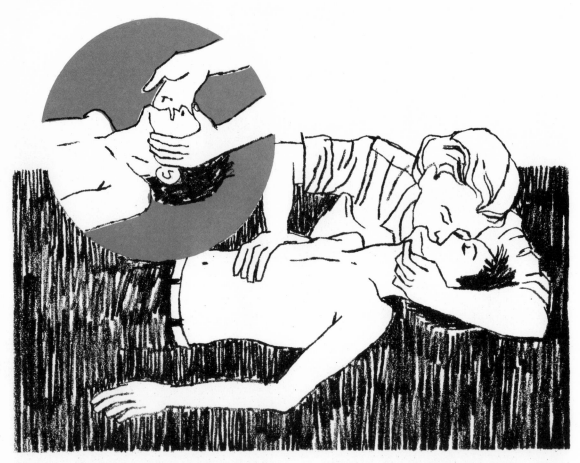

Mouth to mouth respiration: 1. Be sure chin is up. 2. Clear mouth with fingers—tongue in proper place. 3. Block nose. 4. Take a deep breath, blow in patient's mouth. 5. Remove your mouth, let patient exhale. 6. Repeat about every 2 to 5 seconds.

mouth to be sure the tongue is in its proper position and that there are no foreign bodies present.

The operator then places the thumb and forefinger of one hand on the patient's nostrils and closes off that airway by pinching it. He then places his open mouth over the patient's open mouth and blows his breath into the lungs of the patient in a forcible manner.

The operator then takes a deep breath and blows into the patient's mouth again. If this.is properly done, the patient's chest can

be seen to rise a little with the introduction of each breath. This should be repeated about every two seconds until the patient starts breathing of his own accord.

If the patient's heart continues to beat, sometimes it is necessary to repeat this mouth-to-mouth breathing for a period of one-half hour or longer. It should be kept up as long as there is any indication of a heart beat.

Many lives have been saved using this method—sometimes over rather prolonged periods.

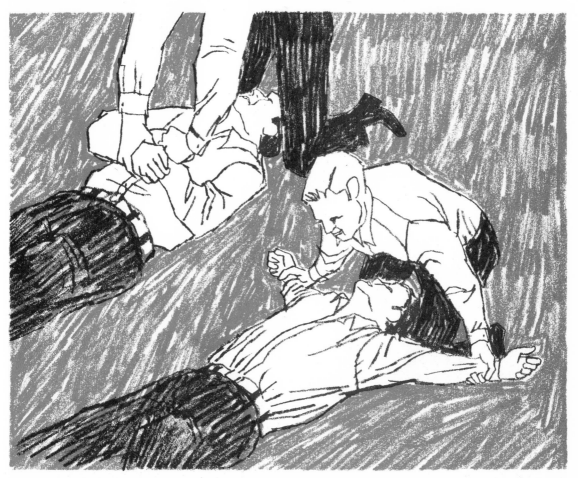

Manual method of resuscitation is shown above. This process should be repeated about every five seconds. Not as effective as mouth to mouth.

If the patient has almost drowned, it is best to turn him on his face at first to clear the upper airway of water before turning him on his back for the mouth-to-mouth breathing.

Before each breath the operator should breathe in deeply in order to obtain a new supply of oxygen which is to be breathed into the patient's lungs.

GLOSSARY

Oxygen   air
Resuscitation   restoring life
Technique   method of procedure

THE CLOSED METHOD OF CARDIAC OR HEART MASSAGE

This is another first aid measure of great importance which is often life saving.

Some years ago, surgeons found that when a patient's heart stopped beating during an operation, they could quickly open up the chest, grasp the heart in one hand and by squeezing it in a rhythmic manner, could sometimes start it to beating again. This life saving procedure was called the open method of cardiac massage.

The same results can be obtained by a closed method—that is, without cutting into the chest cavity and exposing the heart. The closed method may be done by anyone who knows how and should be started until a doctor can be called to take care of the patient. The method to be used is as follows:

If a person's heart stops beating due to an electric shock, or from any other reason which is not a natural one, the person should be placed on his back and mouth-to-mouth breathing as described in the previous chapter should be started.

Another operator should place the flat part of his left hand over the lower part of the patient's breastbone and then place the palm of his right hand over the back of his left hand. Keeping his elbows straight, he should press down on the patient's chest in a forcible way so as to press the breast bone in. This causes the heart to be squeezed between the breast bone and the back bone, forcing the blood out of it much as you would squeeze water out of an ear syringe.

The pressure should be released suddenly and then reapplied in the same manner. This pressure should be applied about every second and should be kept up until the heart starts beating by itself again and the patient starts breathing. Remember that mouth-to-mouth breathing must be performed at the same time the heart is being massaged. This will usually take two people, although if only one person is present he must do both.

When the doctor arrives, and he should be called at once along with an ambulance if possible, the patient is placed in the ambulance or some other vehicle and taken to the nearest hospital.

During the transfer by ambulance, the cardiac massage should be kept up at about the same rate and the mouth-to-mouth breathing should also be continued.

When the patient arrives at the hospital, doctors take over. One of them continues the intermittent pressure and release on the lower anterior chest. Another will hook up an anesthetic machine and place an airway into the patient's mouth by pressing on a rubber bag full of oxygen. He can force oxygen into the patient's lungs at regular intervals, thus taking over the mouth-to-mouth breathing part of the job. A third doctor will probably place a needle in a vein of the leg and start dripping some intravenous fluid, which will contain a drug such as wyamine, that will cause the blood pressure to rise. People in the state of shock always have low blood pressure and it needs boosting.

In the meantime the nurses will be busy getting instruments and medicines for the doctors. One of these machines which the nurses will bring in is called a defibrillator, and this is very important in restoring the normal heart beat. This is the way it works:

In cases of cardiac arrest, that is, when the heart stops beating, the heart muscles instead of contracting in a rhythmic way will just quiver all over like a bowl of jelly, and of course this quivering will not deliver blood to different parts of the body. This is why the heart has to be pressed or massaged from the outside of the body. But the fact that it is quivering shows that the heart muscle is still alive. This irregular action is called ventricular fibrillation and if it continues the patient will die. The defibrillator is used to send a strong electric current or shock through the heart muscle by placing two pads or conductors on the anterior chest wall, one at the top and one at the bottom of the heart. When these pads are in

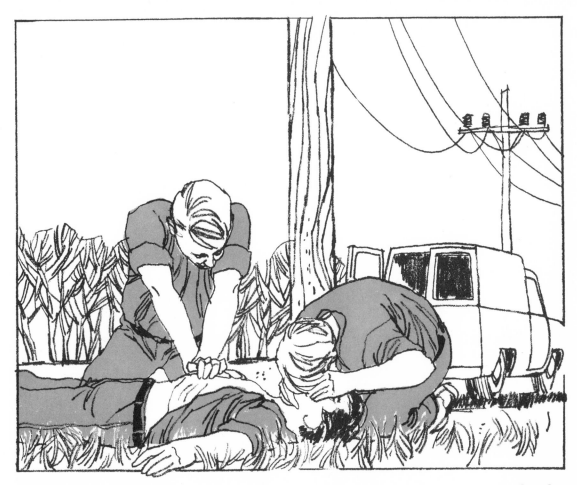

This illustration shows two men performing what may be life saving procedures, i.e., external cardiac massage and mouth to mouth breathing. The patient has apparently received an electric shock which caused his heart to stop beating.

place, the doctor steps on a pedal and sends a strong electric current through the heart muscle. In many cases this will stop the quivering or irregular contractions of the heart and it will start beating in a regular way. The patient is then placed in bed, and with his breathing and heart action restored, will recover.

Many patients are alive today who have been administered this cardiac massage and mouth-to-mouth breathing, sometimes followed by several uses of a defibrillator.

Some of them have been worked on for many hours and show no ill effects in later life.

Several facts must be remembered about the above procedures. They do not work after a heart stops beating following disease, or the so-called natural causes of death, and they do not work in all cases of accidents where they are usually employed. But they are successful in enough cases to warrant the effort of trying to keep a person alive after an accident such as near drowning or accidental electric shock. This method should always be tried, and every hospital should have a defibrillator.

One other word of explanation is needed. The ventricular fibrillation described is not to be confused with auricular fibrillation. Life cannot exist in continued ventricular fibrillation as described above. However, a person may have auricular fibrillation and recover from it or may live in comparative comfort while he has auricular fibrillation.

The heart has four chambers—two auricles and two ventricles. The auricles, which are the upper chambers, have thin walls and do not have much function in pumping the blood through the body. When the auricles get off in their timing and auricular fibrillation occurs, this doesn't do much damage and in most cases can be corrected. If the ventricles or the thick-muscled lower chambers get out of timing, however, they can no longer pump the blood to the body and the patient dies. That is why we have stated above that if ventricular fibrillation persists, life cannot be maintained.

GLOSSARY

Fibrillation   muscle fibers beating independently and without rhythm
Intravenous   into the vein

Chapter 28

Poisons

WHEN THE POISON which has been swallowed is known, specific treatment may be started by a doctor. However, there are certain non-specific treatments which should be carried out at once, before the doctor arrives.

If the poison is taken by mouth, the stomach should be emptied. When the patient is conscious, vomiting can be induced in any of the following ways:

1. One tablespoon of mustard to eight ounces of warm water
2. Strong suds of laundry soap in a large glass of water
3. Have patient tickle back of throat with finger, after giving either of the above drinks

After emptying the stomach, give the following mixture: two parts powdered burnt toast, one part strong tea, one part milk of magnesia. Mix these in water—one teaspoon of the mixture to a glass of water. After each dose, the stomach should be emptied by vomiting. This may be repeated several times.

The patient should then drink a mixture of milk and raw egg.

Save the bottle so that the doctor will know what poison has been taken.

When acid has been taken, give strong solution of bicarbonate of soda and water.

When an overdose of sleeping pills has been taken, empty stomach and give stimulant such as strong coffee, while waiting for the doctor.

For phosphorus poisoning, such as matches, rat or roach paste, empty stomach and give dilute solution of hydrogen peroxide or oil of turpentine (one part of the medicine to ten parts of water).

In all cases, empty the stomach as directed above. The patient should be taken to a hospital emergency room, where a doctor will wash out the stomach using a "stomach pump."

For food poisoning, empty the stomach and give dose of castor oil or epsom salts. Call a doctor.

POISONOUS SNAKE BITES

Cause and Nature

In the United States there are four kinds of snakes whose bite may cause death. 397

These are:

1. The rattlesnake
2. The cottonmouth moccasin
3. The copperhead moccasin
4. The coral snake

During the period 1950-1954, there were only seventy-one deaths reported as having been caused by snake bites, and only one percent were caused by coral snakes.

The venom introduced through a puncture wound, when the snake bites, is the cause of death in most cases. However, in some cases of snake bite, shock and fright may cause a fatal heart attack.

Treatment

First of all, keep cool. Do not become excited. Keep the patient at rest. Undue exercise may cause the venom to spread faster. Whiskey will increase the rate of circulation, and hence, is not good for snake bite.

The first step in treatment, is to tie a tourniquet (lightly) just above the bite, or between the bite and the heart. The tourniquet should be tight enough to stop the venous and lymphatic flow, and should be released about every five minutes and tied again. It should not be tight enough to stop the arterial blood from reaching the part.

Multiple incisions (five or ten) should be made around the puncture wounds and suction applied, either by mouth or by suction cup. The incisions should be from ⅛ to ¼ inch deep, and should be spaced through the area of swelling. If possible, suction should be maintained for about two hours.

The patient should then be seen by a doctor, who will give injections of antivenin, followed by injections of antibiotics and antitoxin. The antivenin contains horse serum, and people who are sensitive to horse serum should be treated with care. Most

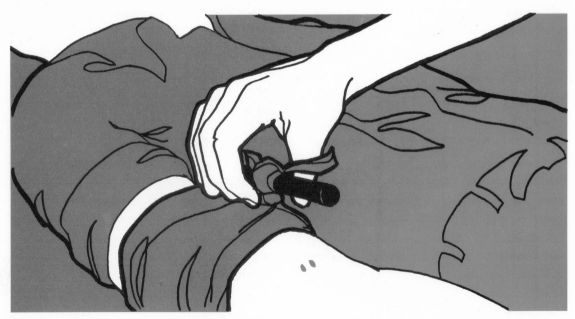

The first step in treating a poisonous snake bite. The fang marks are shown and a tournequet is being placed above the bite.

snake bites are not fatal, as will be noted by the fact that only seventy-one deaths were reported in four years.

GLOSSARY

Antivenin   medicine for treating snake bite
Arterial   of the arteries; deep
Circulation   flow of blood in the blood vessels
Incisions   cuts
Lymphatic flow   glandular flow just under the skin
Stimulant   something that peps you up
Tourniquet   a tight bandage around a limb to slow down the circulation
Venom   poison
Venous   of the veins

CHEMICAL BURN

If the burn is caused by acid, wash off at once with water and bicarbonate of soda. If caused by an alkali, wash off with a dilute solution of vinegar, after washing with water while the solution is being prepared.

POISONOUS PLANTS

Cause and Nature

Poisoning by plants is very common and may cause symptoms ranging from skin irritations as in poison ivy and poison oak to upset stomach and even to convulsions and death when the poison plant is eaten in sufficient quantities. Death has been known to follow the consumption or eating of just a few poisonous mushrooms.

This chapter will emphasize the poisonous plants that are planted and cultivated by many of us who do not even know that they are dangerous. The children, who are the only ones who are liable to eat enough of one of these plants to cause damage, should be taught by their parents to never place any part of a plant in their mouth—much less eat a plant. To teach the children properly, the parent should know which plants are poisonous.

Because of the bitter, burning taste of most of these plants, very few children will eat enough of them to cause serious damage; however, there has been a reported case of death in a child who was dared by her older brother to eat a number of castor beans.

As has been noted in another chapter, the consumption of common household substances such as flavored aspirin, ammonia, bleaches, cleaning fluids, and insecticides causes a great many accidental deaths, while eating poisonous plants causes relatively few casualties.

There are over two hundred common plants which may cause symptoms when eaten. These symptoms will vary with the plant and the amount eaten. Some of the most common plants will be described here because they are ornamental and as a rule planted and cultivated. The portion of the plant which is poisonous will be designated. One or more of these plants may be found in most gardens or surrounding environment.

Signs and Symptoms

These will vary with the amount eaten and vary all the way from nausea and vomiting, a burning feeling in the mouth, and diarrhea, to convulsions and death. The signs consist usually of a small piece of the ingested plant in the child's mouth and the parent should taste this small piece carefully in order to determine the kind of plant. Fortunately the child will usually stop before eating too much because of unpleasant taste.

Treatment

This should be in the hands of a physician. The stomach should be emptied at once by inducing vomiting. The only real way to prevent this type of an accident is to teach the child never to eat any kind of a plant.

Plant   Poisonous Part

ACONITE, *roots and seed*
BITTERSWEET, *berry only*
BLUEBONNET, *seed only*
BURNING BUSH, *all of the plant*
CASTOR BEAN, *beans only*
CYCLAMEN, *tuber only*
DAPHNE, *bark, leaves, and berries*
DUMB CANE, *all of the plant*
ELEPHANT EAR, *all of the plant*
FOUR O'CLOCK, *the root and seed only*
FOXGLOVE, *roots and seed*
IRIS, *stem of the plant*
IVY, *leaves of the plant*
JIMSON-WEED, *all of the plant*

LARKSPUR, *all of the plant*
LILY OF THE VALLEY, *all of the plant*
MOCK ORANGE, *fruit only*
MONKSHOOD, *roots only*
MOUNTAIN LAUREL, *all of the plant*
NARCISSUS, *bulb only*
OLEANDER, *leaves only*
PIMPERNEL, *all of the plant*
POTATO PLANT, *seeds and sprouts*
RHODODENDRUM, *all of the plant*
SCOTCH BROOM, *seed of the plant*
SPANISH BAYONET, *root only*
SWEET PEA, *stem only*
TULIP, *bulb*

GLOSSARY

Bicarbonate of soda   baking soda
Conjunctivitis   inflammation of the lining of the eyelid
Ingested   having taken food or drugs into the stomach
Milligram   a unit of measure
Nonspecific   not limited to one disease or condition
Pallor   paleness; wan appearance
Regurgitate   to vomit
Susceptibility   lack of resistance

Chapter 29

Diseases Caused by Effects of External Physical Agents

ABNORMALITIES DUE TO CHANGES IN ATMOSPHERIC PRESSURE

Cause and Nature

Pain in one or both ears during a flight in an airplane is due to compression or pressure on the eardrums when the atmospheric pressure is increased too rapidly. This increase of pressure occurs when the plane is in descent or landing. The increased pressure on the eardrums is not noticed when the Eustachian tubes are open. These are the tubes that lead from the middle ear, that is the cavity back of the eardrums, to the space back of the soft palate in the throat. When these tubes are open, the atmospheric pressure on both sides of the eardrum is equal and the drum is not pushed in by increased pressure on the outside. Hence, if a person is subjected to rapid descent in an aircraft while this person has a cold or sinus infection, the possibility of his having pain in one or both ears is greater because more than likely one or both of his Eustachian tubes are stopped up. That is the reason a passenger is given gum to chew while the aircraft is landing. The act of chewing may open up the Eustachian tubes and equalize the pressure on both sides of the eardrums. This is also the reason why most commercial aircraft are not allowed to descend rapidly. The usual limit of descent permitted these aircraft is about three hundred feet per minute, and even with the plane coming down gradually, a certain percentage of passengers will experience pain in one or both ears while landing. This pain may continue several days after the flight, especially if the passenger has a cold which has stopped up his Eustachian tubes.

Pain in the sinuses and even in the teeth has been noted from rapidly increasing atmospheric pressure. When deep sea divers go down too rapidly this same effect of increased pressure may be noted.

Signs and Symptoms

A dull aching pain is noted in one or both ears as the aircraft lands and the pressure is increased. This pain may be accompanied by a decrease in hearing, and both of these effects may disappear rapidly as the Eustachian tubes open up. The pain may be mild or quite severe. At times the pressure is so great that small hemorrhages occur in the tissues of the ear.

Treatment

The best treatment is prevention, that is, by not descending too rapidly in an aircraft and by seeing to it that the Eustachian tubes are open when descending.

No active treatment is needed after you are on the ground for this condition clears up by itself. However it may be hastened by seeing a doctor if the pain has lasted for some time, and the pain, of course, can be lessened by taking the pain-killing drugs such as aspirin.

The hearing nearly always returns to normal as soon as the otitis has cleared up. This is exactly opposite to the effect which has been noted upon men who are exposed to the firing of big guns as in the artillery. These men exposed to repeated concussion or suddenly increased pressure to their eardrums may suffer a loss of hearing which will not return to normal.

GLOSSARY

Atmospheric air
Hemorrhage bleeding
Otitis inflammation of the ear
Sinuses cavities in the bone of the face

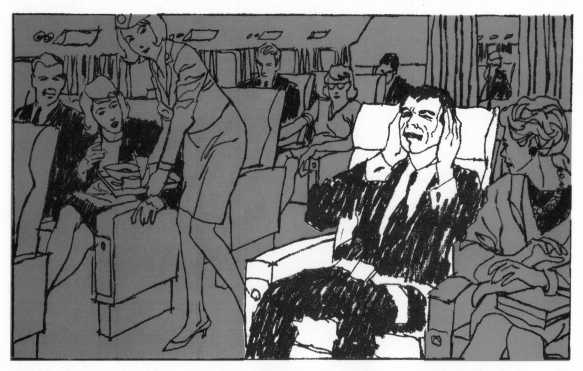

Pain in the ears caused by increased air pressure, such as when an airplane is landing, can be avoided if the Eustachian tubes in the ears are kept open. Chewing gum will help to do this.

PAINFUL OR ACHING FEET

Cause and Nature

In America today we often hear the remark, "My feet are killing me," and usually this statement is made by people who should know how to correct the causes of painful feet. The causes of these hot, aching, sweating feet can often be corrected. Some of these causes are: 1. Poorly fitting shoes. 2. Poor ventilation to the feet. 3. Socks which are too short. 4. Socks made of the wrong material.

Signs and Symptoms

Poorly fitting shoes may cause blisters, which in turn become infected. The feet are hot and sweating and as the day progresses they tend to swell and become more painful.

Some people have a tendency for their feet to sweat more than others. This is called hyperhidrosis. Others have a tendency to exude an odor from their sweating feet; this is known as bromohyperhidrosis. Both of these conditions can be corrected with the proper care.

At pressure points many people develop corns and calluses and these prove to be very painful. The cause for these pressure points is usually improperly fitting shoes.

Plantar warts on the sole of the feet do not go away as other warts do. The longer they persist the more painful they become and gradually a thickening of the skin or callus is formed around them.

Soft corns between the toes are very painful, especially if they become infected.

A painful heel may be due to a spur on the heel bone or os calcis, but most often it is a simple bursitis. The difference between the two can be determined by X ray. How-

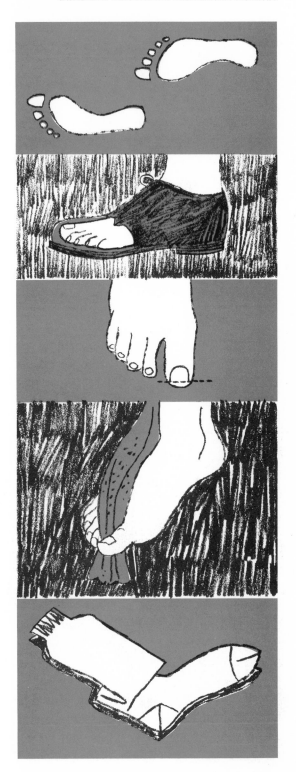

Foot care: Proper walking, well fitted shoes and socks, squarely cut nails, and dry toes.

ever, the treatment for both of these conditions is just about the same and will be noted below.

As we get older the circulation in our feet begins to slow down and this contributes to the foot discomfort. It is surprising how many older people have as their chief complaint painful feet.

Not all of these conditions are caused by poorly fitting shoes and socks, for some of them are due to the structure of the foot itself. Some of us are born with feet which are not properly formed.

Many of these conditions are known by different names. Flat feet which may cause foot strain and pain; this condition can be helped. Hammer toe and claw toe produce discomfort. The bones in our feet may be shorter in some places and longer in others causing undue pressure and callus formation on the soles of the feet or on the tops of the toes.

Foot strain and discomfort is often caused by not walking properly. This is most often seen in women who wear high heels.

Treatment

The single most important part of treatment is prevention. By this we mean properly fitting shoes. The shoe should have a broad heel, a soft top, and in summer or hot weather, it may be well for the tops to have some form of ventilation. The shoe should be long enough and the toe should not be pointed. The shoe should also be broad enough and to obtain shoes of this kind it may be well to buy shoes at the end of the day so the feet will be swollen if they tend to swell and a good fit can be obtained. The socks should be longer than the longest toe. In hot weather socks should be made of

wool or cotton if the wearer tends to perspire a lot. Wool or cotton materials tend to offer better ventilation and to absorb sweat. If the feet perspire more than usual the socks should be changed once a day; that is use two pair of socks daily.

Women will find these recommendations hard to live up to as their shoes usually have too high heels, are too narrow, and the toes are too pointed.

Often aching feet can be helped by simply resting and elevating the feet. Then using a good antiseptic soap, the feet should be washed, dried well, and sponged off with rubbing alcohol.

When people are older and the circulation is not good they should use alternate hot and cold soaks to stimulate the circulation. After these soaks dry the feet thoroughly and while lying down exercise the toes and ankles for about five minutes.

People who suffer from bromohyperhidrosis or excessive odor, may help this by taking a teaspoon full of mild bleaching powder to a pint of water and washing the feet once a day. After drying the feet thoroughly, a dusting powder composed of two parts talcum powder to one part boric acid can be used to benefit this condition.

Hyperhidrosis or excessive sweating can be helped by bathing the feet in rubbing alcohol or sponging them with rubbing alcohol. After drying, use foot powder, being certain that the powder goes between the toes.

For feet which are not properly formed an orthopedist or a good podiatrist, that is a foot doctor, should be consulted. The patient should not try to trim his own calluses or corns because this is a very common cause of infection and someone else should perform this duty for him.

The painful heel is often relieved by soaking the feet every night in hot water with Epsom Salts. Then apply a soothing or pain-killing ointment. The next step in relieving a painful heel is to apply a pad which has a small hole just over the painful area.

These things should be done by a podiatrist the first time because much discomfort is caused by self-treatment—that is, by placing pads, arch supports, and other devices in a shoe.

Burning or hot feet are often caused by improper dietary habits. The vitamin B complex will at times relieve this, especially by doses of nicotinic acid and riboflavin. Since these are part of the vitamin B complex, a less expensive way of obtaining them may be to go to the drug store and buy some brewers yeast. This contains all elements of vitamin B complex and is inexpensive. Take two tablets, three times a day.

Feet which persist in giving off a bad odor may also be caused by the wrong diet and if this condition does not clear up a doctor should be seen to rule out diabetes.

Remember if you have foot pain, burning, or odor, the family doctor is the man to see and he may refer you to a good foot doctor or podiatrist.

GLOSSARY

Spur a projecting piece of bone
Calcis pertaining to lime or to calcium
Hammer toe shaped like a hammer
Claw distortion of the toe

BLAST INJURIES

Cause and Nature

Blast injuries are caused by rapidly expanding gases from an explosion. They may occur in the air or under water. The sudden wave of pressure striking the human body has very little effect on the solid parts of the body but may cause internal injuries to the tissues containing air such as the lungs, the intestine or bowels, and the ears. People or animals suffer from blast injuries if they are near an explosion of great magnitude, such as would follow an atomic bomb explosion.

Signs and Symptoms

The patients may be dazed or unconscious. When they revive there is usually pain in the ears. If the lungs have been injured they will complain of shortness of breath and, rarely, painful breathing. There may be blood-flecked sputum, and after severe injuries pure blood may be coughed up.

The blast wave under water causes injuries most often to the intestines, and these small hemorrhages into the bowel may cause abdominal pain. If the blast is strong enough, there may be a rupture of the bowel. Blast injuries following explosions in the air usually affect the lungs more than the intestines.

Treatment

The best way to treat injuries to the lung is by administering oxygen to relieve shortness of breath, keeping the patient at rest, and cleaning out the throat by suction so he can breathe better.

If there is considerable loss of blood the patient should receive blood transfusions, and if there is a ruptured internal organ, surgery should be performed to repair the injury if possible.

GLOSSARY

Flecked spotted
Rupture tear
Sputum saliva

ELECTRIC SHOCK

Cause and Nature

Most human beings receive an electric shock at some time during a lifetime, and since some of these shocks may cause death or serious disabilities, it may be well to understand something about the nature of such shocks.

The electric shock is caused when any part of the body comes in contact with an electric current in such a way as to allow the tissues of the body to become a conducting medium of the electric current. In other words, the body becomes in effect an electric wire. Conducting the current not only implies coming in contact with a current but it also means the body must be grounded so the current can flow out the other end.

This grounding is a very important factor. For instance, if a body receives a shock while in a bathtub or while standing in water, this shock might well prove fatal, although the same shock received while standing on dry ground would not injure the patient too seriously.

If the body is wet from perspiration or rainfall when the shock occurs, this will also increase the damage.

Two other factors may determine the extent of the damage. The first and most important is the nature of the current, the voltage involved, and the frequency of alternation.

The second factor is the length of time the body is exposed to an electric current and is forced to act as a conductor of this current.

Concerning the first factor, an alternating current will ordinarily do more damage than a direct current. High frequency alter-

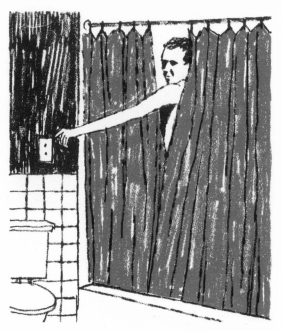

Danger: Never touch any electrical outlet while in contact with water.

nations are the most dangerous. A direct current of less than three hundred volts will seldom cause death, while an alternating current of much less voltage may prove fatal. The longer a person is exposed to an electric current the more damage will be caused.

Signs and Symptoms

Burns are caused by electric current and the visible burns are usually seen where the current enters the body as well as where it is conducted out of the body. As a rule, current of low voltage may cause the heart to stop beating and current of a high voltage is more likely to paralyze the muscles which control respiration and the patient will cease breathing.

Death may be sudden, almost instantaneous, or it may occur a few hours after the shock. People who are not killed by an electric shock may suffer from headaches, nervous instability, fatigue, and in some cases, cataracts in the eyes, causing gradual loss of vision. The rule is, though, that if a person survives an electric shock he will have no permanent ill effects.

Treatment

The immediate treatment of the electric shock victim is to free him from the current. This should not be done by touching him, for if you are well grounded and touch the victim you will also become a wire to conduct the current. Use some nonconductive material to pull him free. An example of this might be the leather belt you wear.

Artificial respiration should be begun at once if the patient is not breathing. The mouth to mouth method of artificial respiration is now considered the most effective.

The length of application of artificial respiration is very important. Some people have been known to survive and start breathing again after several hours of artificial respiration. Efforts to revive a victim should not be abandoned until he becomes stiff and cold—that is, not before rigor mortis sets in.

The burns should be treated in the customary way and the pain should be relieved by aspirin or aspirin and codeine.

GLOSSARY

Rigor mortis   stiffening of the body after death

SHOCK

Cause and Nature

The causes of shock are many and this is one of the most inadequately understood conditions encountered by doctors today.

One of the frequently seen and easily treated causes of shock is fainting. This is usually a psychogenic affair. For instance, some people will faint if they see a needle and think it is going to be used on them. Other more serious causes of shock are:

1. Loss of blood (usually any amount of a quart or over will cause shock)
2. Trauma or injury
3. Infection
4. Heart conditions such as a heart attack
5. Adrenal insufficiency
6. Overuse of drugs which lower the blood pressure

Signs and Symptoms

The skin is pale and cool. There is either loss of consciousness or extremely slowed up mental reactions. The skin may be damp from sweating or just pale and dry. The blood pressure is usually low and the urinary output is decreased.

Treatment

In simple cases of shock such as fainting, the patient will recover automatically if placed in the horizontal position; that is, lying flat without a pillow under his head. The patient should be kept warm. If bleeding is present it should be stopped if possible. When the cause is more complicated and the patient does not recover in a short period of time, a doctor should be called.

This is a serious condition in most cases, except the very simple one of fainting, and a great deal of careful and intensive treatment may be needed. Therefore, the treatment should not be delayed.

GLOSSARY

Adrenal insufficiency   Addison's disease (not enough secretion from the adrenal glands)
Psychogenic   caused by mental influences
Trauma   wound or injury

DECOMPRESSION, THE BENDS, OR CAISSON DISEASE

Cause and Nature

This condition is caused by a too rapid or too sudden decrease in atmospheric pressure such as would be experienced by a deep sea diver who is returned at a fast rate to the surface of the water, where the pressure is less than where he was working deep below the surface.

When aviation workers are decompressed too rapidly by ascending from the ground to very high altitudes, they experience the same symptoms.

The cause of pain and disability in this disease is said to be caused by formation of bubbles of gas in the blood vessels or outside the blood vessels in the joint spaces or

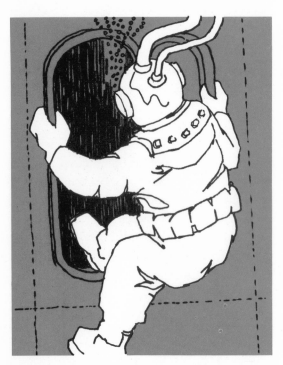

This illustration shows a deep sea diver entering a decompression chamber where the pressure will be slowly reduced.

muscles. The sudden change in atmospheric pressure has interfered with the exchange of gases.

Hence it has been noticed that a diver with good circulation is less likely to get the bends than one with poor circulation. A man under eighteen years of age is less likely to be affected because his circulation is usually better. People who have had severe injuries so that the circulation is impaired may be easy victims of decompression sickness.

Signs and Symptoms

The first symptom noted during decompression sickness or the bends is a dull throbbing pain which may be felt first in one part of the body and then in another. The joints and muscles are the most common sites of pain. This pain comes on gradually and may be preceded by a feeling of numbness or tingling. The patient becomes pale and his skin cools off. In some instances dizziness, deafness, and even paralysis of the legs occur.

Along with these manifestations the patient may feel difficulty in getting a good breath. The early deep sea divers described this feeling as "the chokes."

Treatment

The only treatment for this decompression sickness is immediate and prolonged compression. The person should be placed in a chamber and have the pressure elevated until it stimulates the pressure at which he was originally working. In some cases more pressure than this may be required. This increased pressure should be maintained for a long time, sometimes for several days, and should be very gradually reduced.

ALTITUDE SICKNESS

Cause and Nature

When a mountain climber goes above eighteen or twenty thousand feet the atmospheric pressure is much less than at sea level and the supply of oxygen in the air is greatly decreased; hence, he may show symptoms of decompression sickness. These symptoms may be increased because the mountain climber, in contrast to the airplane pilot, is exposed to cold and muscular exertion.

People who live in high altitudes are accustomed to the lack of oxygen and hence can do work at altitudes which the man who comes up from sea level could not even tolerate. Men who are going to climb high mountains sometimes live at higher altitudes, such as sixteen to eighteen thousand feet, for several months before they attempt their climb, in an effort to become accustomed to the lack of oxygen and to the decreased atmospheric pressure.

When a climber goes above twenty-five thousand feet he may need additional oxygen and he will not be able to stay and climb above this altitude for more than ten or twelve days. The men who climbed Mount Everest (29,002 feet) had to work fast after they passed 25,000 feet because their time up there was limited.

Signs and Symptoms

Very few of us will try to climb high mountains, but the symptoms may be noted by all of us who go from sea level to a much higher altitude. There will be noticed at first a difficulty in breathing (shortness of breath), the sleep may be disturbed at night, and there is a feeling of laziness and inability to perform manual labor. In going

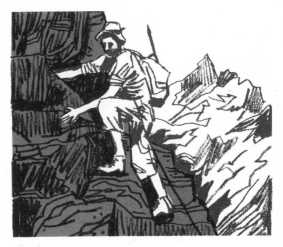

Climbing to extremely high altitudes may cause altitude sickness.

to a moderately high altitude the body gradually adjusts itself and we no longer feel symptoms.

If a doctor should take a blood count after a person has moved from sea level to a high altitude he would note that the red blood cells would be greater in number and the patient would show an increase in the percent of hemoglobin.

Treatment

The treatment of altitude sickness consists of prevention—that is, work up to the higher altitude slowly. If this is impossible, then the person who goes to a higher altitude should rest more and give his body time to adjust to the change in atmospheric pressure and the oxygen content of the air.

People with heart disease or badly impaired circulation should not cause a greater load to be placed on the heart by going up too high.

GLOSSARY

Atmospheric air
Decompression release from pressure
Impaired having less value or strength

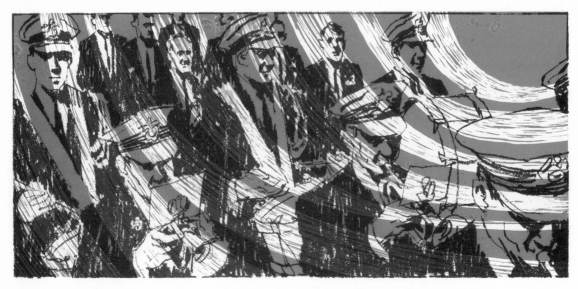

Heat prostration and heat stroke may be caused by exercise in hot weather.

HEAT EXHAUSTION OR PROSTRATION

Cause and Nature

When exposed to high temperature, especially when associated with high humidity, some people show symptoms of heat exhaustion or heat prostration. The person usually has been sweating profusely, thus losing water and salt. Other symptoms are restlessness, headache, nausea, dizziness, throbbing, and a rapid pulse. He may later collapse, and the skin become cold and clammy, in spite of a slight elevation in body temperature. There may be muscular twitching and cramps.

Treatment

Treatment consists of rest and removal to cooler surroundings. Prevention is more important than treatment. This is accomplished by avoiding hard work in high temperatures, and by taking large quantities of salt and water.

Salt can be purchased in tablets, which are easier to take than table salt. These tablets are called thermotabs.

HEAT STROKE

Cause and Nature

Heat stroke is more severe than heat prostration, and is a very serious condition which, if not treated promptly, may result in death.

The symptoms are dramatic, marked by sudden collapse and a rapid rise in body temperature—up to 105 or 106 degrees. The skin is very dry and very hot.

Treatment

The treatment is to reduce the body temperature promptly by immersion in cold water until the temperature is down to 102 degrees. Then use fanning, etc. Large quantities of water and salt should be given the patient. A doctor should be called for this condition.

FROSTBITE

Cause and Nature

Frostbite is caused by overexposure to cold, and is usually noted in the hands, feet, or ears. Being exposed to cold first causes the part to turn red, and if exposure persists the part turns white. This indicates a contraction of the small vessels. If the exposure lasts too long, gangrene may be the result.

After the exposure to cold ceases, red areas which burn and itch may occur on the hands and feet. These are called "chilblains."

Treatment

The treatment of choice is the gradual warming of the frostbitten area. If the freezing has been severe, some doctors advise rapid warming by immersion in hot water.

The areas should not be rubbed, as ulcers may be caused by rubbing off the skin.

RADIOACTIVE FALLOUT

The testing of atomic weapons which is accompanied by nuclear detonation has made it important to ascertain the effect of the radioactive particles which fall to the ground after these tests. A very exhaustive and careful study has been made of this fallout material, in a hope that accurate determinations may be made as to the effect of radioactive fallout on our health, and upon the health of future generations. There is no way at present to make an exact determination of these effects because of the constantly changing nature of the tests, and the widespread or world-wide distribution of some of these particles. This makes it impor-tant for us to understand some of the simpler facts about this radioactive fallout in order to protect the health of our families.

When a nuclear explosion takes place, the radioactive particles, or debris, fall to the earth in three different patterns.

1. Local fallout: The particles reach the earth within a few hours and usually within a few hundred miles of the point of detonation. The pattern of the fallout will depend upon how hard the wind is blowing and in what direction

2. The finer particles will go up in the bomb cloud and remain in the troposphere, which is not as high as the stratosphere. These particles will be carried by atmospheric circulation all the way around the earth in a narrow east-west band, and most of the particles will settle to the earth within a month or two

3. The real large bombs or small bombs, detonated at high altitudes, will send most of their particles high into the stratosphere where they may remain for years after the explosion, depending upon the size of the particle and the atmospheric circulation. It has been estimated that fifty percent of this debris settles out in each five to ten year period following the detonation. This stratospheric fallout is distributed over the entire earth

Most of the particles in all three patterns lose their radioactivity in a very short time; after two weeks the radioactivity is very small, and after two months has ceased to exist. But a small percentage of the radioactive fallout has a long life—up to forty years, and this long-lasting radioactivity, which may be distributed over the entire world, has to be studied closely in order to prevent the accumulated effect of assimilating small amounts into the body over a period of time—long enough to become a serious health hazard.

The local fallout following weapons testing can be and has been very carefully controlled, but world-wide fallout presents a more complicated problem. The effects of this fallout will be studied for years to come, and now samples of earth and water are being collected all over the world and examined for their radioactivity.

There are two types of radiation from fallout with which we have to cope:

1. Gamma radiation, which is similar to X ray and will penetrate matter of some thickness
2. Beta radiation; these electrons travel at high speed and cannot penetrate. They may be stopped by a few inches of air.

The gamma radiation presents a hazard both to the body and the genes; that is, it may cause deformities in unborn children if the genes in the sperm or ova of the parents have been damaged by radiation. This result has never been proven conclusively in human beings, but extensive animal experiments are under way and our knowledge of the results is growing rapidly. This much we do know, that we should have a great deal of respect for radioactivity, and this respect should be built upon knowledge rather than guesswork.

The principal danger from world-wide fallout may come from the eating or drinking of food or water which contains some of the long-living radioactive materials. The two which live the longest (for years) are:

1. Strontium 90
2. Cesium 137

Strontium 90 gives off beta radiation to a great extent and cesium 137 emits gamma radiation.

As noted above, gamma radiation penetrates deeply and may cause a great many disabilities, ranging from death a few hours after exposure to leukemia, or bone cancer, which may occur many years later.

Now, we want to know how much radiation it will take to cause the human body to be harmed. The dose of radiation is measured in a unit called a roentgen or R; sometimes this is cut down and spoken of as a milliroentgen or MR, which is one thousandth of an R. To judge the effect one must know the number of Rs in a dose, and the length of time to which one is exposed to radioactivity.

We know that all of our bodies are exposed to a certain amount of radioactivity—cosmic rays from the sun and rays from the ground where there are quantities of uranium; and from our own bodies which have been exposed to radiation, and have retained some of the radioactivity in the calcium of our bones such as the strontium 90, which has a life of about forty years.

This natural radiation has been measured and amounts to a total of .1 to .2 (one-tenth to two-tenths) R per year, depending upon the location and altitude; those who live at a higher altitude get more natural radiation from the sun or cosmic rays because they are nearer to it.

The effects of this radiation upon future generations of children has not been measured accurately on human beings, but from experiments on plants and animals it is felt that about ten percent of the genetic mutations (this means the abnormal changes, or in other words, the babies born with abnormalities or changes from normal) may be caused by natural radiation. But remember, this is an estimate and has never been proven. Then we know that the fallout from the testing of nuclear weapons amounts to a very small radiation dose of about 0.005 R per year; but this is cumulative, and if weapons tests are carried out over a long period of years, or if atomic weapons are used in warfare, this cumulative amount may grow into a larger dose which could cause genetic mutations in future generations. Another form of radiation to which we are exposed is medical radiation, and this is in very small amounts which do not do any harm. It is very important that X rays be taken in many cases so that a diagnosis may be made, such as in pulmonary tuberculosis or cancer of the lung. Such medical X rays are usually taken by a person who knows his business, and the patient is never exposed to a dosage that will harm him. So it cannot be emphasized too strongly that necessary medical X rays are not harmful, and should be used to aid in diagnosis. On the other hand, X ray machines which are used to fit shoes in some stores, can be very harmful, because there is no way of regulating the dosage as is done in medical X rays. Most states have passed laws prohibiting the use of these X ray devices in shoe stores.

It has been estimated that if a group of people were exposed over their whole bodies to about 450 R of gamma radiation, fifty percent of these people would die. This is what we have to worry about in the local fallout which would occur in the event of a nuclear war.

The aspect of this question which has caused the most serious worldwide concern, is the amount of strontium 90 and cesium 137 which may fall to the earth following the explosion of atom bombs.

Strontium 90 is chemically very much like calcium, and if it falls to the earth it will be taken up into plants; cows eating the plants will receive this calcium-like substance, which in turn will be taken into human bodies by drinking the milk. It is then stored in the bones, just as calcium is, and over a period of time may cause leukemia or bone cancer. This strontium 90 emits no gamma rays, and is no threat to future generations because these rays do not cause genetic mutation.

The strontium 90 is not taken into the muscles of cows, so that if a feeding range were known to be contaminated by strontium 90, the cows on this range could be used safely to produce beef—but their milk would be dangerous to drink.

Tests done on the bones of young children show that these bones have received about .002 R a year of strontium 90 since the weapons testing began. We must remember that this is a very small amount, not as large as the natural radiation to which we are all exposed; but we also must be watchful and keep testing soil and vegetables all over the world as long as the practice of testing nuclear weapons is carried on. This is to prevent the cumulative level of strontium 90 from becoming too high.

Cesium 137 has a chemical structure something like sodium, but it lives for forty years, and must be carefully watched to determine the amount falling out in different parts of the world. This substance emits gamma rays and so could cause genetic mutation; but fortunately, being like sodium, it is not retained in the body permanently as strontium is, but passes out of the body in about six months. The present level of this substance in bones is about .0015 R per year, which is smaller than the level of strontium 90.

The question is important as to what steps a person may take to protect himself and his family in the case of war, when an atomic bomb or nuclear weapon could cause dangerous fallout.

The simplest method would be to do a little reconstruction on existing cellars or basements, which would protect the occupants adequately from local fallout. Since the place would have to be lived in for several days after the explosion, it should be supplied with food, water, and sleeping quarters. The next step would be to erect public shelters which can be put up at a reasonable cost. A steel-shell shelter, which would accommodate about 120 people, could be erected for about $2,500.

In order to take advantage of the shelters, we must be warned in time to be able to reach them before the explosion occurs. This warning would probably come over the radio and every family should have a radio, preferably one powered by a battery, since the electric lines may be down. This battery radio should be transistorized for long lasting life, and if possible each radio should have an inexpensive radiation meter attached to it. It is to be sincerely hoped that an inexpensive battery-powered, transistorized radio with a radiation meter attached will be made available to every family in the United States soon.

The above discussion has been written in the hope that a great many people will get to know something about radiation. It must be remembered that we do not know all there is to be known about world-wide fallout; for instance, it is comforting to understand that a very careful program is being carried out to estimate the amounts of fallout in different parts of the world.

Above all, we should know that the small amount of radiation we receive from diagnostic studies, such as X rays of the chest, will have no harmful effects if they are taken by a properly trained person. The information gained from them is very important. As a matter of fact, a lifesaving diagnosis may be made in some cases only by taking X rays. So do not be afraid to take the advice of your family doctor when he advises some X ray studies.

GLOSSARY

Altitude height
Assimilating taking in
Atmosphere the layers of air surrounding the earth
Cosmic rays radioactive rays from the sun
Cumulative adding to
Debris leavings
Detonation explosion
Electron a kind of electrical charge
Emits sends out
Genes elements in parents' sperm or ovum that determine the child's growth and appearance
Genetic mutation an inherited abnormality
Nuclear detonation explosion of an atom bomb or hydrogen bomb
Particles tiny pieces
Radiation emission of rays
Radioactive containing active rays
Roentgen measurement of radiation
Sodium salt
Stratosphere upper layer of air surrounding the earth
Troposphere layer of air under the stratosphere

Chapter 30

Addictions

HALLUCINOGENIC DRUGS

Cause and Nature

A drug which causes people who take it to have hallucinations is called an hallucinogenic drug.

These drugs are not new. They have been used for many thousands of years. Only recently we see a great deal of publicity given to them in the press and other news media.

These drugs are taken by man to cause himself to be transported to an artificial paradise. He has wonderful dreams and experiences flashing sensations of sound and color.

One of the newer drugs of this nature is called L.S.D., which is short for lysergic acid diethylamide and is said to produce a state similar to schizophrenia. Some researchers in this field think that the use of these drugs in experiments will lead to the discovery of methods of treating schizophrenia and other psychotic states.

Hashish and marijuana are obtained from Indian hemp and have been used for centuries. It is said that the word "assassin"

Potent hallucinogens illicitily used in the United States	Source
Lysergic acid diethylamide	Fungus
Psilocybin	Mushroom
Mescaline	Cactus
Dimethyltryptamine (DMT)	Readily synthesized
Bufotenin (rarely used)	Toad skin
Hashish (pure cannabis resin)	Cannabis sativa

Some characteristics of 114 L.S.D. users	
Average age	23 (range 15-43)
Male	68.4%
White	88.4%
L.S.D. 1-3 times only	72.8%
Overwhelming panic	13.1%
Violence	12.3%
Homicidal or suicidal	8.6%
Underlying overt mental disease	34.2%
Requiring extended hospitalization	15.8%

Hallucinogenic drugs used indiscriminately have dire consequences as shown above.

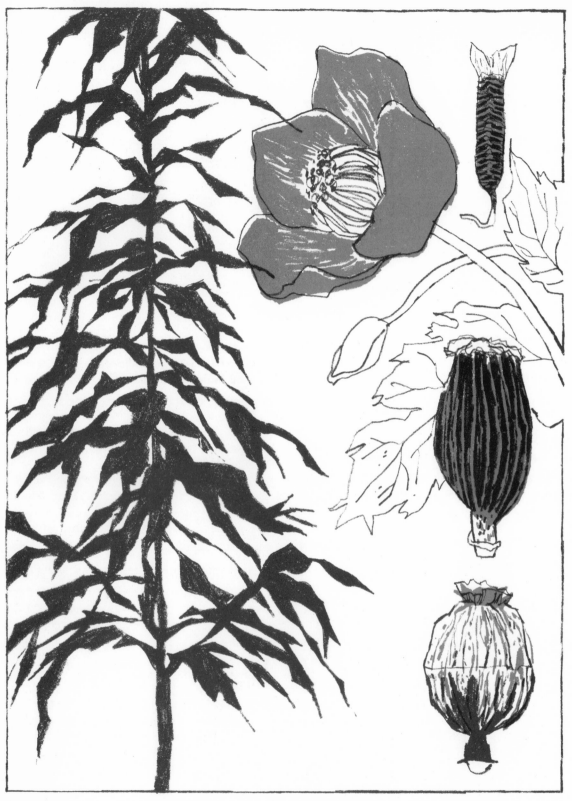

The marijuana weed (at left) and the opium poppy and pods from which narcotic drugs are made.

was derived from an ancient order, the members of which were persuaded to commit murder while under the influence of hashish.

Symptoms

This is an escape mechanism which is used to get away from reality. The use of these drugs can lead to habit formation which is called addiction and will be discussed in more detail below.

Some of these drugs like L.S.D. cause in the user a state of subacute schizophrenia. Most of them if used long enough will undermine the health and moral fiber of the individual user.

Treatment

The treatment of addiction to the hallucinogenic drugs varies with the type of drug used and must always be in the hands of a physician. The method used is withdrawal and the means for accomplishing this vary greatly with the drug.

GLOSSARY

Hallucinations   seeing objects with no reality, or experiencing sensations with no external cause
Hashish   intoxicating substance
Psychotic   any serious mental derangement
Schizophrenia   a type of psychosis characterized by loss of contact with environment and by disintegration of personality
Subacute   somewhat acute. Between acute and chronic

MARIJUANA

(Hashish or Cannabis Indica)

Cause and Nature

Marijuana is a dangerous drug made from the flower at the top of the hemp herb. This hemp grows wild in a great many countries and it is cultivated in some countries. In the United States it may grow wild by the roadside or in gardens. The legal growth of hemp in the United States is regulated very carefully by the Federal Government.

The hairs on the top of the flower of the female hemp plant have a resinous substance on them which contains the active ingredients and this is usually dried and smoked in cigarettes called "reefers" by the users in the United States.

For many centuries the effects of this weed have been known all over the world. In addition to being smoked, it sometimes is swallowed and snuffed.

Since it has a very great psychic effect it is a very dangerous drug and has been the cause of much suffering to its users and their families.

Signs and Symptoms

This weed is used mostly by young people who are frustrated and emotionally unstable, and who seek release or escape from these feelings by smoking marijuana. Many users feel inadequate and try to build up their morale by becoming intoxicated on marijuana.

The effects vary greatly with the person who uses it and with the route of administration as well as the amount used. The user gets a feeling of well-being, a reddening of the eyeballs, and he may start giggling or laughing and have an increase in appetite. There also may be a dryness of the mouth and nausea. The addicts may become restless and talkative or they may enter into a state which is marked by exaltation and happiness. There may be a marked tremor, a loss of the sense of balance, and increased sensitivity to pain. This may be followed by a sense of drowsiness which leaves the user greatly let down after he loses the effect of the drug.

Treatment

The drug should be withdrawn immediately. There are, as a rule, no severe withdrawal symptoms as suffered by opium addicts. The emotional instability which has caused the person to use the drug should be treated to prevent further use.

GLOSSARY

Resinous   a plant substance, soluable in water
Psychic   pertaining to the mind
Tremor   a trembling, from disease or weakness

BARBITURATE ADDICTION

Cause and Nature

The addiction to barbiturates is very common in the United States. It is caused by prolonged use of one of the derivatives of barbituric acid, and since these drugs are commonly prescribed by doctors, nearly everyone has been exposed to a certain amount of this drug.

The drugs most commonly used are barbital, phenobarbital, amytal, nembutal, and seconal. The first two act slowly and the effects go away slowly, while the latter two, nembutal and seconal, act rapidly and the effects wear off rapidly. That is the reason nembutal and seconal are used most often by doctors to produce sleep.

There are many people who will not take these sleeping pills because they are afraid that they will get the habit or become addicted. Doctors know that small doses of nembutal or seconal taken at night to produce sleep will not produce addiction, and they feel that the danger of habit formation is much less harmful than the loss of sleep night after night. Some people may become addicted to most anything. Coffee drinking and cigarette smoking are very common forms of addiction. However, these habits may be terminated or broken off, if the person really wants to stop, without any great suffering or withdrawal symptoms.

People who use small doses of barbiturates at night in order to sleep may do so almost indefinitely without becoming addicted and may stop using them without too much trouble. However, if large doses are taken over a long period, then a true addiction results and it may be difficult to break this habit. If the doses needed to produce the required effects become larger and larger, then the person may suffer from chronic barbiturate poisoning. This is a serious disease and may well lead to death.

Acute barbiturate poisoning is a common occurrence. This is caused by taking large doses of barbiturates in an attempt to commit suicide, or by accident; in either case it is a serious condition that requires immediate treatment. It has been estimated that between fifteen hundred and two thousand deaths caused by acute barbiturate poisoning occur in the United States every year. This is one reason why sleeping pills or any other medicine containing barbiturates should never be left where children can get them. Since the use of alcohol and barbiturates may go hand in hand, it must always be remembered that a person confused by alcohol or by previously taking an unknown amount of barbiturates may continue to take the sleeping pills until an overdose of barbiturates will result, which may lead to death.

In summary it should be remembered that the barbiturates are useful and harmless drugs when taken under the supervision of a doctor, but they may become habit forming and very harmful if taken over a long period in large doses. The size of the dose needed to cause addiction varies from person to person.

Signs and Symptoms

The signs and symptoms of barbiturate poisoning may resemble those of alcoholic intoxication, but there is no odor of alcohol on the breath and the face is not flushed. The person loses the ability to think clearly, may become very talkative, and cry or laugh easily. These symptoms gradually progress into a loss of control over muscles, then confusion, drowsiness, sleep, and coma. The breathing becomes shallow and the coma becomes deeper, finally leading to death if not treated.

Treatment

People who have taken large doses recently should have their stomachs pumped or washed out to remove any drug that remains in the stomach. They should not be allowed to go to sleep. Large doses of coffee may help in this respect. A doctor should always be in charge of treating these cases and he will know that in attempting to treat a case of chronic barbiturate poisoning the drug should never be completely withdrawn suddenly. The person being treated should be under the absolute control of the doctor—preferably in a hospital where regular doses of barbiturates can be administered at intervals, and in gradually reduced doses until they can be withdrawn altogether. This will take days or weeks, and other drugs must be used. The person who has been cured of this habit may expect to live a perfectly healthy life if barbi-

turates are left alone. In cases where the barbiturates have been taken because of emotional instability or some form of psychoneurosis, the patient should be treated by a psychiatrist until the condition which caused the use of barbiturates in excess has been cured.

GLOSSARY

Addiction   inability to discontinue a habit, such as taking drugs
Barbiturates   a group of drugs used to quiet nerves or induce sleep
Coma   unconsciousness caused by disease, injury, or poison
Derivative   a substance made or obtained from another substance
Psychiatrist   an expert in that branch of medicine that deals with disorders of the mind
Psychoneurosis   a nervous disorder which presents the symptoms of a disease
Terminate   to end

AMPHETAMINE POISONING OR ADDICTION

Cause and Nature

Chronic amphetamine poisoning is seen among people who consume large amounts of benzedrine, desoxyn, or dexedrine over a long period. There are other amphetamines but the above three are the most commonly used. The people who use these drugs to the point of addiction or chronic poisoning are quite often alcoholics or barbiturate addicts. Prisoners in some of the larger penal institutions are frequent users when they can obtain pills. One of the little recognized but larger groups of persons who use amphetamines to excess are truck drivers who have to stay awake over long periods and use the pills to prevent drowsiness while driving long distances. These drugs are nearly always taken by mouth.

Signs and Symptoms

The immediate effect of the pills is a sense of alertness and loss of feeling of fatigue. The person who uses more and more of these stimulative pills becomes an addict, and the signs of addiction or chronic poisoning are jerkiness, nervousness, loss of appetite, and inability to sleep.

The amphetamine addict may develop a rapid pulse, high blood pressure, and will usually show a fine tremor of the hands. Anyone who uses the pills over a long period and in large amounts may develop a psychosis with hallucinations and deliriums.

Treatment

The treatment consists of abrupt withdrawal of the amphetamine pills and administration of sedatives to combat the withdrawal symptoms which will appear. In case the person who is using these pills to excess is found to have severe personality defects he should be treated by a psychiatrist.

BROMISM

(Chronic Bromide Poisoning)

Cause and Nature

Chronic bromide poisoning is caused by taking too many bromides. This often occurs because many nerve tonics, which can be obtained at drug stores or soda fountains without a prescription, contain bromides.

This is a very common disease and often goes undetected. It has been noted that as high as twenty-one percent of the patients admitted into the psychiatric divisions of some large hospitals were suffering from bromide poisoning.

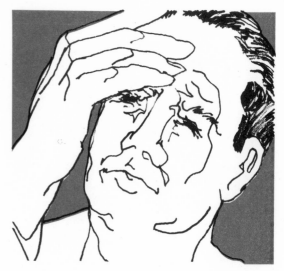

This illustration shows a man suffering from Bromide poisoning. He is disoriented and has a severe headache.

The symptoms for which bromides are taken, such as headache and nervousness, are the very symptoms which go along with bromide poisoning and are relieved temporarily by taking bromides. Hence, people take more and more of this dangerous drug thinking that they are being helped by it.

One other reason for the great number of cases of bromide poisoning is that people who have arteriosclerosis, or use alcohol to excess, are very susceptible to bromide poisoning, and relatively small amounts of bromides taken to relieve the symptoms of these two conditions may result in bromide poisoning.

Signs and Symptoms

These may vary greatly from patient to patient. In a small percentage of cases a bromide rash may be seen. In other cases there may be headaches, weakness, slurred speech, irritability, emotional instability, loss of memory, disorientation, and in some cases, hallucinations.

Treatment

The use of bromides must be stopped at once. The patient is given a large amount of fluids daily to wash the bromides out of his system. This may be helped by taking large amounts of salt or sodium chloride along with the increased fluids.

Symptoms such as irritability or restlessness may persist after the bromides have been removed from the body, and these may be controlled by using a mild sedative such as Equanil.

A doctor should be in charge of all cases of bromide poisoning as there may be some underlying disease which caused the patient to take bromides, and this disease will also need treating.

GLOSSARY

Arteriosclerosis   hardening of the arteries
Hallucinations   sensations with no real external cause

NARCOTIC ADDICTION

(*Chronic Opium Poisoning*)

Cause and Nature

Narcotic addiction is caused by taking drugs which are derived from opium. These drugs, in the order of their strength or potency are heroin, morphine, dilaudid, methedrine, meperidine or demerol, and codeine.

Opium itself is used by smoking it, most frequently in the Orient, and the habit of opium smoking is quite common there.

People who have become addicted to the opium derivatives find that it takes more and more of the drug to satisfy them, and sooner or later they may get into the habit of using heroin which is one of the stronger forms. Since the narcotic addict must have the drug and it is quite expensive to obtain, most addicts sooner or later resort to crime in order to obtain enough money to buy the drug. This is one of the reasons that narcotic addicts are found quite often among criminals. The user often resorts to selling the drug or "pushing" it in order to get money to buy his own supply. In order to create a market he takes pains to teach other people how to use the drug. This is especially true among students in large city high schools, in members of gangs, and in other susceptible persons.

This teaching of other people to use narcotics in order to create a market is one of the most serious crimes with which our nation is confronted. The user of narcotics soon becomes so intent on securing enough of the drug to satisfy himself that his every thought and action is concentrated upon getting enough money to buy more narcotics. He loses all feeling of social responsibility. A narcotic addict cannot be expected to tell the truth about anything.

Since the sale of narcotics is illegal, the product which is sold is usually greatly diluted in order to make more money and it usually is contaminated by bacteria and fungi. Since the habitual user in this country most often takes the drug by injection, and sometimes the injections are made directly into the veins in order to get quicker results, there is a high percentage of infections at the site of injection.

Many people have tried to determine just why a person becomes a narcotic addict, but no clear picture has been developed. It is often thought that many people became chronic users because a doctor had prescribed or given a person narcotics for the relief of pain. As a matter of fact, only a very small percentage of narcotic addicts

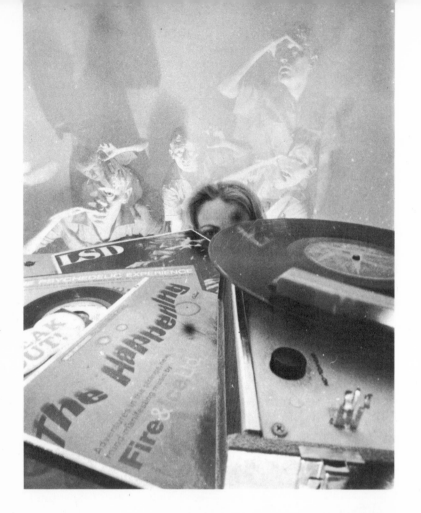

Psychedelusion: Young people carried away by doubts and conflicts are deluded into believing that a "trip" or some "pot" will make things right.

Coffeehouses, where young people can find sympathetic understanding and redirection are springing up in "hippie" centers.

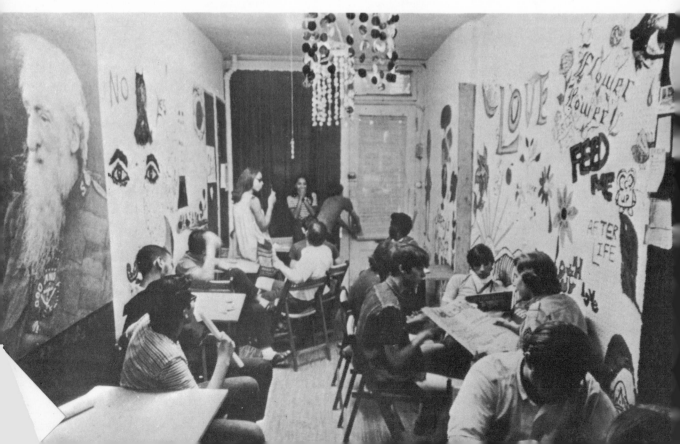

are started out in this way. Usually there is some weakness or abnormality of character which causes a person to seek escape from the realities of life by using narcotics.

The person who becomes a slave to this habit will suffer untold miseries, will cause great damage to himself and other members of society with whom he comes in contact, and will sooner or later end up in the lowest state of degradation. For these reasons, law enforcement officials and other conscientious persons are continuously waging a determined fight to wipe out narcotic addiction. So far there does not seem to be any decrease in the number of narcotic addicts.

Signs and Symptoms

The addict will say that the initial effect of taking narcotics is a pleasurable tingling feeling, relief from pain, and sense of increased drive. There is a general feeling of well-being, but with a chronic user it takes more and more of the drug to accomplish this end. Before a person develops a tolerance to the drug it may cause nausea or an itching of the skin.

After a person has become addicted it is almost impossible to detect the condition. He will always lie about it, and about the only way to be sure that a person is a narcotic addict is for a doctor to perform a test by the use of another drug called N-allynormorphine. The expert use of this drug by a physician will accurately establish whether or not a person is an addict.

After using the drug for a long time the puncture marks can be seen in the skin, often over the superficial veins, and the user may become pale and undernourished because of the neglect of food in favor of narcotics.

Treatment

The withdrawal symptoms are very severe and the treatment of a narcotic user must be in the hands of a physician in a special institution. When a narcotic addict is deprived of the drug he becomes restless and nervous, he yawns a great deal, his eyes run tears or water, and he begins to perspire. These symptoms are followed by a feeling of chilliness alternating with warmth. Diarrhea and vomiting may appear, and there will always be severe pain, muscle cramps, and an inability to sleep. Stopping the narcotic habit is one of the most terrible experiences that a person can imagine, and should always be in the hands of a physician.

The outlook for a permanent cure of a narcotic addict is poor. Although they may go without the drug for years, they usually sooner or later resume the habit. Everyone should be taught the terrible nature of this habit so they will know better than to take the first step in narcotic using.

The final step in the treatment of a narcotic addict is to have a psychiatrist attempt to correct the character defect which led to addiction.

GLOSSARY

Abnormality   something strangely irregular
Amphetamines   a synthetic drug which stimulates the central nervous system
Delirium   temporary mental disturbance
Derivative   something obtained from something else
Psychiatrist   an expert in that branch of medicine which deals with disorders of the mind
Psychosis   a mental disease
Stimulative   having power to quicken
Superficial   lying on or affecting only the surface
Susceptible   having little resistance
Tolerance   the increasing resistance to the effect of a drug due to continued use.

ALCOHOLISM

(Alcohol Addiction)

Cause and Nature

Alcoholism presents one of the most serious problems in public health to be found in the United States.

There are millions of so-called social drinkers who drink in moderation, but when a person drinks enough to have it interfere with his relationship with other people and with his mental and physical health, he then becomes an alcoholic.

There are many different stages of alcoholism, and very intensive studies are being carried out to curb this great menace to the health and happiness of so many Americans.

It has been estimated that perhaps sixty million people in the United States use alcoholic beverages. Of these, maybe one million are real alcoholics. Chronic alcoholism has come to be considered as a character disorder. A "problem drinker," that is, one who cannot control his drinking, must certainly be classified as a psychoneurotic.

People who are moderate drinkers appear to suffer very little in the form of physical health or mental health. However, chronic or heavy drinkers usually suffer from deficiencies of food and vitamins and this faulty nutrition affects their health and shortens their lives.

The effect of alcohol is seen mainly in the central nervous system or brain. A few minutes after drinking an alcoholic beverage, alcohol can be detected in the blood and if the concentration in the blood is 150 milligrams per 100 cc. of blood, or 1.5 percent, the person is said to be legally under the influence of alcohol.

Because alcohol knocks out the inhibitions and restraints, many people become violent and even commit violent crimes when sufficiently under the influence of alcohol.

Some people think of alcohol as a stimulant, but actually it is a depressant, as may be seen when a person who has had too much to drink gradually becomes more sluggish and finally passes out.

Signs and Symptoms

This part of the discussion will be confined to the signs and symptoms of chronic alcoholism.

A chronic alcoholic, after taking one drink, is unable to refrain from drinking more until he finally comes to rest in a hospital, at home, or in jail. There are two types of chronic alcoholics—the spree drinker, who may remain sober for weeks between sprees, and the steady drinker, who consumes large amounts of alcohol every day. These people are seldom able to recognize the fact or to admit that drinking is a problem with them.

The symptoms of chronic alcoholism are almost too numerous to mention. There may be chronic gastritis or diarrhea, loss of weight, nausea, and vomiting. A coarse tremor of the hands is usually present, especially if they have been without a drink for some time. The liver may be behind in its duties because of the heavy load placed upon it in detoxifying the alcohol and because proper food elements and vitamins are missing. This may lead to cirrhosis of the liver, with swelling of the legs, and fluid in the abdominal cavity. The person becomes less efficient in his work, his mentality slows down, and he may become emotionally unstable.

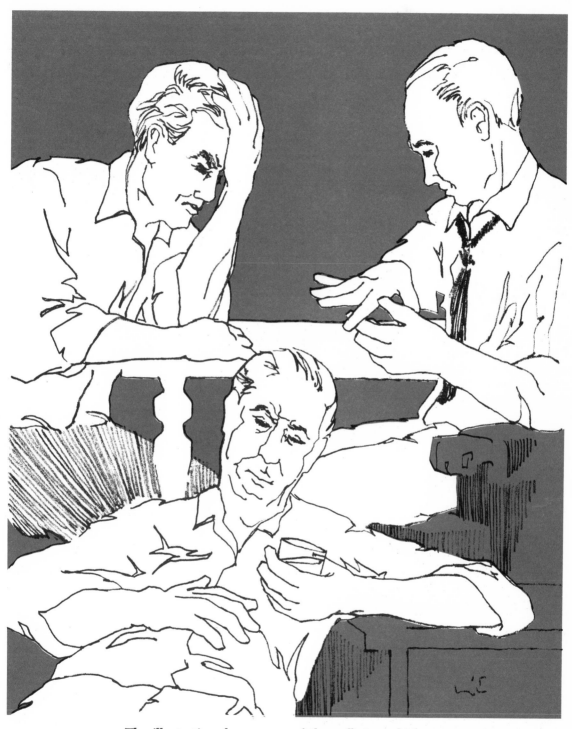

The illustration shows some of the suffering which results from the abuse of alcoholic indulgence—headache, a coarse tremor of the hands, and abdominal pain.

If this excessive drinking is continued, the brain will suffer great damage, which at times cannot be repaired. There may also be convulsive seizures and delirium tremens.

Delirium tremens is characterized by disorientation, confusion, delirium, and hallucinations. These hallucinations may be either visual or auditory. Most often visual hallucinations predominate; the patient sees pink elephants, snakes, etc. With the auditory hallucinations the patient hears nonexistent voices.

Korsakoff's syndrome occurs in alcoholics who have abused themselves by excessive drinking over a long period of time. It is recognized by memory loss, disorientation, and amnesia. Victims may have neuritis and they like to tell amazing untrue stories. Some patients may recover from this type of damage in two or three months, while in others, this psychosis may last forever.

Treatment

The treatment of these patients can only be carried out successfully if they admit that drinking has become an uncontrollable problem. They must admit that they are licked and come asking for help. Alcoholics Anonymous is an organization of former alcoholics who are able to help some problem drinkers who admit that they are unable to control their drinking.

The best form of treatment for chronic alcoholics is in a state psychiatric hospital. They must go into these hospitals because they know and admit that they need help, and they must be prepared to stay in the hospital for one or two years.

While under treatment in the hospital, they are given drugs, vitamins, and psychiatric treatment, which may help to correct the character defect which caused them to be alcoholics.

PART 6

Emotional Disorders
and Mental Diseases

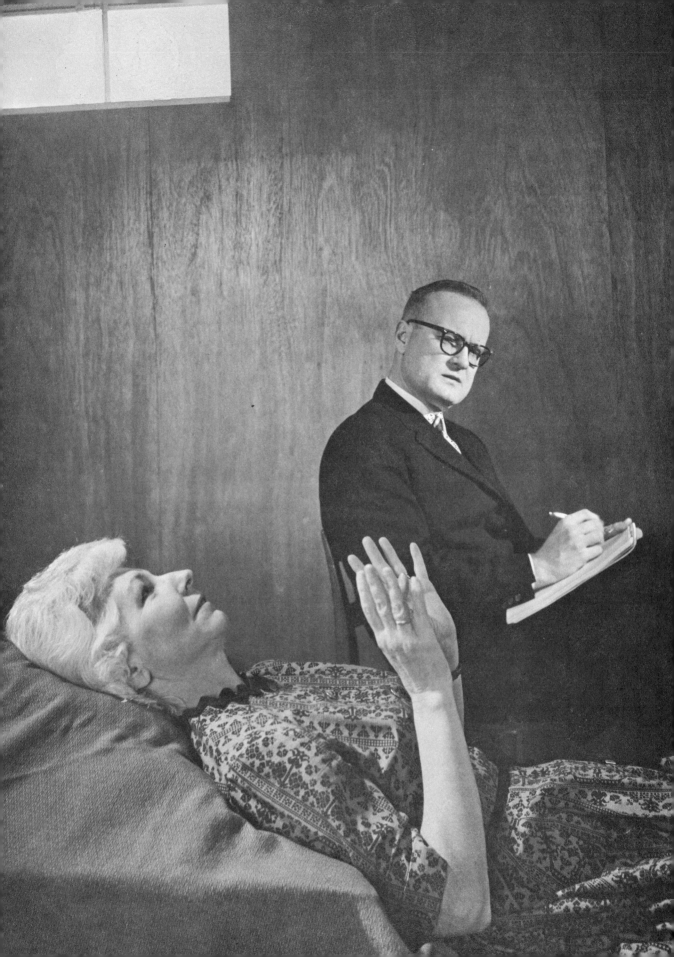

Chapter 31

Neurosis or Psychoneurosis

PEOPLE are said to be neurotic or suffer from a neurosis when they exhibit symptoms for which no organic lesion, that is, no disease of the organs of the body, can be blamed. This is called a functional disorder, in contrast to an organic disease.

In recent years doctors have learned more about the neuroses than was ever known before, but there are still a great many unknown facts to be learned about the mind and the nervous system. It is to be hoped that some day our knowledge of the workings of the mind, along with its relation to the functioning of the different organs of the body, will be more complete. When this knowledge is obtained and properly used, a great deal of needless suffering will be done away with.

Cause and Nature

Since our understanding of the mind and its interaction with the body is not complete, this chapter on neurosis must be restricted to some of the fundamentals which are accepted by the medical profession and which are used in the diagnosis and treatment of nervous conditions.

A doctor who treats diseases of the mind is known as a psychiatrist and he is especially trained in the field of mental disorders. A general practitioner or family doctor can recognize character or personality defects, and in some cases he can help the patient by discovering the underlying cause of his trouble and in that way do away with most of his symptoms.

We must understand that there is a little bit of the neurotic in all of us and know that the discussion in this chapter will pertain to the nervous conditions which cause marked symptoms.

It has been estimated that about sixty out of every hundred patients who go into a doctor's office for treatment are suffering from some functional disorder and have no organic disease.

It therefore becomes very important for all of us to try to understand some of the factors which cause the distressing symptoms seen in people who are said to be suffering from some form of neurosis.

Every person develops character or personality which is influenced, first of all, by inheritance (the type of nervous system and mind which is given to them by their parents). Secondly, the environment in which a person is raised has a great influence upon his character formation. The number of brothers and sisters in the family, the relationship between the mother and father, and lastly, the love and attention which is given to the baby by its mother, are all very important. Not to be overlooked is the amount of stress and strain to which the young child is exposed during its growing years. To try to understand the neuroses, it is very important to keep in mind the way in which every personality or character is developed.

When the baby is first born it has a set of unconscious drives or biological instincts which at first are manifested only in hunger, need for warmth and comfort, and need for love. These drives or instincts become more complicated later on, and they are always unconscious. These are called the "id."

It is of great importance for the mother to give the baby food, comfort, and love during the very first months of life, for if he is deprived of these, the child will develop a sense of frustration or insecurity which may affect its later life. If the mother does a good job, she will build up in the child a sense of trust in others, and the concept of giving and sharing with others.

As the child becomes older, say three or four years old, it develops a second important part of its character called the "super-ego" or conscience. This is to keep on developing throughout life, and in a way it can be called the person's or child's ideal picture of himself. This super-ego or conscience is greatly influenced by the parents, by what the child thinks his parents expect of him, and the things he sees them do

which, of course, he thinks at that time are socially acceptable. In other words, the child begins to develop his own idea of what is right and what is wrong.

It is easy to see how this super-ego can be affected in its formation by excessive criticism on the part of the parent and especially can it be influenced by an overambitious parent who, after the child starts to school, expects him to be perfect and to get good grades which he may not be able to make. Failure to live up to this ideal of the parents builds up in the child a sense of shame or guilt. Do not push the child too hard or expect too much of him.

This formation of the super-ego or conscience is influenced perhaps to the greatest extent after the baby is about one year old, when he begins his first experience in socialization. This is the time of toilet training and the way in which this is carried out may have a great effect upon the child's future life. The mother should not be too strict or too critical. The process of toilet training should be carried out in a friendly, casual, and not too demanding fashion. Any feeling of guilt or shame which the parent instills in the child during this period may be stored up in his subconscious mind and give rise to feelings of insecurity, shame, and guilt in later life.

The third and perhaps the most important part of the child's personality make-up begins to form in the first few days of life and continues to grow or change throughout life. This is called the "ego." The first two components of the child's nervous make-up are largely unconscious, but the ego is largely conscious.

Its function is to test reality—that is, conditions that exist in the child's environment—and to manage a satisfactory adjustment between his own instinctive drives or id, his conscience or super-ego, and conditions that exist in the outside world in which he lives. This adjustment should manage to protect or preserve the personality of the child and at the same time permit him to obtain gratification of his instinctive drives in such a manner as to keep intact and satisfy his conscience or super-ego.

Much has been said about how important the first few years of life are. As a matter of fact, some great teachers have stated that if they could have the child during the first seven or eight years of its life, they would have no fear about its satisfactory personality development. This may be overstating the case, but there is no doubt that the first few years are extremely important.

We have commented on the child's or baby's need for love, food, warmth, and comfort. However, a child must learn to master the stresses of life and if in these first few formative years the baby is subjected to over-protection and over-solicitousness on the part of the mother and father, he may be greatly handicapped in developing a satisfactory personality and may exhibit symptoms of neurosis later on. There are no authoritative statistics available to prove this statement, but it is entirely possible that as many or more neurotic, maladjusted personalities are caused by a domineering, overprotective mother or father, as are due to a lack of love, warmth, and understanding on the part of the parents.

One of the ego's most important functions is to distinguish and modify any unreasonable demands of the instinctive drives so that they become acceptable to society or to the outside world of reality.

Now we have discussed the three factors in life which are responsible for the formation of a satisfactory personality. These are the id or instinctive drives, the super-ego or conscience, and the ego which controls these two more or less unconscious traits so that they perform in such a way as to conform with reality.

We have noted the extreme importance of a mother's relations to a baby during the first few years, and how the father and mother, in their relation to each other and their attitude toward the child, may affect his later life. We have stressed the fact that a baby should have lots of love and affection but should not be over-protected or over-restricted by domineering parents so as to prevent his developing an adequate personality of his own. We will discuss some of the various forms in which the symptoms and signs of neurotic behavior appear in later life.

The neuroses or psychoneuroses usually appear in early life and very seldom do they make their first entry upon the stage after a person is about fifty years old.

Before discussing the signs and symptoms of the neuroses it may be well to have it understood that there is a definite difference between psychosis or insanity, and the neurosis. Insanity or true mental disease will be discussed in another chapter.

Psychoneurotic reactions occur when the ego is not strong enough to control or adjust the biological drives to the moral restrictions which exist in the environment or in reality.

Although the most important period in the development of personality or character occurs during the first years of life, other periods are also filled with unusual strains and stresses which may result in symptoms. These periods are puberty and adolescence, when the sexual drive begins to complicate the problem; and young adulthood, when the choice of a vocation and the choosing of a marital partner (with the subsequent responsibilities attendant upon raising children and earning enough money to support them properly) may bring out feelings of anxiety and insecurity in some people. As the span of life becomes longer we have more and more older people who exhibit neurotic symptoms when they are subjected to the strains of being without their old friends, filling their time when they are forced to retire, and in general setting up a new way of life.

It should not be implied that the stresses and strains of life are in themselves harmful, because everyone is and should be subjected to these forces. The proper handling of difficult situations is the thing that gives us strength and helps develop a strong personality. This is one of the reasons why a mother should not over-protect her child but should allow him to make his own decisions.

The hospitals are full of patients who have been unfortunate enough to have an imbalance between the ego, super-ego, and biological drives, for it has been shown that continued stresses and strains such as anxiety, guilt, anger, etc., improperly handled, will cause physical sickness or at least contribute to it.

The jails and penitentiaries are also largely populated by unfortunate people who, in some cases, have failed to develop a conscience or super-ego. In other cases they have had a poor home life as children; some may have had an alcoholic father or no father at all; others for some unknown reason have not developed a strong ego. You have heard the expression, "He just never grew up," and this explains some criminals who have never learned how to pass up a chance for immediate pleasure or gain.

As we have stated above, all of us show some signs of being neurotic; but when the signs and symptoms are so great as to cause real trouble, then definite patterns appear and some of these will be discussed below.

Signs and Symptoms

The signs and symptoms of the various psychoneurotic disorders are very seldom clear cut; that is, the different neurotic syndromes or illnesses have many features in common with other psychoneurotic disorders.

The ego has a difficult time in maintaining harmony between the instinctive drives (id), the conscience or super-ego, and the outside world or reality. When this proper balance is not kept the ego calls upon various defense mechanisms and this attempt to keep harmony by the use of some defense reaction results in symptoms.

It must be remembered that this turmoil and strife usually takes place in the unconscious mind, and the person who suffers from these symptoms or neurotic syndromes is very seldom aware of the causes.

The various defense mechanisms used by the ego in an attempt to maintain harmony may be classified by placing them in groups which are symptom pictures of certain neurotic disorders. These result in abnormal conditions called reactions. Again it must be stated that these reactions seldom occur in the pure form and that each one of them may contain some of the same emotions or elements found in the other reactions. The predominant or outstanding component of such disorder is often used to classify it.

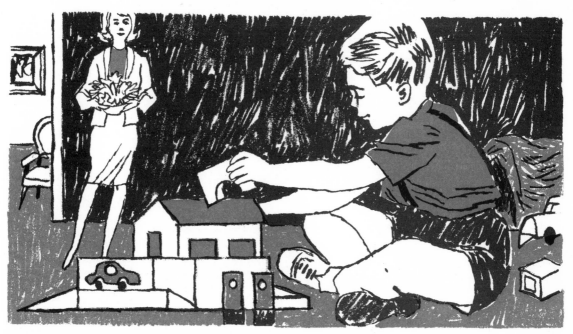

Mentally retarded children may be helped greatly with special attention and help.

MENTAL RETARDATION

(Mental Deficiency)

Cause and Nature

The failure of a child's brain to develop to its full capacity may have many causes such as injury, disease, and the inheritance of certain genes from his family.

This mental retardation will make itself felt before the child is full grown and any mental deficiency noted in an adult is usually called dementia.

This condition may make itself known in many different forms and degrees, with or without physical characteristics.

Signs and Symptoms

The recognition of true mental deficiency is nearly always made by psychometric tests. There are many of these tests and they will not be named here as a psychologist or psychiatrist must administer the tests. Usually they give a test to determine the intelligence quotient (I.Q.). The difference between the mental age of the child and his chronological age, or age in years, is often used to calculate his I.Q. A person with an I.Q. of sixty or seventy and below is considered mentally retarded.

Many other things are taken into consideration, such as the child's ability to get along in school, his emotional reactions, and his behavior. These children require supervision in order to protect them and to see that they do no harm to others.

Treatment

A great amount of interest has been shown recently in detecting these children and giving them special instruction. Operation Head Start is one of these programs.

Many children are considered mentally deficient when they may not be deficient at all. It may be the parents or some other influence in their lives, such as a deprived environment, that causes them to seem to casual observers to be retarded. Indeed some of them may be just the opposite from deficient and may be geniuses.

Therefore a great deal of investigation must be carried out before the diagnosis is made. First a thorough examination should be made by a pediatrician. This will include the family history, many laboratory tests (such as an electroencephalogram), a history of injury or accidents, and a knowledge of the diet, and other factors in the home life to which the child is subjected. Many of these children are in the low-normal group of our civilization. Just as many of our children are in the high-normal or genius class. Therefore a great deal of care and study must be used in differentiating or diagnosing them.

Special Mental Retardation Clinics are now being held in many parts of the country where the suspected mentally retarded are studied and the appropriate form of help is given.

Most of the infantile forms which are inborn are severe in nature, and are caused by a combination of genes which the baby has inherited. The classification of these babies is rather crude, but it is the only one we know of now. There are different names applied to them which are not entirely accurate. Those born with an I.Q. of below twenty are called idiots. The ones with an I.Q. of from twenty to forty-nine are designated as imbeciles, and those from forty-nine to sixty-nine are called morons.

As a general rule these children do not live very long. Most of them die before the age of fifteen.

It is the children in the upper limit or upper part of this classification that we hope to help by classes for the mentally retarded.

Remember that a child is not to be considered mentally retarded until he has had a thorough examination as outlined above, and that a great number of such children can become useful citizens with the proper care and treatment.

GLOSSARY

Psychometric   measurement of the action of the brain

Electroencephalogram   a graphic tracing made by encephalography which is a recording by means of electrodes applied to the scalp of electric currents developed in the brain similar to an electrocardiogram used in examining the heart.

ANXIETY REACTION

Perhaps the emotion which causes the most trouble when it is stored away in the unconscious mind is anxiety. The anxiety reaction may be classified as either an acute anxiety reaction or chronic anxiety reaction.

Acute attacks of anxiety are characterized by a sudden feeling of dizziness and light headedness; there may be palpitation of the heart with some discomfort in the chest; there is shortness of breath, and coldness. There is a feeling of weakness and tingling of the hands or feet, and there also may be a desire to go to the bathroom frequently. Sometimes these acute attacks are brought on by overbreathing; that is, by breathing too rapidly. This is called hyperventilation. These attacks may recur at various times and are usually caused by some deeply hidden feeling of hostility or rage at some person who is important. There are other causes, but it is hard to define them because they are buried in the subconscious mind; among them are frustration, threats of loneliness, and at times, forbidden sexual desires which are not recognized at all.

Any threat to a person's security may precipitate such a reaction if the person is predisposed or susceptible to this form of reaction. The patient usually complains of a feeling of tension to begin with, and this may be accompanied by a feeling of apprehension, impending disaster, fear, and excitement.

The chronic anxiety reaction may result in any of the above symptoms in a milder form. This type of person is usually sensitive, easily embarrassed, and may be described as having an inferiority complex. As the anxiety becomes more pronounced, the patient may complain of restlessness and an inability to sleep.

SEXUAL DEVIATES

Cause and Nature

One of the most commonly seen types of personality disorders is the so-called sexual deviate. These deviates from normal fall into many classifications. The most often seen is the homosexual. In a woman these people are called lesbians. Their male counterparts are known as homosexuals. These people all act out their personality problems by particular sexual acts with someone of their same sex.

There are many causes of this condition. One is the failure of the child to identify with a parent of the same sex.

In the case of the male homosexual the father may be weak or he may be brutal so that the son hates or fears him; or the father may be absent. Other cases may be caused by isolation or separation from persons of the opposite sex as in prison.

Some of the other forms of sex deviation are known as pedophilia. These people show sexual interest in young children because they fear that they will be inadequate in attempting the act with people of their own age. This type is often an elderly person, or an incompetent person who is fearful of acceptance by his peers.

In many cases there is a destructive or sadistic element involved which leads these people to become murderous or to inflict punishment or wounds upon the children they attack.

One other form of sexual deviate is called an exhibitionist. These persons expose their male characteristics to the public to prove that they are masculine.

In many cases the person who does this has identified with his mother who may have been very dominant and aggressive while the father was either absent or weak and ineffectual. So the son has a compulsion to prove that he does not have a feminine identification.

Signs and Symptoms

The behavior of these people varies greatly but by far the most dangerous ones are the sadistic type who will often mutilate or murder their victim.

The homosexual will usually have sexual relations with his or her own sex, although some of these people may marry and be at least partially heterosexual.

Treatment

The best treatment for a person with one of the personality disorders mentioned above is prevention.

Sometimes a psychiatrist can help by exposing the cause for this socially frowned-upon behavior; psychoanalysis may help uncover the cause.

Sending these people to jail where they are confined with people of their own sex seldom does any good. The only thing prison achieves is to isolate them from the public so they cannot do harm to some innocent person.

GLOSSARY

Sadistic   one who derives pleasure from hurting other people

Heterosexual   normal sex relations with the opposite sex

CONVERSION REACTION OR HYSTERIA

The defense or method of adaptation used by the ego in some patients is called a conversion reaction or hysteria. This is one of the most common reactions seen in the neurotic person, and its outstanding characteristic is the way in which anxiety, hostility, or fear is converted into body symptoms. The hysterical person may inhibit body functions until he suffers from tremors, convulsive movements, feeling of anesthesia (numbness), and even loss of function in some parts of the body. This loss of function may be expressed in hysterial blindness, paralysis of the arm or leg, inability to talk, and in some cases, inability to hear.

The patient unconsciously resorts to this reaction because he has an uncontrollable and unconscious desire to escape from the effects of some deeply hidden emotional conflict.

It is thought that women suffer from this form of reaction more often than men. Some women who are inclined to hysterical episodes have been spoiled in childhood by over-protective relatives and later rejected.

In the man, neurotic symptoms are most often seen when he has to protect himself against unconscious threats to his self-esteem. This does not mean that men are not subject to hysterial episodes, only that they do not exhibit this form of behavior as often as women.

OBSESSIVE-COMPULSIVE REACTION

This type of behavior usually occurs in a person who is suppressing unwelcome or unacceptable thoughts or impulses by substituting for them some other ritualistic thoughts or acts.

The obsession or suppressed thought is compensated for by repeating the same act over and over again. This is a compulsion to perform this act which cannot be overcome. Some of these persons wash their hands continually; they may insist on counting or touching the same object every time they pass it; they may have to check and relock the doors several times before they leave home. This form of reaction is usually related to a feeling of guilt but is most often seen in people who are suppressing feelings of guilt or depression.

A hypochondriac may be placed in this classification. His obsessive-compulsive actions take the form of concern about the state of his health or the condition of one of his organs, for instance, the heart. He may be sure that the illness exists even though reassured by the doctor that his body is in good condition. He has a compulsion to magnify his symptoms. The feeling of fatigue is one of the hypochondriac's common complaints. This symptom may be out of all proportion to any cause which can be discovered.

PHOBIC REACTION

A person with a phobia is attempting to detach some undesirable thought from his mind by displacing it to some other object or situation.

There are many types of phobias, the most common being fear of high places, fear of confined places (claustrophobia), fear of dirt, and an abnormal fear of bacteria. The people who exhibit these phobias are not able to prevent the anxiety and fear which arise when they come in contact with the phobia stimulating situation.

Some people with this type of personality may give a history of having been exposed to a domineering, insistent mother and they try to hide or suppress the thoughts which they think their mother would not approve. Hence, they may grow up with a large number of suppressed undesirable thoughts.

DEPRESSIVE REACTION

This form of reaction is very common and the patient usually complains of moods of depression, fatigue, sleeplessness, and loss of appetite. There may be a lack of ambition and a complete loss of interest in family or friends. This type of patient usually has an over-developed conscience and he is punishing himself for some hidden feeling of anger or hate toward some other persons. People who exhibit this reaction may have been raised by parents who would not tolerate any form of anger on the part of the children towards the parent. Hence, the child, being afraid of losing the affection or good opinion of his parents, hides or suppresses all feelings of anger or hate in his unconscious mind, and later on suffers from depression. It is much better to permit the growing child to express his anger or displeasure and get it off his mind.

These people are usually very dependent upon others, and when they are separated from a member of their family or some friend, they suffer from severe depression.

PSYCHOSOMATIC OR PSYCHOPHYSIOLOGICAL REACTIONS

This form of reaction is one in which the conflict in the emotions is expressed by its effect upon some part of the body instead of by some behavior pattern.

Many books have been written on psychosomatic medicine and it is a well-established fact that functioning of the mind and body is closely related and any disfunction in one will have some effect upon the other.

A simple expression of this is to say that periods of long continued stress or anxiety may have the effect of tightening some of the muscles in the organs. This may decrease the circulation in these organs and if maintained over a long time will cause actual changes to occur. High blood pressure may be influenced in this way.

Another example is the anxiety reaction which may cause a feeling of tremulousness. The patient, to stop this trembling, will tense the muscles of his back and neck. This may lead to headache or backache.

There is a condition which is known as

"neuro-circulatory asthenia," which may be used as an example of a psychosomatic reaction. In this condition there is weakness, fast pulse, shortness of breath, dizziness (may be caused by over-breathing or hyperventilation), headache, easy fatigability, and a consciousness of the heart. There is no disease of the heart, but immature and dependent people seem to be subject to this form of reaction.

DISSOCIATIVE REACTION

(Amnesia)

Periods of amnesia may last for a short time or over a period of years. This reaction results from an overwhelming anxiety which may completely disorganize the personality and cause the patient to forget who he is.

This is called dissociation and is known as a dissociative fugue. A person suffers from this reaction because he needs to suppress the feeling of shame, rage, or guilt. He may wander away from home and assume another name and another personality in which he can act out the repressed impulses which his conscience would not let come to the surface in his original personality. After varying periods of time the patient may remember his name or return to his home to live a normal life.

Sometimes these periods of amnesia may be brought on by a head injury.

Treatment

All of us exhibit mild forms of psychoneurosis but when these symptoms become so marked that they interfere with a person's life, then a doctor should be consulted.

As pointed out above, the best form of treatment is prevention. The kind of a home a child is raised in makes all the difference, and in order to give the child a well-rounded personality, he should have lots of love but should not be dominated. He should be required to do the things he is able to do but should not be expected to perform above his abilities. All children cannot make A's in school and they should not be scolded if they do not reach perfection. A child should learn to give and take, to share with his brothers and sisters and parents.

If the symptoms of psychoneurosis appear in the form of one of the reactions described above (and remember these reactions are seldom seen in the pure form and one person may have symptoms of several different kinds of reactions) then he should see a doctor.

There are a great many good drugs on the market today for the relief of tension and anxiety, and when needed, they can be used by a doctor to great advantage. A word of caution should be inserted here. A certain amount of stress and strain is good for us; it makes us strong, so don't try to get a doctor to prescribe tranquilizers for every little flare-up of tension.

When people are being severely handicapped by their nervous condition or by emotional turmoil, a psychiatrist should be consulted. In some cases, he will use the process of psychoanalysis for treatment, and this is a very important and successful form of treatment in cases to which it can be adapted.

Psychotherapy or treatment of the mind takes a long time and is sometimes quite expensive, but is certainly worthwhile if carried out by a well qualified doctor. Patients

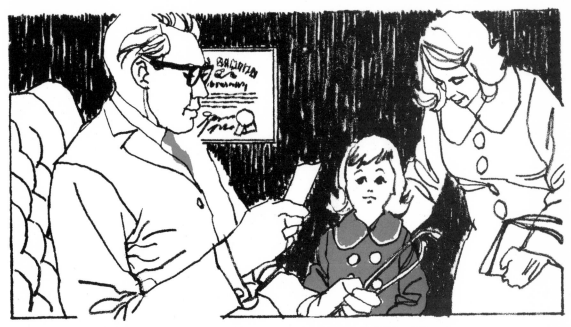

A psychiatrist performs most of his treatment by the proper use of "Words".

with psychoneurosis do not often need hospitalization but it may help in some cases.

Some doctors prescribe a change of scenery such as an ocean voyage or a long vacation. This will often help relieve the symptoms of psychoneurosis.

None of these treatments can make over the personality of the patient, so the time to prevent psychoneurosis is when the personality is being formed; and that is in childhood, from the very first day of life.

PSYCHOSOMATIC MEDICINE

A great deal has been written lately about psychosomatic medicine, and one would think from this emphasis that it is a new subject. However, good doctors have always practiced psychosomatic medicine—even before the term was invented.

The word "psycho" has to do with the mind or brain, and "somatic" has to do with the body. Therefore, psychosomatic medicine is that which takes into consideration the effects of the emotions upon the body.

As stated above, all good doctors have always known about the effect of the emotions upon the body, and have taken this into consideration when treating diseases or ailments of the body.

There is no way to separate the two, and when someone tells you, "It is all in your head," he is as wrong as he would be if he told you, "It is all in your body." For instance, when a person is working under a nervous tension most of the time, his body is tense, and his blood vessels may be constricted by this tension. Hence, he may develop high blood pressure in order to force the blood through smaller vessels. The pressure must be higher and the heart must work harder. Hence, sooner or later this strain may show up in symptoms which are related to the body only. This example may be oversimplified, but it will convey the general idea.

Just as emotions may give rise to bodily symptoms, so may bodily symptoms have an effect upon emotions. For instance, a person with a crippling disease, such as rheumatoid arthritis, may find that his personality undergoes a distinct change.

The important fact to remember is that the mind and the body both affect each other, and we must take into consideration all of these facts when a person is beset by symptoms.

HYPNOSIS

as used in the treatment of emotional disturbances and certain character defects

Many of the above described conditions can be treated successfully by a psychiatrist, and some psychiatrists use the process of hypnosis in their treatment.

At the beginning it must be emphasized that all psychiatrist do not use this method, but most of them agree that it is a useful tool. By the same token all psychiatrist do not use psychoanalysis or the old couch approach.

They have many different systems just as a doctor has many medicines. Some of them use group therapy, others family therapy and a few confine their treatment to individual interviews.

The role of psychiatry in our modern society is growing rapidly and many people are beginning to realize how in some cases they can be helped or cured by this form of treatment.

It would not be an over statement to say that most psychiatrists use all the tools at their command including hypnosis, always keeping in mind that different cases need different forms of treatment.

Hypnosis has been defined as "a state resembling normal sleep, differing in being induced by suggestion and by the operations of the hypnotizer with whom the hypnotized person remains in rapport, that is in an intimate and harmonious relation." The person who is hypnotized is therefore responsive to the hypnotizer's suggestions during the time he is in the trance and is even at times responsive to so called post hypnotic suggestion.

This means that after he comes out of the trance he will consciously perform acts which have been suggested to him during the treatment.

It can be understood from the above that this can be an important form of treatment when used by a properly trained and motivated therapist. On the other hand it can be dangerous when used improperly.

Doctors P. J. Bohnert and J. A. Smith who are well known psychiatrists have pointed out that hypnosis has not been used as often as it should be, especially in its application to short term treatment.

The cost of going to a psychiatrist's office is quite expensive and many patients simply cannot afford to keep up their treatment over a long period of time, hence short term therapy when it is effective becomes very important.

One of the uses of hypnosis may be to search out a patients inner conflicts while he is under hypnosis. He may be unaware of this conflict.

As an example, a man who was subject to anxiety attacks which resulted each time in severe headaches, visited a psychiatrist. Under hypnosis he revealed the fact that these attacks were preceded in every case by a report of one of his fellow salesmen that he had been very successful during last week in making sales. The patient subconsciously saw in this a threat to his own job and in that way a threat to the comfort and safety of his family.

After revealing this subconscious reaction and having it explained to him he was able to prevent the anxiety attacks and the severe headaches. This is an example of using the search for the cause of the attacks as a method of treatment.

Another method of treatment is to use hypnosis to relieve the symptoms rather than to look for the cause. This means that by suggestion while under hypnosis, the patient can have his symptoms entirely removed, have them lessened, and allow some less severe symptoms to take the place of a severe symptom.

As a rule anxiety plays a major role in many illnesses and the simple fact the anxiety can be removed by suggestion under hypnosis is a very important result of this form of treatment. This can be borne out by the fact that anxious and nervous people can be helped by taking tranquilizer pills.

Many cases of real illness may have a real psychogenic component. These are called psychosomatic illnesses. One example often used is bronchial asthma. This can be a really crippling disease and it has been said that attacks of asthma may be triggered by some conflict or emotional disturbance in a patient. A psychiatrist using hypnosis may be able to discover the particular set of circumstances which bring on an asthmatic attack and by suggestion, prevent future attacks, or at least make them occur less frequently.

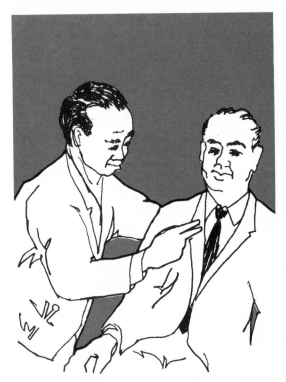

Some of the methods used to induce hypnosis are very simple as shown above.

The anxiety state is a condition which brings many people to a doctor's office and hypnosis can be used to relieve these patients.

Another neurosis which can successfully be treated at times by hypnosis is depression.

It is a well known fact that depression often leads to suicide and we must recognize the fact that depression in the form of a neurosis is different from depression in the form of a psychosis or true mental illness, as in the case of manic depressial psychosis. The true mental illness may be treated by giving shock treatments and the neurosis can be helped at times by hypnotic suggestion.

It has been stated that two of the causes of suicide are anger at oneself and being lonely. One psychiatrist has said that if a potential suicide has just a single real friend it may prevent him from self destruction.

Under hypnosis the potential suicide can by suggestion be taught to vent his anger on something other than himself and can be made to think that he has a friend and does not need to be lonely.

We have discussed the advantages to be gained by suggestion while under hypnosis. Now let us consider suggestion as an instrument to be used in self help.

Many years ago it became a fad to repeat several times a day the sentence, "Day by day, in every way, I become better and better." This was suggested by some person who did a great deal to help many people.

Today this same technique can be used to help our general health through power of suggestion in many ways.

For instance, if a person wants to lose weight he could keep repeating to himself that he isn't hungry, or could suggest to himself that he doesn't like certain types of fattening foods or drinks.

The habit of smoking cigarettes which we all know is unhealthy, could be broken if a person would suggest to himself every day that this is a dirty, expensive, unhealthy habit and one of these days I am going to stop it. Sure enough he may stop smoking without too much of a strain.

Never under estimate the power of suggestion.

Hypnosis is not a useful or successful technique in the treatment of all patients.

In order to be effective, the person who is being hypnotized must be a willing subject and cooperating fully feel that he can be hypnotized.

Some patients resist this treatment and it is impossible to hypnotize them.

HYPERVENTILATION

Cause and Nature

Hyperventilation is the act of breathing too fast. Through blowing off too much carbon dioxide, the person experiences symptoms which are due to alkalosis. The cause most often is reaction to pain or to some important conflict within himself. In the latter case this is one of the symptoms seen in neurosis. One simple cause of hyperventilation is climbing to a very high altitude.

Signs and Symptoms

Hyperventilation or overbreathing may result in many symptoms such as tightness of the chest, a feeling of not being able to get a good breath, and hence the person will find himself taking a long breath quite frequently. Tremors and twitching movements are frequently experienced. Tachycardia or rapid pulse, chest pain, and dryness of the mouth may become troublesome. In addition there may be difficulty in swallowing, bloating of the abdomen, belching, flatulence, dizziness, a disturbance of the vision, and finally, a fainting or a loss of consciousness.

Treatment

The most obvious treatment for hyperventilation or breathing too rapidly is to slow down the rate of breathing. The quickest method of restoring the carbon dioxide balance in the lungs is to place a paper bag over the mouth and nose, hold it snugly, and repeatedly breathe into the bag and then breathe in the same air. This will cause you to take in some of the carbon dioxide which has been breathed out, and thereby restore the proper amount of carbon dioxide.

After stopping the acute attack and the symptoms, the next and most important step is to readjust to the problems of life which are causing nervousness or neurosis.

THE ANXIETY STATE

Cause and Nature

The anxiety state is probably one of the most common conditions which afflicts modern man. It is seen in many forms and has been called by many names; one of the older and more often used names for it was "a nervous breakdown." For the purpose of this discussion, the anxiety state is one of the neuroses, or psychoneuroses which do not show any organic disease. It is to be considered as entirely separate from true mental illness or psychosis.

The causes have been described by many doctors who come in contact with this disease and are different according to the person who describes them. Some doctors speak of anxiety as the main characteristic of all neurosis; some say it is caused by a "strong desire which is likely to miss its goal."

Many psychiatrists believe that anxiety is a response to danger and in the anxiety state this danger is nearly always in the mind of the person affected. In most cases the person does not know what the danger is. In other words, in the subconscious mind there may be some primitive drive which is not compatible with the conscience.

Anxiety neurosis may occur in many different forms. The attacks may be acute, subacute, or chronic, and these attacks have been called by many names in the past, such as hysteria, nervous breakdown, neurocirculatory asthenia, and just plain nervousness. In nearly every case there is no physical cause, although the patient may think there is. Some patients in the acute episodes think they are dying, others think they are having a heart attack. Some people have repeated operations to cure some vague abdominal pain; others are hospitalized on numerous occasions and no physical defect can be found. These are called conversion symptoms in which a patient may convert some imaginary fear into an actual physical symptom such as nausea and vomiting, or pain in any part of the body. In many cases, usually in men, there is a desire for some material gain on the part of the patient. As an example, a man may have these attacks if he thinks in his subconscious mind that they will keep him from being drafted into the army.

The anxiety state syndrome usually has its onset after the age of eighteen and very seldom begins after the age of forty, although there may be exceptions to these age limits. It is found most often in women; almost twice as many women as men are said to exhibit these symptoms.

The attacks may occur at any time of day or night. A person may awaken from a sound sleep with a feeling of anxiety and doctors say that many night calls are made by them because of this condition. These cases are often misdiagnosed, and are seen most often during a war.

In the so-called neurocirculatory asthenia, which has been called a nervous heart or effort syndrome, there is usually excessive fatigability, the patient becomes tired when he tries to work, he cannot participate in games, usually cannot swim, becomes short of breath when he tries to run. These symptoms may constitute a chronic lifelong illness. In other cases the attacks may be of short duration, lasting five or ten minutes with apparently complete recovery.

There are more signs and symptoms in the anxiety syndrome than in most any other condition, and only the ones most frequently seen will be mentioned here. There is usually a feeling of fear or apprehension, nervousness, palpitation, and shortness of breath. These are the most frequently encountered symptoms.

Next on the list are fatigue on effort, headache, chest pain, trembling, dizziness, and sweating. Others are loss of appetite, sighing respirations, strange feelings such as tingling of the hands or feet. These are called paresthesias.

Tightness of the throat and difficulty in swallowing are symptoms of the so-called "globus hystericus."

Many other symptoms could be listed but the above are the most commonly seen. The physical examination very rarely reveals any actual disease.

The acute anxiety attack usually occurs in a given person under almost exactly the same conditions. In other words, a peculiar set of conditions may bring on an attack, such as riding in a car, being closed in a small room, seeing an exciting scene in a movie, going through a tunnel, or riding in an elevator. These acute attacks may last only five or ten minutes and the patient may feel well afterwards except for a feeling of being tired out and worrying about the attack.

Treatment

The treatment of this condition will vary with the type and severity of the attack. In every case a thorough medical examination with laboratory tests should be carried out to rule out any physical disease. The pa-

tient should be told that he has a nervous condition which is very real and he should avoid the circumstances which bring on the attacks. Often the use of sedatives or tranquilizers for a short period of time is effective and in some cases when the patient realizes just which subconscious drives or thoughts are responsible for the attacks he will be relieved.

In every case, the thoughtful and sincere help of a doctor is advisable.

GLOSSARY

Compulsive caused by an irresistible desire
Disorganize any change in organization
Dissociation split off from the conscious
Environment external surroundings
Fatigability showing fatigue
Flatulence the effect of gases in the alimentary tract
Fugue removal from consciousness; flight
Function normal action of an organ
Globus hystericus sensation of having a lumb in the throat
Hyperventilation overbreathing
Imbalance lack of balance
Immature not fully developed
Inferiority below standard
Inhibition restraint effected by nervous influence
Interaction between mind and body
Maladjustment defective acceptance to environment
Neurosis nervous disease
Palpitation rapid action of the heart which is felt by the patient
Paresthesia an abnormal prickling sensation of the skin
Phobia dread or fear
Psychiatrist an expert in mental disease
Subconscious unconscious
Symptoms evidence of disease
Syndrome a set of symptoms
Tremor trembling or quiver

BRAINWASHING

Most all of us have heard of brainwashing—a term which is used to describe the treatment which was given to our soldiers who were captured by the communists during the Korean War. The term "brainwashing" is not a good one for it would be hard to properly define it.

When we heard that some of our boys had been overcome by continuous preachings of all the good points of communism, which they heard day after day and sometimes night after night, we were shocked. We could not believe that anyone could be persuaded that our way of life—"The American Way"—was inferior to any other way. But some of these boys were persuaded, went over to the other side, and became communist or Red.

The people at home at first could not understand how it was possible for such a thing to have happened; and many of us tried to find a cause. It has been suggested, and I believe with a great deal of truth, that these boys were talked into accepting communism because they did not have any answers to some of the questions that were asked them. This was because they did not know what they were fighting for—what the American way of life really is.

In my opinion, the most important and the least known document in the United States is the Bill of Rights—the first ten amendments to the Constitution of the United States. I believe that if these boys had read and memorized the Bill of Rights, they would have known the answers to the brainwashing which they received. Knowing these answers, they probably would never have allowed their captors to persuade them to join the side of the communists.

How many of us know what this Bill of Rights guarantees us? It is with a feeling that we would all be happier, healthier, and better citizens if we studied the Bill of Rights, that I have included a copy of these amendments in this book on health.

THE BILL OF RIGHTS

First Ten Amendments to the Constitution of the United States

Article I

Congress shall make no law respecting an establishment of religion, or prohibiting the free exercise thereof; or abridging the freedom of speech, or of the press; or of the right of the people peaceably to assemble, and to petition the government for a redress of grievances.

Article II

A well regulated militia, being necessary to the security of a free State, the right of the people to keep and bear arms shall not be infringed.

Article III

No soldier shall, in time of peace, be quartered in any house, without the consent of the owner, nor in time of war, but in a manner to be prescribed by law.

Article IV

The right of the people to be secure in their persons, houses, papers, and effects, against unreasonable searches and seizures, shall not be violated, and no warrants shall issue, but upon probable cause, supported by oath or affirmation, and particularly describing the place to be searched, and the persons or things to be seized.

Article V

No person shall be held to answer for a capital or otherwise infamous crime, unless on a presentment or indictment of a grand jury, except in cases arising in the land or naval forces, or in the militia, when in actual service in time of war or public danger; nor shall any person be subject for the same offense to be twice put in jeopardy of life or limb; nor shall be compelled in any criminal case to be a witness against himself, nor be deprived of life, liberty, or property, without due process of law; nor shall private property be taken for public use, without just compensation.

Article VI

In all criminal prosecutions the accused shall enjoy the right to a speedy and public trial, by an impartial jury of the State and district wherein the crime shall have been committed, which district shall have been previously ascertained by law, and to be informed of the nature and cause of the accusation; to be confronted with the witnesses against him; to have compulsory process for obtaining witnesses in his favor, and to have the assistance of counsel for his defense.

Article VII

In suits at common law, where the value in controversy shall exceed twenty dollars, the right of trial by jury shall be preserved, and no fact tried by a jury shall be otherwise re-examined in any court of the United States, than according to the rules of the common law.

Article VIII

Excessive bail shall not be required, nor excessive fines imposed, nor cruel and unusual punishments inflicted.

Article IX

The enumeration in the Constitution of certain rights shall not be construed to deny or disparage others retained by the people.

Article X

The powers not delegated to the United States by the Constitution, nor prohibited by it to the States, are reserved to the States respectively, or to the people.

It is hoped that we will all read, study, and understand these articles, and teach them to our children.

Chapter 32

Psychosis or Insanity

THE CAUSES of insanity or psychosis are many, and they are not fully understood. When a person is no longer able to adapt himself to other people and has serious and persistent faults in judgment, he becomes a danger to himself and to other people. This person is then said to suffer from a psychosis or insanity.

Cause and Nature

Because the insane person presents a danger to society and to himself, most states have laws permitting these persons to be committed to mental hospitals in order to treat them and to protect the patient as well as society.

It has been estimated that there are more patients in mental hospitals in the United States than there are beds in all other types of hospitals put together, and it has also been estimated that about one out of twenty people may suffer from a psychosis at some time during their lives. A common misunderstanding which should be cleared up is that once a patient is sent to a mental hospital he is incurable. This is not true, for about seventy percent of these people can

be successfully treated and returned to their homes. Some of these patients may need treatment for only a few weeks or months and about half of the patients admitted to large mental hospitals are sent back to their communities as cured after one year of treatment.

One of the differences between a neurosis or psychoneurosis and psychosis or insanity is that the person with a neurosis is considered legally sane, while a person with a psychosis does not know right from wrong, and is legally insane.

Signs and Symptoms

One of the outstanding symptoms in a psychosis is the presence of delusions and hallucinations, which are not present in a neurosis. A delusion is a false belief which cannot be corrected by reason. For example, a delusion of grandeur is an insane conviction that a person possesses great power or wealth when this is not so at all.

Hallucination means a sensory perception which is not based on fact. For instance, a visual hallucination would mean seeing "pink elephants" or seeing people

447

who are not really there. An auditory hallucination consists of hearing voices which do not exist.

The most commonly seen types of insanity will be discussed briefly in this chapter considering the outstanding features of each type.

SCHIZOPHRENIA

(Dementia Praecox)

About one fourth of the patients admitted to the mental hospitals are suffering from this form of insanity. It occurs most frequently in younger people and has a tendency toward gradual mental deterioration rather than recovery as seen in other types.

SIMPLE SCHIZOPHRENIA

The simplest form of this condition is seen in the cold, withdrawn type of person who does not react to advances made by his friends and family. He is said to be odd. These people usually do not have delusions and they are not as a rule dangerous, although they are frequently antisocial and may become involved with the law because of vagrancy. They are sometimes considered poor citizens although their real trouble is a mental disease called simple schizophrenia. It is possible for simple schizophrenia to develop into the serious form.

SERIOUS SCHIZOPHRENIA

The more serious forms of schizophrenia do not offer a very favorable outlook for improvement under treatment. These people can be recognized easily by anyone and they fall roughly into three main types.

1. Catatonic Schizophrenia

This type is tense and stiff. They may sit for hours in one position without moving, or if moved by someone else, they may hold the same position in which they have been left for a long time. These patients pay no attention to things that are going on around them. They may suffer from hallucinations which are usually auditory. These hallucinations may take the form of hearing someone say he is going to attack the patient. The catatonic patients may become suddenly violent and they may be very destructive in these wild outbursts.

2. Hebephrenic Schizophrenia

These patients may appear to be very silly and childish. They will giggle and carry on crazy conversations with themselves. These conversations may have no relation to reality, and often these patients will break out in a cold laugh which does not have any element of humor in it. At times they may be dangerous, attacking some nearby person without any apparent cause.

3. Paranoid Schizophrenia

This type of mental illness is not always as easy to detect as the other types. These patients may appear normal at times and they are not entirely out of touch with reality. They do suffer from delusions and hallucinations. They often appear to be frightened because people are always threatening to do them great harm. They have delusions of grandeur and imagine that they occupy a very important position in some wonderful undertaking. Their hallucinations may be directed toward some particular person who they think is persecuting them and this feeling of being picked on or persecuted may lead these people to commit murder. They are liable to commit suicide and so may be considered dangerous to themselves and others.

The various types of mental illness do not often appear in the pure form and often one type may have characteristics of one of the other types. The main thing to remember is that if a person shows that he is out of touch with reality and is suffering from delusions and hallucinations, he may be a danger to himself and to others. This person should be treated by a psychiatrist and preferably in a mental hospital.

MANIC-DEPRESSIVE PSYCHOSIS

The other large group of people with psychosis or insanity can be called the manic-depressive type. This form of insanity is characterized by alternating periods of mania, in which the person feels fine. He is very active, does not need much sleep, and can think very rapidly. This manic phase may change rapidly and the patient will suddenly become surly and suspicious. He may suffer from delusions and hallucinations.

The depressive stage of manic-depressive psychosis sees the patient suddenly becoming very gloomy, depressed, and downhearted. He may be very restless and walk the floor wringing his hands. These patients become very sensitive to the opinions of other people, especially to the people they love. In the depressive stage of manic-depressive psychosis, suicide is very common and constitutes a grave threat because

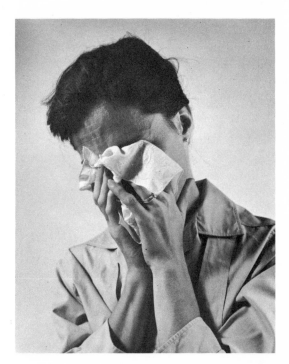

In manic-depressive psychosis the patient often crys for no apparent reason, later the same day be happy and active.

this is the type of person who commits suicide.

Manic-depressive psychosis may suddenly clear up, only to have the patient go into another spell in a short time.

ACUTE TOXIC PSYCHOSIS

There are many other forms of psychosis less frequently seen than the two major groups which have been described. One form is seen in toxic states or major illness with a high fever. This form is called delirium and is of short duration. Most people have seen others who were said to be out of their head with a high fever. After the illness is over the patient recovers with no after effects as far as the mind is concerned.

CHRONIC ORGANIC PSYCHOSIS

This form of insanity may follow infection with syphilis which has attacked the brain. It has been called general paresis or "softening of the brain." Other diseases which cause psychosis in some cases are encephalitis, multiple sclerosis, Huntington's chorea, and brain tumor. These conditions do not always cause psychosis.

TRAUMATIC PSYCHOSIS

(Psychosis Caused by Injury)

This form of delirium may follow a severe head injury. Most of us have seen a person who has been knocked out by a head injury. He doesn't remember where he is or how he got there.

Sometimes a patient will receive a severe head injury and will not go into delirium or be knocked out. He may suddenly change in character, become forgetful, untidy, antagonistic, and easily fatigued. This sudden change in personality should make one suspicious of post-traumatic psychosis and a doctor should be consulted.

SENILE PSYCHOSIS

This is sometimes called senile dementia and is often seen in older people. They become forgetful, childlike, untidy, suspicious, and at times, highly agitated or confused. The only thing that can be done for this type of person is to try to relieve the symptoms and to protect him from himself by careful supervision. Now that our general population is living to an older age more of these cases are seen.

ARTERIOSCLEROTIC PSYCHOSIS

This form of psychosis is caused by hardening of the arteries in the brain and a resulting decrease in blood supply to the brain tissue. It usually comes in the age group younger than that which is classified as senile. This type of insanity or psychosis is far more common than generally believed. Some doctors think that arteriosclerotic psychosis may account for about twenty percent of all psychoses.

Arteriosclerosis may cause a psychosis in persons between fifty and sixty-five if they suffer from severe arteriosclerosis. They are not violent nor do they constitute a danger to themselves or others, but they do show an alteration of personality. The habits may change; they become forgetful, suspicious, and irritable. These people may gradually begin to show an inability to concentrate and gradually become less and less mentally efficient.

Some of the tranquilizing drugs such as Sparine often will help to curb the restlessness and insomnia in these patients.

ALCOHOLIC PSYCHOSIS

(Korsakoff's Syndrome)

About ten percent of the patients treated in mental hospitals may be there because of the unwise use of alcohol. It is not known whether the alcohol itself causes the condition or whether because of the prolonged over-use of alcohol the patient deprives himself of food and vitamins, causing his brain to deteriorate.

The acute case of alcoholic psychosis is called delirium tremens. This is characterized by hallucinations, seeing "pink elephants" or other animals, extreme restlessness, a coarse tremor, and marked agitation. Many patients, if untreated, die in this stage of the disease.

Korsakoff's syndrome or chronic psychosis may follow a prolonged case of delirium tremens. The patient may suffer from lasting brain damage which shows itself in loss of memory (amnesia), dirorientation, and general loss of mental powers. The patients in this category, after it has lasted for some time, have very little chance of improvement under treatment. These symptoms may be improved by the use of sedatives and large doses of vitamin B_1 or thiamine chloride.

FEEBLE-MINDEDNESS

(Mental Deficiency)

There are some unfortunate people who are born with defects in their brain or with very little brain. These people are called by various terms according to the type of brain deficiency which they exhibit. They are called morons, imbeciles, or idiots and there is very little that can be done for them. People who suffer from mongolism, cretinism and microcephaly (undeveloped brain) are classified as idiots.

It has now become possible in many cases to predict when an expected baby is going to be mongoloid, or mentally deficient. This condition which has many names, one of which "Downs Syndrome," is one that may have a hereditary inclination.

If suspected, some of the amniotic fluid (the fluid that surrounds the fetus or growing baby in the mother's uterus) can be withdrawn early in the pregnancy and a study of the chromosomes will indicate whether or not the child may be affected with mongolism.

Although laws regarding abortion have not been brought up to date, it is possible that in the future we may be able to perform an early abortion to prevent the birth of a child with this serious condition.

Treatment

The treatment of psychosis should be in the hands of a competent psychiatrist and preferably in a mental hospital. As has been stated above, many of these people (about fifty percent) in certain types of mental illness can be helped or cured. In the meanwhile, they are in the hospital and cannot damage themselves or others.

Doctors use various forms of treatment; one of the most effective is called shock treatment, in which a heavy electric shock is passed through the patient. Several shock treatments will often cause enough improvement to allow the patient to return home.

Psychotherapy (treatment of the mind), as in psychoanalysis, is often used, and the tranquilizing drugs such as Compazine, Thorazine and Sparine are often used. There are hundreds of drugs on the market now which may be used by psychiatrists in the treatment of mental disorders. These have become too numerous to be named in detail, but the doctor or psychiatrist now has a wide variety of drugs from which to choose. His choice will naturally depend upon the condition he is treating and the response of a given patient to a certain drug. At times a combination of drugs will be successful.

In summing up, when a patient becomes disoriented and out of touch with reality, he may be a danger to himself and others and he should be hospitalized for treatment.

One other word of warning: a patient who is severely depressed is in danger of committing suicide. In the manic-depressive psychosis this depression is easily recognized. On the other hand, the patient who is suffering from schizophrenia may not show symptoms of depression, yet he may be just as likely to commit suicide. These people should be watched carefully and be treated by a good psychiatrist.

The tendency now is to try and treat as many of these people as possible in the local community. There have been formed many local mental health clinics, staffed basically by three types of people. These are a psychiatrist, a clinical psychologist, and a psychiatric social worker. In this way the pressure can be taken off mental hospitals, which are overcrowded.

GLOSSARY

Auditory   pertaining to hearing
Compulsion   an irresistible impulse
Deteriorate   to become worse
Disorientation   the loss of bearing; mental confusion
Mania   insanity
Phobia   dread or fear
Psychoanalysis   method of learning nervous and mental symptoms
Society   companionship or association with people
Suppressed   kept to oneself
Syndrome   set of symptoms
Toxic   pertaining to poison
Vagrancy   wandering about; waywardness

PART 7

Newer Drugs and Techniques

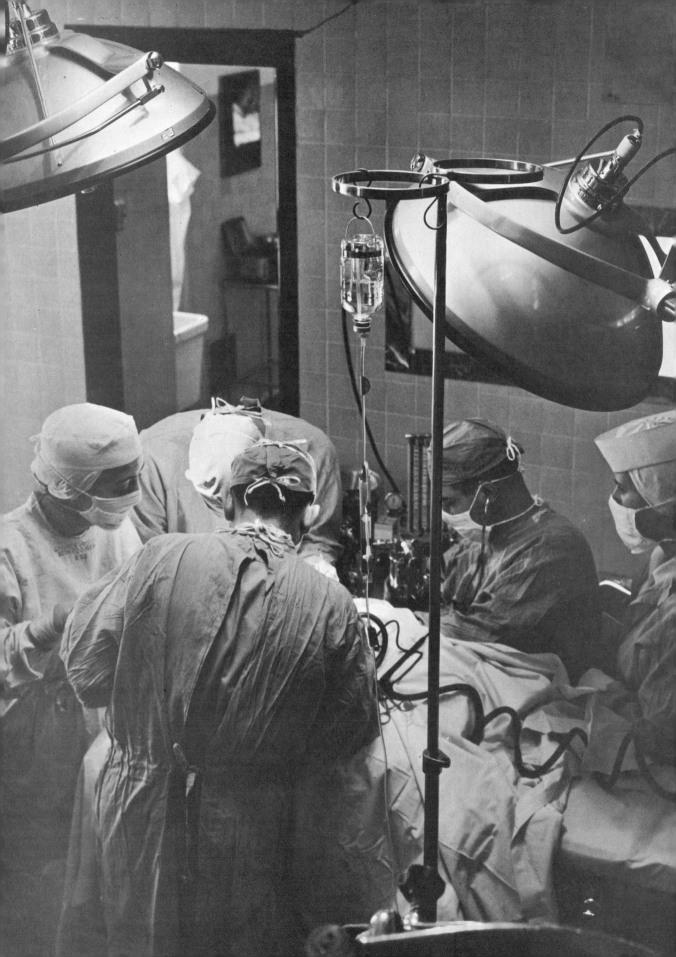

Chapter 33

Some of the Newer Drugs

DURING THE PAST twenty years enormous strides have been made by the drug companies in placing on the market new remedies. Some of these are very fine and indeed have been called "miracle drugs"; others are not so good and many are worthless.

The drug companies are spending millions of dollars every year in an effort to produce new remedies and also to improve upon the remedies already known. In many cases, the government contributes millions of dollars to drug companies in order to assist them in their search for new drugs. This cause is also helped by contributions from the estates of wealthy persons who contribute money for research in drugs.

This ever-increasing flood of new drugs constitutes one of the greatest challenges which confront the medical profession today. Each doctor must be sure that he is prescribing for his patient the most useful drug and at the same time he must be very careful not to use harmful or useless drugs. The cost of these new products is often great, and it becomes the doctor's duty to obtain the best drug at the most reasonable price for his patient.

Many of the more powerful and more useful new drugs produce side effects which may be dangerous as well as disagreeable. These must be watched closely by the doctor.

When we speak of side effects we mean results produced by the drug which are not the result for which the drug was given. Some of these may be drowsiness, fatigue, gastric irritations, nausea, headache, emotional depressions, skin rashes, restlessness, and anxiety.

Fortunately the Federal Government keeps a very close watch on new products which are placed on the market, and through its Food and Drug Laws can protect the public or the consumer of the drug.

There is not the slightest doubt that a great deal of suffering is being done away with, and that diseases such as the acute infections are being rapidly cured by the proper use of these new agents. This is one of the main reasons why the span of life has been lengthened in recent years, and all of us can expect to live longer than we would have many years ago before the new drugs were discovered.

Some of these drugs may be described by speaking of them in groups, such as the tranquilizers, the antibiotics or antibacterial drugs (these are the so-called wonder drugs), and the steroids. There are many other smaller classes of new drugs which will not be described at this time, and the reader must realize that this is a constantly changing picture; in other words, the drugs which are popular now may not be in favor several years hence.

For many years the barbiturates have been used as hypnotics, that is, to relieve tension states, reduce anxiety, and help produce sleep. Because of the fact that these barbiturates, such as phenobarbital, seconal, etc., may become habit forming and a person could become addicted to them, they have been used with extreme caution by both physicians and patients. In recent years a great many non-barbiturate drugs have been introduced to be used as sedatives and hypnotics; these have been called tranquilizing drugs. They have become very popular, and the number of prescriptions written for these drugs is second only to the number written by doctors for the antibiotic or antibacterial (miracle) drugs.

The drugs do alleviate tension states, anxiety states, and nervousness. It has been felt by most doctors, especially the psychiatrists, that the use of tranquilizers has been overdone. They state that a certain amount of tension is good for a person—that it helps develop strength of character and purposefulness. So the use of a crutch or some drug to lessen the normal tensions only weakens a person. This is probably true, and the tranquilizers should be used sparingly and only when there is real need for them.

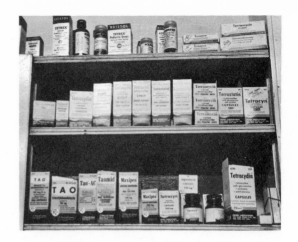

It would be difficult to give a list of all the tranquilizing drugs, but a partial list of some of them is given below with the action which they produce. (all trade names.)

1. Psychotherapeutic antihistamine—example: Atarax
2. Central muscle relaxants (non-sedative)—example: Avosyl, Dioloxol, Mephenesin, Mephson, Myoten, Myoxane, Oranixon, Prolax, Saseral, Sinan, Tysosmolyn, Tolonsin, Tolaolosate, Tolserol, Tolseram
3. Central muscle relaxants (Skeletal muscle relaxants) sedative—example: Equanil, Miltown, Ultron, Demithylone
4. Central parasympathetic suppressants—example: Suavitil
5. Central sympathetic suppressants—example: Thorazine, Pacatal, Trilafon, Compaxine, Sparine
6. Central sympathetic suppressants—rauwolfia derivatives—example: Rauwiloid, Raudixin, Hormonyl, Reserpine

The above examples are just a few of the tranquilizers in use now; when properly used they can be of great benefit in lowering high blood pressure, and can be very valuable in treating mild cases of mental illness. However, they should be used intelligently and with caution.

Because trade name drugs at times tend to be more expensive than the same drug when called by its generic, or scientific name, there have been efforts to request doctors to use the generic name when writing the prescription. Since some of these generic names are so long and complicated the doctors get into a habit of using the shorter or trade name. Example of this is Equanil—trade name, Meprobamate, trade name; tigan—generic name, trimethobenzamide, HCL.

GLOSSARY

Antibacterial destroying the reproduction of bacteria

Antibiotic a chemical substance to destroy bacteria

Barbiturate a quieting drug

Tranquilizer drug having a quieting effect

THYROXIN

Thyroid preparations which have been used for many years have been studied and new products have been manufactured, which because of the changes in their chemical structure, can be used in cases where certain effects of thyroxin are thought to be harmful, or to accentuate other desirable effects. Thus the thyroid hormone—thyroxin—has been changed so as to make it into a very useful drug. This has been done in some cases by taking out the portion of the drug which stimulates the heart and using the part which helps patients who have thyroid deficiency—so-called myxedema. Some of these products are used to treat patients with goiter.

A few of these products will be named here, but no attempt will be made to include all of them. Some of the better ones are called Tetrac, Diac and TF₄. These are the trade names.

MIRACLE DRUGS

Perhaps the greatest development in drugs during the last few years has been the production of the antibiotics or antibacterial drugs which have been of untold value in the treatment of infectious diseases. The first of these were the sulfa drugs which did a great deal toward curing acute infections. These were soon overshadowed by the introduction of penicillin, which is apparently far more effective and less dangerous to use. Then came a veritable flood of new and powerful antibiotics: chloramycetin, erythrocin, terramycin, albamycin, achromycin, auriomycin, bacitracin, cathomycin, streptomycin, dihydrostreptomycin, ilotycin, ilosone, mysteclin, neomycin, panmycin, signemycin, cosa-signemycin. These are just a few of the new drugs, and more are coming out every week. Some of them are synthesized—that is, made artificially, but most of them are derived from molds found in the earth. The various drug companies each come out with their particular brand, and each tries to outdo the other by placing on the market a better product. This is good because it gives the doctor better tools to work with, and the patients a better chance to get well.

There are certain drawbacks to the use of these drugs. One is that the bacteria which have been killed easily by, say, penicillin, may develop a tolerance to penicillin and soon a strong tough strain of bacteria may become entirely resistant to penicillin and not be affected by it. For this reason, these powerful drugs should not be used indiscriminately. That is, a person should not take penicillin for every little cold he gets, for as a matter of fact, we do not know what causes colds and penicillin does not cure a cold. The patient should not insist upon getting a shot of penicillin for a cold and the doctor should refuse to give it, for at some later date this patient may have a serious infection which *can* be cured by penicillin, and he will take it then with the assurance that it may do some good. One of the side effects of penicillin is an allergic reaction characterized by a swelling of the tissues, itching, etc. This may be dangerous, and should be treated at once. Injections of ACTH or cortisone will usually cause this so-called penicillin reaction to subside. For the above reasons, the antibiotics or miracle drugs should be used with caution.

Some of the antibiotics are better in certain types of infections, and others may prove more efficient in a different infection. For instance, penicillin is very good against streptococcus infections and against gonorrhea and syphilis.

The so-called broad spectrum antibiotics such as ilosone, may be effective against a great variety of bacteria, and for this reason many doctors make what they call a sensitivity test—that is, they grow the bacteria which they are treating, and test it with different antibiotics to see which one will be the most effective against this particular infection.

Tuberculosis has been treated very successfully with a combination of streptomycin or dihydrostreptomycin, para-amino salicylate, called P.A.S., and isoniazid. The combination of these three drugs has really had a miraculous effect in curing or arresting pulmonary tuberculosis

Here again, care should be taken to use the drugs cautiously, for streptomycin and dihydrostreptomycin may cause irreversible deafness, or a disturbance of the organs of equilibrium.

In one type of case it is excusable to use the antibiotics quickly and in adequate doses; that is, in a very sick child, who has a high fever and is toxic. Children can become worse so rapidly that it is good judgment to treat them at once, rather than to wait until the kind of organism can be determined. One of the broad spectrum antibiotics should be used.

To illustrate how rapidly these new antibiotics are being developed, at a recent antibiotic symposium three hundred new studies were submitted for review, and among the new antibiotics reported were colistin, aspartain, fervenulin, paramycin, streptozotocin, refomycin B and potassium penicillin.

Let us be thankful that the drug companies are so energetic in getting new products on the market, and never lose sight of the fact that these are powerful weapons with which to fight disease; therefore, we should treat them with respect and use them with discrimination.

The broad spectrum antibiotics have not been very successful when used against infections caused by a virus. We now have a drug called Interferon. High hopes are held out for this drug, but it has not been proven yet.

Too much attention cannot be directed toward the fact that these powerful new drugs may have extremely dangerous side effects and must be used under the supervision of the doctor who knows about these side effects.

The Food and Drug Administration has been very careful about protecting the public. For instance, they investigate a drug so thoroughly before it can be placed on the market, that some drugs like Zyloprim, which is used in the prevention of gout, have been used in foreign countries for a year or more before being placed on the market in this country.

Recently Approved Drugs

Some of the newer drugs which have been proven to be effective are listed below.

Tigan—for the control of nausea.

Elase Ointment—Attacks and removes old dead tissue in chronic ulcers while having little effect on living tissue.

The list of stool softeners and mild laxatives is long. It includes *Dialose* and *Dialose Plus; SenoKaps.*

Some people as they grow older do not absorb food as well as younger people do. This may be compensated for by taking one tablet a day of any of a number of good vitamin tablets such as *Gevrestin, Peritinic,* and *Mediatric.*

Some better cough syrups and decongestants include *Phenergan* with codeine, *Tuss Ornade;* and when just a decongestant is needed: *Ornade, Sinutab, Co-Pyronil,* and *Triaminic* capsules are considered good ones.

Asthma sufferers may get relief from *Isuprel* inhalant or *Isuprel* compound elixir (a cough syrup). *Amesec* is another good drug for asthmatics.

Among the diuretics, so-called water pills which make a person urinate more, the old favorites are *Hydrodiuril, Naturetin K, Hygroton, Diupres;* many others are on the market.

One of the newer pills to be taken by mouth by older people with diabetes is called *Tolinase.*

A new wide spectrum antibiotic cream to be used on infections of the skin is *Garamycin,* to be applied locally.

It is to be remembered that all of these medicines may cause damage or undesirable side effects in certain people and the medicines should always be used under the direction of a doctor.

GLOSSARY

Broad spectrum   antibiotics affecting many organisms
Synthetic   made artificially

THE STEROIDS

The development and intelligent use of ACTH and the steroids, cortisone, hydrocortisone, prednisone, etc., has marked a great step forward in the treatment of many diseases. This is especially true in the treatment of skin diseases and the allergic diseases such as asthma.

When these drugs were first developed, it was hoped that cortisone and ACTH would be the answer in the treatment of rheumatoid arthritis; for by administering them the patient seemed to improve almost miraculously. However, it was soon noted that when the drugs were discontinued the disease resumed its previous course, so ACTH and the cortisteroids may be considered as anti-inflammatory agents, used only for symptomic relief and not for curing the disease.

In skin diseases they are widely used with great effectiveness.

It must be remembered though, that the use of these drugs is not entirely without danger; among the side effects which may follow their use are edema or retention of fluids, and a rounding of the face (moon face); peptic ulcers may be activated, and a person with quiescent or arrested pulmonary tuberculosis may be faced with a reactivation of this disease.

Allergic reaction to
Anti-inflammatory counteracting inflammation or infection
Arrested stopped; checked
Edema swelling
Peptic ulcer an ulcer exposed to acid gastric juices
Reactivation restoring activity
Rheumatoid arthritis chronic disease of the joints
Quiescent inactive; still

ENZYMES

The human body is the most complex machine in existence and every minute within these bodies of ours, tiny chemical changes are taking place which cause the body to function. These changes take place without our being conscious of them and they are in a large part performed by enzymes.

An enzyme is a chemical ferment formed by living cells, and this wonderful chemical is found in living things—from a virus to an elephant. Enzymes cause plant leaves to turn green and they also cause a lightning bug or firefly to light up. These complex chemical compounds called enzymes usually work by splitting or transforming other compounds. For instance, when you eat a piece of beef steak or cow's muscle, the enzymes in your body change the steak into amino acids which are then used by your body to build human muscle. These changes are performed in a relatively short time in your body and they are going on all the time. To show how quickly enzymes in the body work, this example may be used. If a piece of beef steak was boiled in acid in a

laboratory it would have to be boiled at a high temperature all day long to digest it or break it down into the amino acids. These changes take place in your body in just a few hours and at body temperature.

If you did not have enzymes in your digestive juices, you could eat all the time but still starve to death because the food cannot be used by the body until it is digested or broken down by enzymes.

Another of the million functions enzymes perform is to protect the body from poisonous material. For instance, in digesting two lamb chops, enough ammonia is liberated to kill the person who ate the lamb chops if the enzymes did not break the ammonia down into a harmless and useful product. This is all done very quickly.

If it were not for one certain enzyme there would be no human beings. The sperm of the male could not penetrate the ovum or egg of the female if there was not a minute amount of enzyme on the tip of the sperm which dissolves the shell or outer membrane of the egg, thereby allowing the sperm to enter the egg and fertilize it. This is called conception and is the beginning of human life. There are enzymes which cause blood to clot and other enzymes which prevent it from clotting.

The enzyme is such a complicated molecule that research chemists have not been able to reproduce it in the laboratory. However, millions of dollars and millions of man hours are being used every year trying to solve the mystery of these compounds and to reproduce them. Many research workers feel that the secret to all health problems could be solved if we knew how to use these enzymes and could manufacture them. They feel that even cancer could be cured by using the proper enzymes.

To give an example of how enzymes may be used, the following may be cited. A woman died of pneumonia and the doctors found that her blood would not clot. They found that she was heavily infected with a certain kind of streptococcus which produced an enzyme which prevents the clotting of blood. They grew these bacteria and obtained some of this enzyme. So after many years one of the large drug companies is putting out a medicine which contains this enzyme and doctors use it to clean up pus and blood from old infected wounds and to help them heal more rapidly. This medicine is known as Varidase and is now being widely used by doctors.

The discovery of this enzyme which breaks up blood clots may have an important bearing on the future of medicine. The research chemists working for a large drug firm are trying to find a form of this enzyme which can be used to break up the clots found in coronary thrombosis. If they succeed, many people who now die of heart attacks may be saved.

High blood pressure is another condition which could be helped if the proper enzymes could be found to destroy the pressor substances in the blood which cause the blood vessels to contract and thus the blood pressure to go up.

Since all the cells of our body are dependent upon enzymes to keep them alive and healthy, it stands to reason that cancer cells are also dependent upon some enzyme. If this enzyme can be identified so that a way of destroying it in the body could be found, then cancer could be cured.

Examples of diseases caused by enzyme disturbances in the body are numerous. There are at least forty-four diseases which are thought to be caused by some disturbance in enzyme formation, and when the research chemists and doctors arrive at a method of reproducing enzymes, most of these diseases can be prevented.

All of these possibilities give us a very exciting and encouraging hope for the future. We hope that the research men will have enough money and will spend enough time on the study of enzymes to solve these problems.

At the present time there are at least six hundred and fifty enzymes which we know about, and research chemists think that there are many more which have not been discovered. No one knows how many cells are in the human body, but it must run into the trillions. It has been estimated that in each one of these tiny cells there are over one hundred thousand enzyme molecules busily at work. These enzymes are performing chemical changes and they have been called nature's chemists.

As soon as a piece of food enters the mouth the digestive enzymes start to work. For instance, those enzymes that change starch into sugar start to work on a piece of bread when it is touched by saliva. You can prove this by holding a piece of bread in your mouth after chewing it and you will notice that it begins to taste sweet after a while. These enzymes which change starch into sugar are called amylolytic enzymes and are known as amylopsin, ptyalin and malt diastase.

To give a partial list of known enzymes may be of interest. A bacterial enzyme is secreted by bacteria as in the case of streptokinase. An enzyme which helps to cause blood to clot is called coagulase. An enzyme which converts soluble proteins into insoluble forms is known as rennin and fibrinferment. An example of this is the gelling of gelatin or the curdling of milk which has been in the stomach.

Some of the enzymes split sugars up into simple forms, one of which is known as invertin. Enzymes which split up fats are known as lipolytic enzymes, and there are several of these, one of which is called steapsin. Oxidase is the enzyme which causes oxidation in the body. Enzymes which split up proteins are called proteolytic. Some of these are pepsin, trypsin, and papain enzyme.

Only a few of the digestive enzymes have been named above. There are many others with other duties, but space does not permit naming them all.

The drug companies have placed on the market hundreds of enzyme products and there is no doubt that as the secret of these chemical agents becomes known, more and .more products will become available.

To name a few of the drugs which have enzymes as their principal ingredients we now can buy in drug stores: Alidase, Analeptone, Chymar, Caroid & Bile Salts, Pancreatin, Pepsolac, Typsogen. There are hundreds of these preparations on the market now and some of them are very effective in certain diseases. But the great discoveries in the use of enzymes in medicine are in the future, and we all should look forward to the day when these wonderful chemical agents are put to work fighting disease.

Recently enzymes other than digestive ones have been put on the market. One has been proven to reduce inflammation and pain. It is called Buclamose and is put out by the Rystan Drug Company. When taken early after a sprain or bruise of the muscles and tendons it will hasten recovery by reducing inflammation. The chemical name for this substance is alpha-amylase and it is taken by mouth. Avazyme is the trade name for another anti-inflammatory enzyme that can be taken by mouth. Synthetic enzyme pills for the control of appetite are sold under the names Preludin and Wilpom.

GLOSSARY

Bacteria germs
Coronary thrombosis heart attack
Inflammation condition characterized by pain, heat, redness, and/or swelling
Saliva secretion in mouth
Sperm seed
Streptococcus germ causing disease

NEWER VACCINES

Progressive Vaccinia

Progressive vaccinia is a rare complication which sometimes occurs in children vaccinated against smallpox. The vaccination spreads over the body. A product called "vaccinia immune gamma globulin" will hold the process of spread. This substance is furnished by the American Red Cross.

Rabies Vaccine

A weakened rabies virus has been raised on chicken or duck embryo. This live-virus vaccine is used successfully in treating people who have been bitten by a rabid animal such as a mad dog. The larger the bite and the nearer it is to the head, the more important it is to get the vaccine started soon. Persons who are sensitive to eggs should be given antihistamines along with the vaccine. The early use of anti-rabies treatment is a life-saving measure.

Influenza Vaccine

The viruses which cause influenza have been studied extensively and a vaccine has been developed which, in cases of influenza epidemics, has been known to save many lives.

The influenza virus is known to exist in several strains or types. These are known as Type A, B, C, and D. The epidemics of the past have been caused by Types A, A₁ and A₂ and by Type B. The vaccines used are grown on chicken embryos and the virus is killed before it is used in a vaccine. As a rule polyvalent vaccine (one which contains some of all the types named above) is used. One cc. of the vaccine is injected under the skin and this is followed by another cc. about one or two months later. This gives protection for about one year. The vaccine is usually started about the first of September and is important in older people and people who are suffering from some chronic disease such as heart disease.

Mumps Vaccine

The development of a vaccine against mumps has been unsatisfactory. Such a vaccine has been developed by growing the mumps virus on chicken embryos, but it is not generally used. The protection afforded lasts for only a short period (about six months) and after a person has been exposed the vaccine does not do much good. Therefore, vaccination against mumps is not a routine procedure but is saved to be used in the case of very sick or weak people who are susceptible. These people may be protected for six months in the case of an epidemic. The use of this vaccine in healthy adults and children is not advocated.

Poliomyelitis Vaccines

The Salk vaccine is very seldom used now because of the proven worth of the oral vaccine.

THE ORAL (*Sabin*) VACCINE. Oral vaccine against poliomyelitis as developed by Sabin is now being manufactured and used extensively in this country. As there are three different types of viruses which cause polio, Type I, Type II, and Type III, an oral vaccine has been developed against each one of these types. This oral vaccine consists of a live virus which has been greatly weakened and the person who takes the drops of vaccine actually contracts a mild case of poliomyelitis which gives him immunization against future attacks of polio. Drops representing all three types should be taken because immunization against one type does not protect against the others. It has been proven that when one person in a family takes the oral vaccine all the other

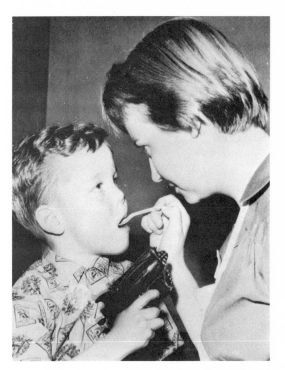

This youngster is taking his first dose of oral Sabin vaccine which will give him immunization against future attacks of polio.

members of his family may catch polio from him and thereby become immune in a secondhand way. They will have mild cases and not even know they are sick. It is thought to be advisable for all members of one family to take the oral vaccine pills at the same time in order to prevent the possibility of the virus changing in strength as it passes from one person to another. This type of change has never been actually noted but to prevent it from happening it is better for all members of the family to take the vaccine by mouth.

The question which now arises is should a person who has been taking the Salk vaccine injections every year and is supposedly immune against polio also take the oral vaccine. The Salk vaccine consists of all three types of the killed or dead virus and has proven highly effective. In other words any person who has been fully immunized or has had all of his shots of Salk vaccine and continues to take one shot every year is considered to be ninety-seven percent safe against polio. He does not need to take the oral vaccine if he keeps the shots up. He may do away with the shots in the future years by taking the oral vaccine. So far as we know now the oral vaccine does not need to be repeated. If a person has not been immunized at all a good way to start would be to take three doses of Sabin oral vaccine with an interval of about six weeks between doses. After that it might be well to have an injection of Salk vaccine about once a year when the person is still young. After middle age a booster dose of Salk vaccine should be given every three or four years. There is one exception to this rule. All nursing infants and all infants under six weeks of age should not take the oral vaccine but should be immunized by the Salk injection.

With the intelligent use of the Salk and Sabin vaccine by the people in the United States the dread disease poliomyelitis will soon be wiped out completely.

Measles Vaccine

(Measles — Rubeola or Red Measles)

This is a highly contagious and dangerous disease. A successful vaccine has been developed against this condition and every baby when it reaches the age of nine months should receive this protection.

A live, weakened vaccine is used and three injections at monthly intervals will give lasting protection.

(German Measles — Rubella or the Three Day Measles)

This is a mild disease and no vaccine against it has been developed.

This is the type of measles which sometimes causes defects in babies if the mother has the disease during the first three months of pregnancy. If a pregnant woman is exposed, she should have injections of gamma globulin which may keep her from having the German measles.

GLOSSARY

Chronic   long standing
Embryo   before birth
Injection   forcing in of a liquid
Oral   by mouth
Virus   a living minute organism

Chapter 34

New Techniques in Surgery

THERE HAVE BEEN great advances in the use of ultrasound in surgery. A piece of copper which was in a boy's eye, very close to the retina, was located by using a small ultrasound device and watching the blips on a phosphorescent screen. When the approximate location of the foreign body was located, another small ultrasound device with a pair of small ophthalmic forceps attached was passed through an incision in the pupil. When the blips on the screen showed the small sliver to be close, the forceps were opened and closed, and when they were withdrawn, the piece of metal came with them, thereby saving the vision in that eye for the patient.

Cyrosurgery, or surgery by freezing has been used successfully to freeze small parts in the brain in Parkinson's disease. It has also been used to remove malignancies of the skin. This type of surgery prevents bleeding at the site of the incision.

The laser beam has been used to repair detached retinas in the eye and is also found to be useful in joining small blood vessels together without clamping them and causing hemorrhage.

SURGERY TO CHANGE SEX

There are some unfortunate people who are born with the body of one sex and the mind of another. Since it is impossible to change the mind, doctors for some time have been operating and changing the body of these people.

For years it has been necessary to go to some foreign country to have this operation performed, but now in Baltimore we have a clinic set up in the Johns Hopkins Medical Institution to help these unfortunate individuals. This clinic is called the Gender Identity Clinic and since it is in one of our very best medical schools it can be considered trustworthy.

A person with the body of a boy and the mind of a girl is called a transsexual, and the name also applies to a person with the body of a girl and the mind of a boy. We do not know what causes this condition but we do know that these people in the past have been forced to go through life suffering a great deal of unhappiness. They are not homosexuals and they get only small relief from dressing like a member of the opposite

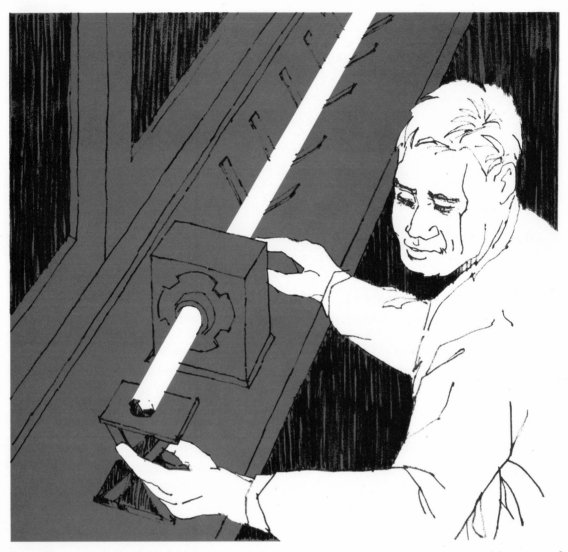

Laser Beam is a powerful light being used often in treating detached retinas, external benign and malignant lesions and birth marks—other uses are predicted.

sex; so the only chance for something that approaches happiness for them lies in surgery. Many of them commit suicide before they can be helped.

No one knows how many of these transsexuals live in the United States, but it is known that the doctors at Johns Hopkins have operated on about ten of these people and they usually have more than a hundred persons on the waiting list.

This clinic accepts only about two applicants a month and the candidates for the operation are carefully screened. They are studied from a psychological standpoint and extensive studies of their metabolic mechanisms are carried out. They must have been on treatment with hormones at least two years and their chromosomes are carefully studied before they are finally accepted for surgery.

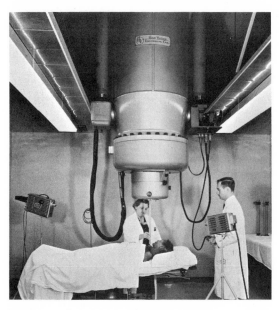

Doctor and woman technician prepares patient for treatment of lung malignancy using the Van de Graff Supra Voltage Unit.

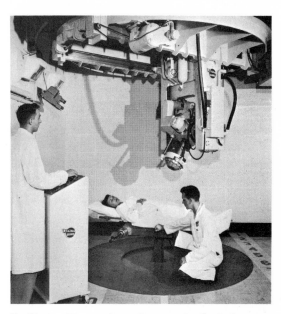

Radiation Beams from Cesium-137 Teletherapy Machine used much like X ray in treating deep-seated malignant tissue.

Briefly this is how the operations are performed. When treating a boy who has the mind of a girl, the penis and testes are amputated. A specialist creates a fossa or cavity about five inches deep between the rectum and the prostate. This cavity has a rubber mold placed in it which stays in place about six months and the resulting cavity acts as a vagina.

The skin of the penis and scrotum are sutured together to form the lining of this cavity and the sensitive skin of the penis permits the person to have more satisfactory sexual relations than an ordinary skin graft would.

With a girl who has the mind of a boy, the uterus and ovaries are removed. The breasts are amputated, but the nipples are sutured back in place.

This type of operation is done in several stages. A penis is constructed from an abdominal graft and this is made to contain a urethra for the passage of urine. A scrotum is constructed from a skin graft from the thigh.

This newly formed penis cannot be used for sexual functions, but it permits the person to urinate while standing up. Psychologically this seems to help.

The male to female patients have to take hormone treatments for the rest of their lives and they have been able to have fairly normal sexual relations. Indeed some of the girls marry, although they cannot have children.

There have been many moral and legal obstacles to this surgery in the United States, but is to be hoped that with success of the Johns Hopkins Clinic these will be removed.

All of the patients operated upon to date have expressed great satisfaction with the results and some of them are extremely grateful.

NEW METHOD TO STOP SEVERE NOSE BLEEDS

Epistaxis is often a very severe condition and a very severe prolonged nose bleed has been known to lead to death.

When the ordinary methods of packing the nose, both anteriorly and posteriorly, are not successful, a new method has been developed, and to date has proven successful.

A small balloon is inserted into the nostril and filled with ninety-five percent alcohol. A hypothermic machine is attached and the temperature of the alcohol is brought down to about seventeen degrees below zero. This temperature is maintained for about six minutes and the cold air flow is turned off. About fifteen minutes later the machine is disconnected and the balloon is slightly deflated, but is left in place for twenty-four hours.

This freezing of the mucous membrane stops the hemorrhage and the patient who receives this treatment seems to have no bad after-effects. No loss of smell or atrophy of the mucous membrane has been noted in patients who have been examined months after the treatment. There is some crusting for about seven days.

This deep freeze method of treating nose bleed was developed in the University of Pittsburg Hospital and it is hoped that its use will be taken up in other hospitals.

PART 8

General Health and Well-being

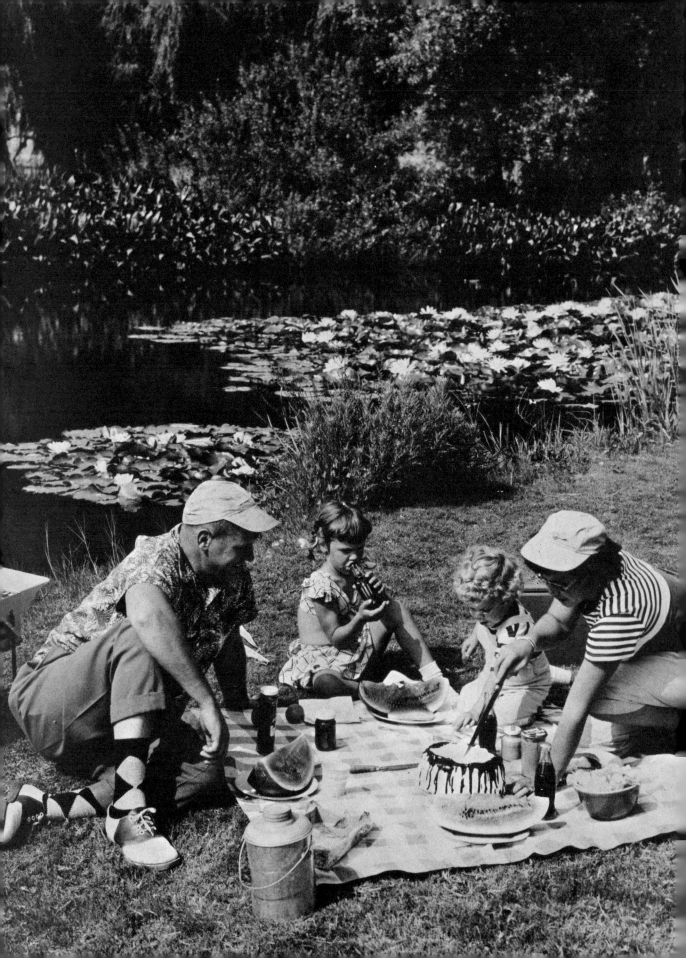

Chapter 35

Hints on Health and Welfare

SUGGESTED CONTENTS FOR A MEDICINE CHEST

The medicine chest, usually located in the bathroom, can be used to great benefit if properly equipped; and it can be misused if the wrong medicines are stored there in an indiscriminate manner.

First of all, the chest should be locked or out of reach of small children, because when the small child begins to climb, he will investigate the chest and may try some of the medicines.

The first shelf could be used for tooth paste or powder, Band-aids, applicators (that is a stick with cotton wrapped around the end), a bottle of some mild antiseptic—merthiolate solution or a stronger one like tincture of merthiolate, to be applied to small abrasions and cuts. The *tincture* of merthiolate has alcohol in it and will burn. The *solution* of merthiolate however, is a clear liquid and does not burn when applied. As a matter of fact, soap and water applied to a fresh cut is just as effective, when it comes to killing germs, so use soap if you have no merthiolate.

The second shelf could have on it a tube of Kip, to be used on mild burns. A small tube of neocortif-opthalmic to be used in mild irritation of the eyes and some mild ointment like zinc oxide ointment for use on mild skin irritations. A roll of one-inch adhesive tape and some sterile flats could be on this shelf, along with a roll of bandage to use, where Band-aids are not large enough.

The third shelf could be used for shaving equipment, deodorants, hair tonic, etc.

The fourth shelf could have various medicines—aspirin for mild headaches or pain, and maybe a few Equanil tablets which have been prescribed by the doctor for insomnia and/or nervousness, and other bottles of medicine which the doctor has prescribed. I think it well to have a few empirin compound tablets with one-half grain codeine (prescribed by a doctor) for use in cases where the pain cannot be controlled with aspirin. They should be used only for severe pain until a doctor can be seen.

The above suggestions are matters of personal preference, and can be arranged in any way the owner of the house sees fit. But always remember to keep the poisons and

471

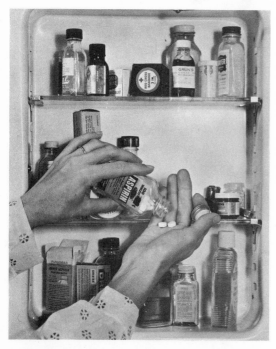

A medicine chest, well organized and maintained will benefit the whole family. Keep medicines out of reach of young children.

medicines safely away from the exploring hands of young children.

GROOMING

When we say that a person is well groomed we mean that he looks well dressed and clean. Although some people just naturally develop the art of looking well groomed others do not and it is so important that children should be instructed by their parents in this phase of living. They should be advised by their teachers as to the mistakes they are making. We feel that this has a certain bearing or influence on the future well being of an individual. A person who dresses well is admired by other people and this gives him a feeling of confidence which helps him in his daily undertakings. When a person is successful in his work he will enjoy better health since he is not handicapped by the frustrations and worries which go with failure or lack of success.

For the above reasons we feel that a short chapter on good grooming should be included in any book which attempts to aid people in enjoying good health.

The most important element in good grooming is cleanliness. A person may be well dressed, and may spend a great deal of money and time in selecting his clothes, but if his body is not clean and the clothes are not kept in good condition he will not be well groomed. A daily bath is important to keep the body clean. Clean hands and well clipped finger nails are important. Dirt under the finger nails should never be permitted. Most grown people need to use a good deodorant, especially under the arms. It is a well-known fact that a person may not be conscious of his own body odor but other people around him will.

The hair should be well cut and properly combed or taken care of. In women this has become a matter of great importance as is proved by the business done in beauty parlors. It is just as important for men to take care of the appearance of their hair.

The shoes should be well shined with heels not run down and the clothes should be kept clean and well pressed.

Care should be taken in the choice of clothes. The color of the tie and suit should blend and not clash. Some men look better in a light-colored suit while others prefer dark clothes. This is a matter of taste but it may be wise when selecting the clothes to consider what the general effect will be rather than to buy clothes of a certain color because you like that color.

Some people are color blind and should have someone else help select their clothes. A man's wife is usually happy to help him select his ties. When a man is not color blind and likes to select his own ties he should do so because he feels better wearing a tie which he has selected himself.

A feeling of confidence which goes with being well groomed will help in maintaining the general health of any person, therefore we feel that instruction in grooming is important and should be emphasized at home and in the schools.

HOW TO CHOOSE A FAMILY DOCTOR

The choice of a family doctor should be made with a great deal of careful thought, and after thorough investigation. In my opinion a family which has obtained the services of a family doctor who suits them and serves them well should be considered a very fortunate family. Certainly with such a doctor their troubles, which go along with sickness such as expense, pain, worry, and loss of time from work, can be greatly reduced.

As a doctor, I am going to tell you how I would go about selecting a family doctor for my own family, and I think you may be helped by taking these points into consideration when selecting a doctor for yourself and your family.

In the first place, the doctor should be well trained, and you can find out quite easily what medical school the doctor graduated from. Most of the medical schools today turn out well-trained people.

I would like to know if the doctor will be available any time I want him. That is, does

he make home calls, and especially does he make night calls; because sometimes at night, during an emergency, you might need the presence of a doctor in your home more than any other time.

If the doctor in question does make house calls, will he be available most of the time, or does he spend a great deal of time out of town, attending conventions, fishing, or hunting?

Do not misunderstand me, for I would prefer to have a doctor who likes to fish and hunt, as long as he doesn't spend most of his time at it; and certainly I would not like to have a doctor take care of my family who does not attend conventions. In that way, he may do some postgraduate study and keep up with the great progress being made in medicine today.

I would like to know who takes the doctor's calls or substitutes for him when he goes out of town. Usually, you will find that the kind of doctor you like and have selected as your family doctor, will use good judgment in choosing someone to take his calls for him when he is out of town.

Now, having determined that the doctor is well trained and available, we come to the most difficult part of the evaluation of our prospective doctor. That is, has he a personality which will cause me and my family to like and trust him. This is very important, because if you trust a doctor and like him he can help you a great deal more than could one in whom you have very little confidence.

In the matter of personalities, we run into complications because the doctor who pleases me, may not please my wife or my son or daughter. However, there are certain fundamental characteristics to look for. The doctor should be kind and gentle, while being firm with his patients. He should be sincere and should show interest in any case upon which he may be called. You will find some doctors who will work very hard on some serious illness, but will show a lack of concern about something which, to the patient, may be very important. He should be truthful, and should go to some pains to explain to the patient just what the condition is for which the patient is being treated. This takes time and patience and, above all, understanding; for instance, a doctor can usually sense that a patient is worried or frightened because he is afraid that the condition which is being treated may be, say, cancer. Then he should take time to reassure the patient that this is not cancer, without the question being asked. That is, if he can truthfully do so.

The doctor should be thorough; this doesn't mean that every time you go to his office he should do a complete examination, but he should have at some time done a complete examination and then on the follow up, or subsequent visits, do enough of an examination to determine the cause for the symptoms which brought the patient to his office.

The question of expense can never be left out of any phase of our lives today, and especially that which pertains to illness. Hospital costs, the costs of drugs, and the doctor's fees are vital, and your ideal family doctor should be glad to talk over these costs with you at any time and at great length. If I were choosing a doctor, I would try to get one who would be careful in prescribing drugs for me, because some drugs are more expensive than others which accomplish the same things, and some illnesses require a longer period in the hospital than others. Your doctor should make every

effort to see that you are spared unnecessary expense. In case of proposed surgery you should talk over carefully with your doctor how much his fee is going to be, and get an estimate of the hospital expenses, including X rays, laboratory fees, and assistants' fees.

If your hospital bill seems too much, be sure to show it to your doctor, for he can easily find out if a mistake has been made. The right kind of a family doctor will be glad to assist you in this way.

Now the last and perhaps the most important characteristic which I would look for in a doctor, is whether or not he is a man of good judgment and common sense. You often read in novels about "the wonderful hands of a surgeon." I would not worry nearly as much about his hands as what he has in his head. In other words, when the surgeon opens an abdomen and finds a very unusual condition which needs correcting, will he have the good judgment to know just how much to do and how much not to do. This applies to all illness (good judgment), and if you are watching for it, you should be able to recognize it in your family doctor.

I realize that all of the above qualifications may be hard to find in one man, but there are many doctors who have all of these and other good points. In choosing a doctor, try to get as many of those qualities as you can, and choose a doctor whom you can consider a friend. And remember that because you have called on a doctor once or twice, does not mean that you must retain him forever. You are at liberty at any time to change doctors. But, both you and the new doctor will feel better if you will notify your previous doctor that you are changing. This is particularly true if your disease is the same one for which one doctor has been treating you. Then the new doctor will almost surely refuse to take the case if the other doctor has not been notified of the change. This notification is not necessary when you have not seen the first doctor for some time, and the disease in question is something different from what he has been seeing you for.

When moving into a strange town or neighborhood, you may ask the advice of some friend whose judgment you respect as to which doctor to call. If you are a stranger and know no one in the town, call the local County Medical Society and they will give you the names of several qualified physicians. You should have these names and their telephone numbers in a convenient place, so the doctor may be called at once in case of a real emergency. If you have not obtained the name of a doctor before an emergency arises, you can ask the telephone operator for the local County Medical Society and they will get a doctor for you.

When you are moving from one town to another, ask your family doctor to recommend some doctor in the town to which you are moving. If he doesn't know anyone, he will be able to find out the name of a good doctor through some of his friends. He will always be glad to do that for you.

Remember, it is to your advantage to be able to consider your family doctor as your friend as well as your physician.

You may be able to find someone who appeals to you as a family doctor on the first trial, or it may take several trys. But be sure to look for most of the points enumerated above, and you will experience a feeling of safety and satisfaction in having a family doctor of your own.

PHYSICAL EXAMINATION OR MEDICAL CHECK-UP

Most of us have heard how important it is to go to a doctor for regular examinations at stated intervals, say once a year. But many of us do not know just exactly what to expect in the way of a complete examination, and when we leave the doctor's office we do not know whether or not we have received a good examination.

With this in mind, a copy of an examination form used by some general practitioners is printed here with explanations as to the various steps. If these steps are understood, then perhaps we would not look upon a visit to a doctor's office as something mysterious, which is to be dreaded. As a matter of act, these periodic examinations may uncover some simple trouble connected with your body which, if discovered, may be corrected easily; but if allowed to go on too long before discovery, may cause a great deal of damage to the body, and be responsible for suffering which could have been prevented.

In the first place, an appointment should be made and the doctor's secretary told that a general examination is desired. Some doctors will do this complete work in one visit, while others may require two or three visits before all the needed information can be obtained.

When you reach the doctor's office, he may have an assistant take the preliminary history.

This part of the examination is very important. It will give the doctor not only an idea of what sicknesses, operations, and accidents you have had in the past, but also information about your parents, your grandparents, and your children.

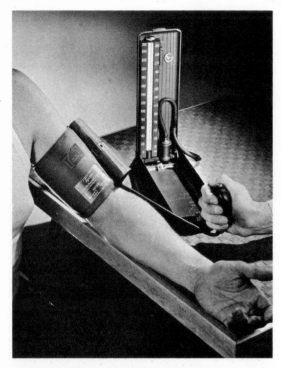

Blood pressure readings are given as *systolic* (contracting) and *diastolic* (relaxing) pressures. (120/85)

After the history, which will include the past performance of your systems, that is for example, your gastrointestinal system, or your urinary system, etc., the doctor will want to know something of your habits—how much coffee you drink or how many cigarettes you smoke, for example. He will want to know if you are at the present time taking any medicine, and if you have taken any considerable amount of medicine in the past.

Then will come the physical examination. There is nothing mysterious about this, and you should not be frightened or apprehensive when you see a great number of instruments or tools in the doctor's office. He is not going to use them all on you, and the whole examination usually can be performed without any pain or discomfort to the patient.

The doctor will consider the patient as a whole, whether he or she seems older than the stated age, seems to be in any pain, etc.

The skin is then noted, warm or cold, dry or moist, ruddy or pale, distribution of hair, and the presence or absence of enlarged lymph glands in the neck, under the arms, or in the inguinal region or groin.

The head will be described and then the eyes; are the pupils equal and regular, and do they react to light and distance. The doctor will then examine the background of the eye, called the fundus, with a light and a special instrument which allows him to note, among other things, what the small blood vessels in the fundus look like. This may give him an important clue as to the presence or absence of hardening of the arteries, kidney, or heart disease.

The nose is then examined to see if there is a good airway, and if not, what is causing the obstruction.

Next come the mouth, the lips, teeth, gums, tongue, tonsils, and throat. All will be carefully observed.

After the mouth is examined, he will usually feel of your neck to see if the thyroid is enlarged or if there is a goiter.

The chest examination is very important and will give the doctor many clues as to your health. He will listen to your lungs, front and back, with a stethoscope to try and detect any abnormality. He may thump your chest with his hands; in this way he can tell, among other things, the size of your heart. Again, there is nothing mysterious about this, as he is using the same procedure you would use to thump a wall to find out where the studs are. When he thumps over the part of the chest where the air-filled lungs are, he will get a hollow sound; but over the muscle of the heart he will get a flat, dull sound, which will tell him approximately the size of the heart. He will listen to the heart sounds with his stethoscope, to see if the sounds are normal or if there are any strange sounds which would indicate a leaking valve.

A careful examination of the abdomen is next. The doctor will look for any scars from old operations, any hernias or ruptures; he will feel carefully to see if there are any masses there that do not belong. He will thump below your ribs to see how far down your liver extends and how large your spleen is. Then he will probe deeply in the upper right hand side of the abdomen to see if there is any tenderness in the gall bladder region. The same deep probing will take place in the lower right hand side of the abdomen to see if there is any tenderness over the appendix. When pressing on the left side he can tell if your colon or large bowel on that side is tender. During these pressings or probing he is looking for unusual masses as well as for tenderness or pain.

If you are a woman he will next do a pelvic examination and from this examination a great deal may be learned, so it is important for the patient to be relaxed and not frightened in order that the doctor may more easily feel the organs in the female pelvis. This is usually called a bimanual or two handed examination. One hand or two fingers are inserted into the vagina and the other hand is placed on the abdominal wall to get the true size of the womb and other organs. The inner hand will first note each side of the vagina to see if there are any masses where the ovaries and tubes are located. The cervix or mouth of the womb is

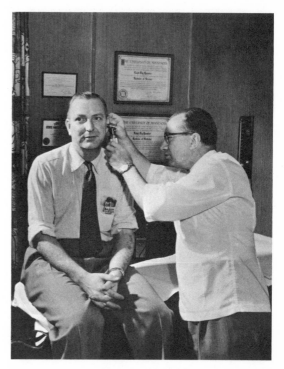

The otoscope with its magnified light source is used to examine the interior of the external ear.

then felt, and with the help of the outer hand the size and shape of the uterus or womb can be determined. Any undue tenderness or pain is noted. Now the doctor will use one of his special instruments, the vaginal speculum; this will not hurt, although it looks as though it might. The outlet of the vagina is noted to see whether there is any bulging either in the roof or floor of the vagina in women who have had babies. Sometimes when babies are born some of the muscles of the roof of the vagina are torn or weakened and the urinary bladder, which is located just above, will protrude through the weak place causing a bulge. This is called a cystocele. If the floor muscles have been weakened there will be a bulge at the bottom where the rectum may be protruding upward. This is called a rectocele. Both of these conditions, if they cause much trouble, can be corrected surgically. After the external examination, the speculum will be inserted and the interior of the vagina will be examined. The cervix or mouth of the womb can be seen, and a smear may be taken by rubbing a cotton applicator in the cervix and transmitting it to a glass slide. This is especially important in women over forty-five as a "Pap" smear can be used to detect early cancer of the cervix. There should be no pain and very little discomfort during this examination, if the patient cooperates.

In the male the external genital organs are carefully examined.

The temperature, blood pressure, and pulse rate are taken at sometime during the examination, usually at first.

The extremities, or hands, arms, feet, and legs are next examined in order to detect abnormalities, such as tremor or trembling of the hands, swelling of the ankles, varicose veins of the legs, and the conditions of the nails, etc.

Then the doctor will strike your knees with a rubber hammer or his hand to test your knee jerks, which is just one of the ways in which reflexes are tested. The only reason for testing these reflexes is to determine the condition of your nervous system, the brain, and spinal cord.

The doctor may then carefully examine your back to obtain information about the vertebrae and muscles of the back.

A rectal examination is next, and any man over forty-five who has an examination which does not include a rectal examination has not been really examined. In this way the doctor can examine the prostate gland with his finger, determining the size and consistency of it, and by pressing on it cause some of the secretion to come out the end of the penis and be caught on a glass slide. This can be examined under a microscope in order to see if there is any infection present, or in some cases to determine the presence or absence of spermatozoa.

A woman does not have a prostate gland, but the rectum should be examined to detect the presence of hemorrhoids.

In order for your doctor to have a complete inventory of your physical status, certain laboratory tests will be needed; these can vary from a few simple ones to a very great number of tests, depending upon the information needed.

In nearly all cases a complete blood count and urinalysis will be done. Some doctors will need an X ray of your chest, and this is very important. The test is absolutely safe, and may give valuable information as to the presence of tuberculosis, which may be present without giving symptoms. In rare cases, a lung tumor can be detected early. An E.C.G. or tracing of the heart (electrocardiogram) is the best way to uncover unsuspected early heart disease, and a gastrointestinal X ray series may show up a stomach ulcer. All of the conditions can be treated if found early, and the earlier the better.

As you may have guessed, it sometimes takes more than one visit to the doctor in order to obtain all of the above information; but after he has this material at hand he can give you a very good estimate as to the state of your health, and can immediately correct any small defects which may have been uncovered. Let me again emphasize that there is nothing mysterious or frightening about this type of examination. It is much the same procedure that you would expect

TYPICAL

PHYSICAL EXAMINATION FORM

NAME John Doe   ADDRESS Quincy, California   DATE

AGE 45 WT. 160 HT. 5'10" SEX M NATIONALITY American OCCUPATION Clerk

CHIEF COMPLAINT:	Loss of weight, generalized weakness, excessive thirst and hunger
PRESENT ILLNESS:	The patient was well until about two months ago when he began to lose weight. He drank a great deal of water and urinated more often than usual. He noted that he became weak although he ate more than was his habit.
PAST HISTORY: DISEASES:	Had the usual childhood diseases. Pneumonia 5 years ago.
OPERATIONS	T&A as a child and appendectomy 2 years ago.
ACCIDENTS	Broken right leg at the age of 21—auto accident.
FAMILY HISTORY:	His mother and father are living and well. One uncle had diabetes. Has two brothers living and well.
MARITAL HISTORY:	Married for 10 years—compatible.
SYSTEMS: E.N.T.	Has had infrequent sore throats but has noted decrease in hearing lately.
RESPIRATORY	Frequent colds
CARDIOVASCULAR	Normal
G.I.	Negative
G.U.	Frequency of urination—no burning
N.S.-N.M.	Negative—negative
CATAMENIA	(In case the patient is a woman) Periods began at age of eleven;-regular-every 28 days;-last four or five days;-no pain.
HABITS:	Drinks 3 cups of coffee a day—smokes one pack of cigarettes and has an occasional highball
MEDICATION:	None. No known allergies.
PHYSICAL EXAMINATION:	
GENERAL APPEARANCE	A well-developed, poorly nourished white male of about 45 who appears to be ill.
SKIN	warm and moist
LYMPH GLANDS	several enlarged cervical glands
HEAD	well formed—hair scanty
EYES	pupils are equal and regular. They react to light and distance.
EARS	both m.t. are normal
NOSE	good airway
MOUTH: LIPS:	no cyanosis
TEETH	marked dental caries
TONGUE	protrudes in the midline
THROAT	posterior pharynx is red—tonsils absent
NECK	thyroid gland is not enlarged
THORAX	symmetrical and well clothed
BREASTS	There are no masses
LUNGS	Lungs are clear throughout
HEART	Sounds and rate are normal—no enlargement—no murmurs—rhythm regular
BLOOD PRESSURE	140/84
TEMPERATURE	98.6
ABDOMEN	Soft—no masses or point tenderness. McBurney scar. Liver or other organs not palpated.
GENITALIA	normal male
PELVIC	
RECTAL	no hemorrhoids
PROSTATE	non-tender, smooth, and within normal limits of size
EXTREMITIES	no pitting edema, contractures, or deformities
REFLEXES	present and equal
SKELETAL	
POSTURE	good
JOINTS	negative
LABORATORY REPORTS:	urine = +++ sugar
IMPRESSION:	Diabetes Mellitus
PROCEDURE:	This patient will be hospitalized for further study in order to stabilize his diabetes.

a good mechanic to follow in checking your automobile. He would check the gas line, ignition, lubricating system, and so on down the line; and the doctor in giving you a thorough physical examination uses a similar approach.

I am presenting here a copy of such a physical examination to give you an idea of what the doctor will record after examining you. All doctors do not use the same technique, but their methods are usually quite similar. The typical physical examination form on page 479 may be considered as showing the results of an average examination.

GLOSSARY

Abdomen   the part of the body between the thorax and the pelvis

Abnormal   not normal

Blood count   a counting of corpuscles in a certain amount of blood

Goiter   enlargement of the thyroid gland

Genitals   reproductive organs

Hemorrhoids   painful swelling at the anus

Hernia   protrusion of an organ or part

Lymph gland   one of the masses of lymphoid tissue

Pelvic   pertaining to the cavity formed by the backbone and hipbone

Penis   male genital organ

Prostate   male genital gland

Reflex   not controlled by the will

Rupture   tissue or organ which sticks out

Spermatozoa   male germ cells

Spleen   glandlike ductless organ in upper left quadrant of abdomen

Thyroid   gland in the neck

Urinalysis   chemical analysis of the urine

Vertebrae   segments of the spinal column

ACCIDENT AND SICKNESS INSURANCE

The costs of medical care and hospital care have become so high that it has become a "must" to carry some form of accident and sickness insurance. In order to obtain a policy which does not cost too much, the head of every family should understand the different kinds of policies available and should purchase the one that fits his situation.

The ordinary case of sickness or small accident does not cost over one or two hundred dollars and this may not cause much trouble with the family budget, but the serious accident or the so-called catastrophic illness, such as poliomyelitis can run into huge costs which may well cause any family to go bankrupt. It is this kind of situation that every person should be insured against, for none of us are immune to catastrophic illness or safe from the likelihood of a serious accident. As proof of this, a recent survey has shown that in one year more than half a million families in the United States were subjected to medical expenses which either equaled or exceeded their annual incomes. Think seriously about this statement!

There are literally thousands of different health insurance plans and it is comforting to know that one hundred and twenty-seven million people in the United States are protected by some program of medical insurance which will help pay the doctor and hospital bills.

Twenty years ago, there were only ten million people so protected. It is to be sincerely hoped that in the near future everyone will benefit from the protection given by some form of health insurance.

There are two large groups into which all health insurance policies can be divided. (See also article on Medicare.)

1. Group plans in which the policies are set up to provide for groups of people who have similar jobs, places of employment,

etc. Some of these cover only the person named on the policy while others include the families as well. Then there are the policies that only cover the employee while he is employed by the sponsoring company

2. Insurance plans for the individual, which are developed to meet special needs of an individual or a family. Some people have company group plan insurance and individual insurance to take up where the company plan leaves off. The individual plan covers a person when he may be between jobs and also after he retires

Whether you buy a group plan or an individual plan, you must be sure that you are protected against three major fields of financial loss.

1. Basic plans to help pay for hospital bills, doctor bills, drugs, special treatment, and other related bills

2. The second program may be called income insurance, or indemnity insurance. It helps replace some of the income lost while a person is unable to work because of sickness or accident. This is extremely important, especially when the wage earner is unable to work for a long period because of a serious accident or disease. It makes it possible for the family to have money for rent, food, etc., while the wage earner is incapacitated

3. This is the most important of all. It is called major medical or "catastrophic" insurance and will cover a substantial portion of the expense incurred while being treated for a major accident or long-term illness; and this is the kind of disability that can wreck a family budget if it is not insured against. Not only could the budget be wrecked but the savings of a life time could be wiped out

There are many different kinds of major medical or catastrophic insurance, but most of them have two features.

1. The deductible clause which is similar to your automobile collision coverage. That is, you pay the first $100 to $200, and the insurance company pays most of the rest

2. The other feature which is nearly always included is called the co-insurance plan. Suppose you have a twenty-five percent co-insurance plan and you or some member of your family has a serious illness which costs $8,000. You pay the deductible part, say $500. The comapny will pay seventy-five percent of the remaining expense $7,500. This would mean that the company would pay $5,625 of the $7,500 owed. This deductible and co-insurance plan makes it possible for you to buy a good policy without paying too high a premium

Major medical policies vary. Some will pay only up to $5,000 while others will pay as high as $10,000 with the deductible and co-insurance clauses described above. A major medical policy will cost from $65 to $120 a year in premiums for a man aged thirty and his family. They are all well worth the price.

Here are some suggestions to a person who is trying to obtain the best possible sickness and accident insurance for himself and his family.

1. See your insurance agent and get his advice as to which policy would be the best for your particular needs

2. Be sure to go over your health insurance periodically, for this field grows and changes so rapidly that a policy which you bought several years ago may be completely inadequate. There may be a better policy on the market now which offers wider coverage for less money. The costs of hospital and medical care are going up and you may not have enough insurance now

3. Be sure the plan you select fits your family and your pocketbook

4. This is the most important of all—carry some form of sickness and accident insurance which is voluntary—that is, one which you select to fit your own needs

PROTECTING YOUR HEALTH

The following paragraphs present specific "do's" and "don'ts" on some important matters of health and safety. A good general rule is to examine every situation that occurs in your household, and anticipate the things to do or not to do in solving each problem and completing each project.

Intelligent Care

We must all realize that our bodies comprise the most delicate and wonderful piece of machinery that was ever devised. It runs automatically, without any thought or effort on our part; but because it is so delicate and complicated it sould be given intelligent care, such as we would give any complicated piece of machinery.

It is difficult for us to give this care to our bodies if we do not understand the body. Since we all cannot study physiology and anatomy, it is wise to have some instructions at hand to follow in case the body does not function properly, and needs help.

How the Doctor Helps

Generally speaking, the body has the power to heal itself—that is, to correct damage which has occurred, as in the case of a broken bone. If this bone is put at rest, it will heal itself. No doctor knows enough to make the broken bone knit, but he can help it by putting it into the correct position, and putting it at rest—as in a cast or on a splint.

In the case of torn muscles or tendons, we put them at rest and apply heat, which brings more blood to the part. This is like bringing more carpenters on the job, because our own blood must repair the damaged tissues.

The Importance of Rest

Rest is the most important single item in helping the body to cure infections. Thus, staying in bed when we have a cold accompanied by a fever will help the body overcome this infection.

In addition to rest, we must see to it that the body has the proper kind of food and plenty of water, and that the functions of elimination, such as bowel movements and urination, are working properly.

Medicines and Immunization

Since doctors and other scientists have been studying the causes of diseases and their proper treatments for hundreds of years, it is possible for a doctor to help the body throw off a serious infection by using certain drugs wisely.

The body can also be encouraged to throw off certain diseases, such as diphtheria, whooping cough, smallpox, poliomyelitis, and many others by immunization in the form of injections which every baby should have as it starts out in life.

Life-Saving Surgery

In many cases, different organs of the body become infected, and the only way to cure this infection is to remove the organ by surgery, such as in appendicitis. Other conditions which require surgery are cancer and gangrene. Never forget that surgery is a life-saving procedure in a great many instances, and if your doctor advises surgery, this may be the means of saving your life. Most doctors will not advise surgery unless they are sure it is really needed.

Treating Infections

Many times when infections become localized, pus is formed, as in the case of a boil or abscess. This pus should always be drained out, and this drainage is usually accomplished by a doctor's making an incision into the abscess, relieving pus under pressure.

The general rules for the treatment of local infections are:

1. Rest
2. Elevation
   (to prevent swelling)
3. Heat
   (to bring more healing blood to the part)
4. Drainage
   (allowing the pus to drain out)
5. Antibiotics
   (drugs used to kill certain bacteria)

Prevention of Accidents

The prevention of accidents should be practiced with care and intelligence. For instance, when going out at night, children and older people should wear white garments or yellow raincoats. People who drink should not drive cars while drinking. Seat belts should be used in all cars.

Medicines and poisons should be locked up out of the way of children.

Remember that accidents now are the fourth leading cause of death in the United States.

Simple Rules of Health

Every person should take the best of care where his body is concerned. There should be plenty of rest, plenty of exercise, a good, well-balanced diet which will contain all the vitamins you need, and sufficient water should be drunk every day. Many people neglect this—about eight full glasses of water or other fluids should be enough and finally, do not neglect nor ignore the bowel movement habit.

The Art of Growing Old

This last, and one of the most important concepts, has to do with the art of growing old gracefully.

After having taken the best care of your body possible during childhood, adolescence, and middle life, then one must realize that the wonderful machine has been used for a long time, and it will show signs of wear and tear.

Growing old should be looked forward to as a privilege—a period of reward for all of the effort and strife which has gone before.

Exercise must be moderated more and more; rest becomes more important, and should be indulged in.

Diet should be watched more carefully, and the habit of regular elimination should be strongly developed.

So, instead of taking more medicine as one grows older, a person should enjoy this period and really live.

To put the above into a simple sentence, we should try to remember that we are not "all American" athletes at this stage of the game, and take things easy.

All people should develop some hobby which can be practiced as they grow older. Golf, hunting, fishing, etc. As one grows older he should try to keep busy, take a moderate amount of exercise each day, and try to remain independent of others.

In order to keep the body in good working order, we should visit a doctor at least once a year in order to have him evaluate our physical condition and make the needed corrections.

HEALTH BILL OF WRONGS

Dangers to Avoid

One should never give a dose of cathartic to a person with a pain in the stomach. This may cause the appendix or some other organ to rupture.

It is very dangerous to squeeze a boil in order to express the pus. This breaks down the tissue around the boil and hinders the healing process. Squeezing an infection around the nose or face is especially dangerous as it may cause some of the bacteria to be forced into the blood stream or lymph channels. This may result in serious disease.

It is wrong to try and work off a cold or any other kind of infection. The body needs rest to aid it in throwing off these infections.

Excesses to Control

Over-eating and over-drinking put a strain upon the system which will result in permanent damage if practiced over too long a period.

Smoking to excess has a harmful effect upon the circulation, especially of the feet and legs. This has been proven, and there is enough proof to indicate that smoking cigarettes may be one of the causative factors in cancer of the lungs as well as heart disease.

The Only Safe Way

Never drive an automobile when you have been drinking and never ride in a car which is being driven by a person who has been drinking. You may know how many you have had, but you never know how many the driver may have had if he has been drinking.

The First Rule of Health

Never eat without first washing your hands thoroughly.

Tell Your Child the Truth

Never evade a question about the human body, sex, and other matters pertaining to the body which is asked by a young child. Tell them the truth.

A Word of Caution

Never go into a doctor's office and ask him for a shot of penicillin in order to try and cure a cold. Penicillin has no effect upon the virus that causes a cold; it is dangerous to take as there are often reactions following injection of penicillin. Sometimes these reactions result in death. There are deaths reported every year caused by injections of penicillin, and perhaps the most important reason for not taking penicillin too often for minor infections is that by doing so bacteria build up a resistance to this drug and when you really need it for a serious infection you may find that it does not do any good.

A Hint for Hikers

After the age of forty never go on a strenuous hike or hunting trip without first getting into condition by taking graduated exercises to prepare yourself for the trip.

GLOSSARY

Bacteria　very tiny living plants, some of which cause disease
Cathartic　medicine that quickens evacuation
Causative　effective as an agent
Lymph channel　a vessel for carrying lymph
Virus　a small living organism which may cause disease

Appendix

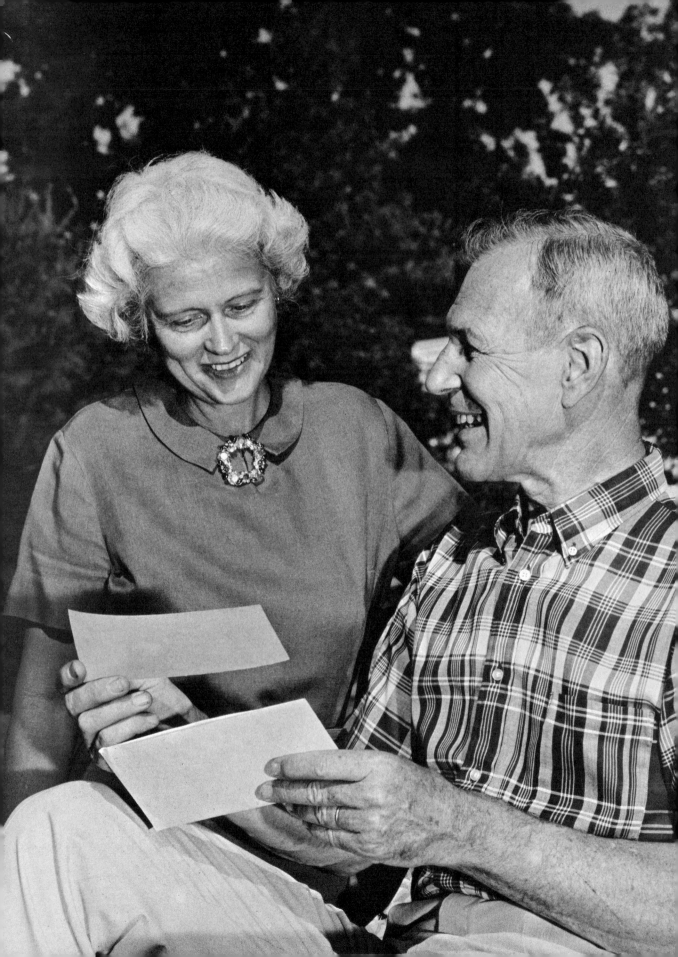

Medicare

HEALTH INSURANCE UNDER SOCIAL SECURITY

THERE HAVE BEEN a great many changes in the practice of medicine during the past twenty years and one of the most significant of these changes is the so-called Medicare Act, passed by Congress.

This is not the correct name for this act since the term Medicare has been used to describe the benefits of medical care to which the dependents of a man in military service are entitled.

Since the name Medicare is short it has caught on and has been used to describe "The Social Security Amendments of 1965."

These amendments are very complex and only the basic parts of the law will be described in this article.

There are two fundamental portions in the law. These are called Title 18 or "Health Insurance for the Aged," and Title 19 or "Grants to States for Medical Assistance Programs."

TITLE 18

We will describe Title 18 first. This part of the law is divided into Part A and Part B.

(For further information see your district social security office.)

Part A

This part is titled "Hospital Insurance Benefits for the Aged" and applies to almost all people sixty-five years of age and over and is paid for from special Social Security Trust Funds. It is applied to:

1. In-patient hospital services up to ninety days for each "Spell of Illness." The patient must pay the first forty dollars in all cases and if he stays in the hospital over sixty days he must pay ten dollars a day for the next thirty days. After this ninety day period is passed the government no longer pays any part of the bill if the patient is still in the same hospital, or in any acute hospital for the same "Spell of Illness."

2. After leaving the hospital, the patient may be cared for in a nursing home or the convalescent section of a hospital for a period of one hundred days. In this long-term facility the patient must pay five dollars a day after the first twenty days.

3. A certain amount of out-patient care is paid for under this section. That is, if a patient has X rays or laboratory services in

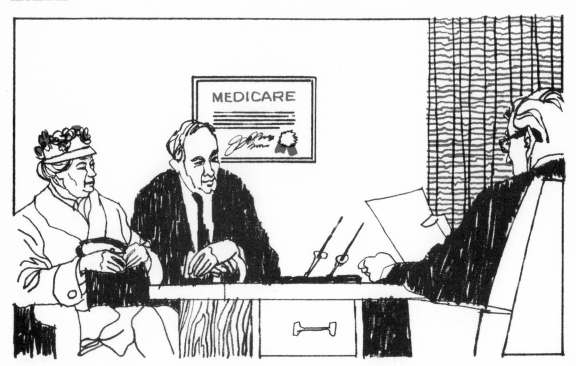

Retired couple meeting with district social security officer—discussing the benefits of the Medicare program and receiving their health insurance cards.

a hospital but is not confined there, eighty percent of the costs are paid for a consecutive twenty day period at the same hospital after the patient pays the first twenty dollars.

4. The next part is called Home Health Services and the services are provided by a team called the Home Health Agency which is under the Public Health Department of the county or state in which the patient resides. These services are made up of one hundred visits in any three hundred and sixty-five day period after the patient leaves the hospital or extended-care facility. Home Health Services must be under the direction of a doctor who writes the orders. The services may be supplied by a visiting nurse, a physiotherapist, a speech therapist, an occupational therapist, a medical social service person, home health aid, or in some cases the visit of an interne or a resident.

These services are all paid for by the Home Health Agency if there is one in that particular locality and they may also include visits to the hospital for out-patient service as in the case of a hydrotherapy treatment which cannot be secured at home.

It will be noted that the term, "One Spell of Illness," has been used several times and it may be well to know what is called a "Spell of Illness." It begins the first day a patient is treated in the hospital and ends after he has been at home for sixty consecutive days after leaving the hospital or extended care facility.

Part B

This part is titled "Supplementary Medical Insurance Benefits for the Aged," and is voluntary; that is the person may or may not take advantage of it.

If the person decides to take out Part B of Title 18 he must pay three dollars a month and the government puts up another three dollars. After the patient has signified his desire to take out Part B, the three dollars is automatically taken out of his social security check every month and in many cases it doesn't cost the patient anything because his social security has been raised three dollars to cover this charge.

Part B pays eighty percent of "Reasonable Charges" for the following services after patient has paid the first fifty dollars.

1. Visits to a doctor's office or a clinic, or home call by a doctor.
2. Visits from Home Health Agency.
3. Diagnostic tests such as X rays, and such things as splints, ambulance service, surgical dressings, and casts.

There are also provided limited services for mental illness.

The payments for visits to a doctor's office under Part B may be made in two ways.

1. The doctor may accept assignment and the fiscal intermediary, or insurance company which has been chosen by the state, will pay the doctor eighty percent of a reasonable charge. That is, if the charge for an office call is $6.00, the doctor will be paid $4.80 by the insurance company, and the patient will pay the remaining twenty percent—in this case, $1.20.
2. If the doctor does not accept assignment he bills the patient for the full amount, say twelve dollars for two office calls. When the patient pays the doctor he is given a receipted bill and he may then send this bill to the Insurance Company and they will send him eighty percent of the money. This also can only take place after the patient has paid the first fifty dollars.

When a patient is in a hospital and drugs are prescribed the insurance carrier pays for them. When a patient visits a doctor in his office and the doctor writes a prescription, the patient must pay for the medicine when he gets it at the drug store.

The only drugs that are paid for under Part B are the ones which the doctor gives in his office as part of his treatment, as in the case of an injection of penicillin.

The fiscal intermediaries or insurance companies vary from state to state. They are nominated by the state and if the government approves of them they are given money from the federal funds or Social Security Trust Funds to pay these bills.

This is a very costly system since the insurance company must be paid for every bill they process.

Railroad retirement beneficiaries are in a separate catagory. This portion of Social Security covers the railroads throughout the United States. Benefits are paid by a single insurance company which acts as a fiscal agent for the Retirement Board.

TITLE 19

The second part of the new law is called "Title Nineteen" or "Grants to States for Medical Assistance Programs." This is also a very complex law and it's implementation varies from state to state.

In order to receive from the federal government money to be used in the State Medical Assistance Program, or money to be used to help take care of the medically indigent, the state must pass a law outlining this kind of a program.

In California this is called the Medi-Cal Program and it is used to take care of the people who are in one class or another of the welfare program. There are many categories, i.e.; Aid to Totally Disabled, Aid to the Blind, Old Age Assistance, Aid to Families with Dependent Children, and Aid to the Children in Families whose Fathers are not Employed.

The Federal Government supplies fifty percent, the state twenty-five persent, and the county twenty-five percent of these funds.

Some states do not have such a Medical Assistance to the Needy Program and they therefore do not receive money from the federal government under Title 19.

From the above it can be seen that in some states it is possible for a person to be eligible under both Title 18 and Title 19. For instance a man sixty-eight years old may be taken to an acute hospital and not be able to pay the first forty dollars. After the first sixty days of his stay he may not have the money to pay ten dollars a day. In states which have passed laws to comply with Title 19, such as the Medi-Cal Law in California, the welfare department will pay the difference since, if he is medically indigent, he falls into one of their categories of aid.

The Medi-Cal law also states that in California all eligible patients must have free choice of doctor and hospital.

In most states there are rigid schedules to define medical indigency. For instance a man with a wife and four children may be eligible for help if his total income is say $4,000 a year. These limits vary from state to state.

Title Nineteen also helps people who are in one of the welfare categories to buy prescription drugs. If a man is on Old Age Assistance and has a county welfare number, this number can be used on the prescription form which the doctor writes and the welfare department pays for the drugs. These drugs are limited for they must be in the formulary or list of drugs which is put out by the government. On the other hand a person may be on Medicare, visit a doctor in his office, and be given a prescription for some drug. If he is just on Medicare and not in one of the welfare categories, he must pay for the drug out of his own pocket.

It is evident that these laws pay only a portion of medical expenses. For instance, in Part A of Title 18, the patient pays the first forty dollars, plus ten dollars a day after the first sixty days in the hospital. In Part B of Title 18 the patient pays the first fifty dollars for calls to a doctor's office. After that the government pays eighty percent of the "Reasonable or Customary Charge" and the patient is supposed to pay the other twenty percent.

For the above reasons it may be wise to carry some additional form of insurance against sickness to fill in the gaps. This is especially true when cases of catastrophic illness are involved, for they will require longer periods of treatment than those provided for in these laws.

To Summarize

Public Law 89-97 or "The Social Security Amendments of 1965" is divided into two parts.

Title 18 which became a law July 1, 1966. Under this law almost all people over sixty-five are entitled to benefits under *Part A*.

1. Hospital in-patient service: up to ninety days for each spell of illness. The patient pays the first forty dollars plus ten dollars a day after sixty days.
2. Post-hospital services: Up to one hundred days of care in a participating nursing

home or convalescent section of a hospital for each "Spell of Illness." Patient pays five dollars a day after the first twenty days. This part of the law became effective January 1, 1967.

3. Hospital out-patient diagnostic tests: Eighty percent of the cost after the patient pays the first twenty dollars in a consecutive tweny day period in the same hospital.
4. Home Health Service: If there is a Home Health Agency in your County, you may have up to 100 visits in a 365 day period following discharge from a hospital or long-term institution.

Part B is a voluntary section of the law and the patient who is sixty-five or over must pay three dollars a month out of his Social Security check. The government puts up a matching three dollars. The plan pays eighty percent of reasonable charges after the first fifty dollars is paid by the patient in each year for the following services:

1. Physicians: calls in clinic, hospital, office, or home.
2. Home health: Up to 100 visits a year.
3. Other: Diagnostic tests, X ray, radiation therapy, some ambulance services, surgical dressings, splints and casts. Limited treatment for mental disorders.

Title 19 provides for agreements with states for assistance in providing health care to the medically indigent.

The provisions of this Title 19 cannot be spelled out as they vary from state to state.

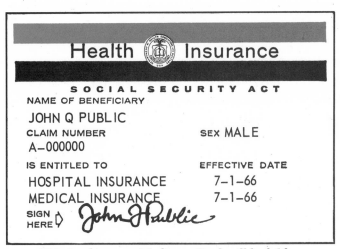

This is what your Medicare Card will look like.

The following pages have been provided
for your convenience,
to help you keep an accurate record
of your family's health,
which can be invaluable to you.

Fill in only those areas which apply
to each individual member of your family.
Keep it up-to-date.

PERMANENT

Family Health Record[*]

Name _____ Relationship _____

Date of Birth _____ Place of Birth _____

Maiden Name _____ Date of Marriage _____

Place of Residence (age, 0-18) _____ (18-26) _____ (26-?) _____

Occupation _____

Pregnancies _____ Miscarriages _____

Number of Children Living _____ Contraceptives Used _____

Periods Began (age) _____ Every _____ Days   Regular: Yes _____ No _____

Pain Before Periods: Yes _____ No _____ Flow: Excessive _____ Normal _____ Scant _____

Change of Life: Periods Ceased (date) _____

Symptoms During Menopause _____

"Pap" Smear Test: Date of Last Test _____ Result of Last Test _____

Tuberculin Skin Test: Date _____ Result _____ Chest X ray: Date _____ Result _____

DENTAL HEALTH

How Many Visits to Dentist per Year _____ Date of Last Visit _____

PAST HISTORY (give date of each)

Childhood Diseases

1. _____   4. _____

2. _____   5. _____

3. _____   6. _____

Adult Diseases

1. _____   3. _____

2. _____   4. _____

Surgical Operations

1. _____   3. _____

2. _____   4. _____

Accidents or Broken Bones

1. _____   3. _____

2. _____   4. _____

[*]In filling out this report, either check, answer "yes" or "no", write in number, date or other information requested.

FAMILY HISTORY

Mother _____ Father _____

Brothers _____ Sisters _____

Any history of: Heart Disease _____ Cancer _____ Diabetes _____ Epilepsy _____

    If yes, name relative and disease _____

REVIEW OF SYSTEMS

1. EENT: Eye _____ Ear _____

    Nose _____ Throat: Tonsils, Present _____ Absent _____

2. Skin: Any Rashes or Eczema _____

3. Neck: Enlarged Glands, Yes _____ No _____ Stiff Neck: Yes _____ No _____

4. Respiratory: Bronchitis, Yes _____ No _____ Pneumonia, Yes _____ No _____ Asthma, Yes _____ No _____

5. Cardio-Vascular: High Blood Pressure, Yes _____ No _____ Heart Irregularity, Yes _____ No _____

6. Gastro-Intestinal: Indigestion, Yes _____ No _____ Ulcers, Yes _____ No _____ If Yes, Type _____

    Unable to Eat Certain Foods, Yes _____ No _____ Bowels Regular, Yes _____ No _____ Cathartics _____

7. Genito-Urinary: Frequent Urination _____ Burning Urination _____ Blood in Urine _____

8. Locomotor: Weakness in Legs _____ Dizziness _____

9. Blood: History of Anemia, Yes _____ No _____ Blood Type _____ Rh Factor _____

10. Allergies: To Medicines, if yes, state which _____

    To Foods, if yes, state which _____

IMMUNIZATIONS (give last date of immunizations)

D.P.T. _____ Tetanus Booster _____

Small Pox Vaccination _____ Measles _____

Polio _____

HABITS

Drink (cups per day): Milk _____ Coffee _____ Tea _____ Water _____ Alcohol _____ Carbonated Drinks _____

Smoke (amount per day): Cigarettes _____ Cigars _____ Pipe _____

Recreation: Bowling _____ Tennis _____ Fishing _____ Hunting _____ Other _____

MEDICATIONS (now being taken regularly)

1. _____   8. _____

2. _____   9. _____

3. _____   10. _____

4. _____   11. _____

5. _____   12. _____

6. _____   13. _____

7. _____   14. _____

Family Health Record*

Name_____ Relationship_____

Date of Birth_____ Place of Birth_____

Maiden Name_____ Date of Marriage_____

Place of Residence (age, 0-18)_____ (18-26)_____ (26-?)_____

Occupation_____

Pregnancies_____ Miscarriages_____

Number of Children Living_____ Contraceptives Used_____

Periods Began (age)_____ Every _____Days Regular: Yes_____No_____

Pain Before Periods: Yes_____No_____ Flow: Excessive_____Normal_____Scant_____

Change of Life: Periods Ceased (date)_____

Symptoms During Menopause_____

"Pap" Smear Test: Date of Last Test_____ Result of Last Test_____

Tuberculin Skin Test: Date_____Result_____ Chest X ray: Date_____Result_____

DENTAL HEALTH

How Many Visits to Dentist per Year_____ Date of Last Visit_____

PAST HISTORY (give date of each)

Childhood Diseases

1. _____ 4. _____

2. _____ 5. _____

3. _____ 6. _____

Adult Diseases

1. _____ 3. _____

2. _____ 4. _____

Surgical Operations

1. _____ 3. _____

2. _____ 4. _____

Accidents or Broken Bones

1. _____ 3. _____

2. _____ 4. _____

*In filling out this report, either check, answer "yes" or "no", write in number, date or other information requested.

Mother _____ Father _____

Brothers _____ Sisters _____

Any history of: Heart Disease _____ Cancer _____ Diabetes _____ Epilepsy _____

    If yes, name relative and disease _____

REVIEW OF SYSTEMS

1. EENT: Eye _____ Ear _____

    Nose _____ Throat: Tonsils, Present _____ Absent _____

2. Skin: Any Rashes or Eczema _____

3. Neck: Enlarged Glands, Yes _____ No _____ Stiff Neck: Yes _____ No _____

4. Respiratory: Bronchitis, Yes _____ No _____ Pneumonia, Yes _____ No _____ Asthma, Yes _____ No _____

5. Cardio-Vascular: High Blood Pressure, Yes _____ No _____ Heart Irregularity, Yes _____ No _____

6. Gastro-Intestinal: Indigestion, Yes _____ No _____ Ulcers, Yes _____ No _____ If Yes, Type _____

    Unable to Eat Certain Foods, Yes _____ No _____ Bowels Regular, Yes _____ No _____ Cathartics _____

7. Genito-Urinary: Frequent Urination _____ Burning Urination _____ Blood in Urine _____

8. Locomotor: Weakness in Legs _____ Dizziness _____

9. Blood: History of Anemia, Yes _____ No _____ Blood Type _____ Rh Factor _____

10. Allergies: To Medicines, if yes, state which _____

    To Foods, if yes, state which _____

IMMUNIZATIONS (give last date of immunizations)

D.P.T. _____ Tetanus Booster _____

Small Pox Vaccination _____ Measles _____

Polio _____

HABITS

Drink (cups per day): Milk _____ Coffee _____ Tea _____ Water _____ Alcohol _____ Carbonated Drinks _____

Smoke (amount per day): Cigarettes _____ Cigars _____ Pipe _____

Recreation: Bowling _____ Tennis _____ Fishing _____ Hunting _____ Other _____

MEDICATIONS (now being taken regularly)

1. _____ 8. _____
2. _____ 9. _____
3. _____ 10. _____
4. _____ 11. _____
5. _____ 12. _____
6. _____ 13. _____
7. _____ 14. _____

Family Health Record*

Name_____Relationship_____

Date of Birth_____Place of Birth_____

Maiden Name_____Date of Marriage_____

Place of Residence (age, 0-18)_____(18-26)_____(26-?)_____

Occupation_____

Pregnancies_____Miscarriages_____

Number of Children Living_____Contraceptives Used_____

Periods Began (age)_____Every _____Days   Regular: Yes_____No_____

Pain Before Periods: Yes_____No _____Flow: Excessive_____Normal _____Scant_____

Change of Life: Periods Ceased (date)_____

Symptoms During Menopause_____

"Pap" Smear Test: Date of Last Test_____Result of Last Test_____

Tuberculin Skin Test: Date_____Result _____Chest X ray: Date_____Result_____

DENTAL HEALTH

How Many Visits to Dentist per Year_____Date of Last Visit_____

PAST HISTORY (give date of each)

Childhood Diseases

1._____   4._____

2._____   5._____

3._____   6._____

Adult Diseases

1._____   3._____

2._____   4._____

Surgical Operations

1._____   3._____

2._____   4._____

Accidents or Broken Bones

1._____   3._____

2._____   4._____

*In filling out this report, either check, answer "yes" or "no", write in number, date or other information requested.

~~~ILY HISTORY

Mother _____ Father _____

Brothers _____ Sisters _____

Any history of: Heart Disease _____ Cancer _____ Diabetes _____ Epilepsy _____

    If yes, name relative and disease _____

REVIEW OF SYSTEMS

1. EENT: Eye _____ Ear _____

         Nose _____ Throat: Tonsils, Present _____ Absent _____

2. Skin: Any Rashes or Eczema _____

3. Neck: Enlarged Glands, Yes _____ No _____ Stiff Neck: Yes _____ No _____

4. Respiratory: Bronchitis, Yes _____ No _____ Pneumonia, Yes _____ No _____ Asthma, Yes _____ No _____

5. Cardio-Vascular: High Blood Pressure, Yes _____ No _____ Heart Irregularity, Yes _____ No _____

6. Gastro-Intestinal: Indigestion, Yes _____ No _____ Ulcers, Yes _____ No _____ If Yes, Type _____

    Unable to Eat Certain Foods, Yes _____ No _____ Bowels Regular, Yes _____ No _____ Cathartics _____

7. Genito-Urinary: Frequent Urination _____ Burning Urination _____ Blood in Urine _____

8. Locomotor: Weakness in Legs _____ Dizziness _____

9. Blood: History of Anemia, Yes _____ No _____ Blood Type _____ Rh Factor _____

10. Allergies: To Medicines, if yes, state which _____

         To Foods, if yes, state which _____

IMMUNIZATIONS (give last date of immunizations)

D.P.T. _____ Tetanus Booster _____

Small Pox Vaccination _____ Measles _____

Polio _____

HABITS

Drink (cups per day): Milk _____ Coffee _____ Tea _____ Water _____ Alcohol _____ Carbonated Drinks _____

Smoke (amount per day): Cigarettes _____ Cigars _____ Pipe _____

Recreation: Bowling _____ Tennis _____ Fishing _____ Hunting _____ Other _____

MEDICATIONS (now being taken regularly)

1. _____	8. _____
2. _____	9. _____
3. _____	10. _____
4. _____	11. _____
5. _____	12. _____
6. _____	13. _____
7. _____	14. _____

PERMANENT

Family Health Record*

Name_____ Relationship_____

Date of Birth_____ Place of Birth_____

Maiden Name_____ Date of Marriage_____

Place of Residence (age, 0-18)_____ (18-26)_____ (26-?)_____

Occupation_____

Pregnancies_____ Miscarriages_____

Number of Children Living_____ Contraceptives Used_____

Periods Began (age)_____ Every_____Days Regular: Yes_____No_____

Pain Before Periods: Yes_____No_____ Flow: Excessive_____Normal_____Scant_____

Change of Life: Periods Ceased (date)_____

Symptoms During Menopause_____

"Pap" Smear Test: Date of Last Test_____ Result of Last Test_____

Tuberculin Skin Test: Date_____Result_____ Chest X ray: Date_____Result_____

DENTAL HEALTH

How Many Visits to Dentist per Year_____ Date of Last Visit_____

PAST HISTORY (give date of each)

Childhood Diseases

1._____ 4._____

2._____ 5._____

3._____ 6._____

Adult Diseases

1._____ 3._____

2._____ 4._____

Surgical Operations

1._____ 3._____

2._____ 4._____

Accidents or Broken Bones

1._____ 3._____

2._____ 4._____

*In filling out this report, either check, answer "yes" or "no", write in number, date or other information requested.

FAMILY HISTORY

Mother_____Father_____

Brothers_____Sisters_____

Any history of: Heart Disease_____Cancer_____Diabetes_____Epilepsy_____

    If yes, name relative and disease _____

REVIEW OF SYSTEMS

1. EENT: Eye_____Ear_____

        Nose_____Throat: Tonsils, Present_____Absent_____

2. Skin: Any Rashes or Eczema _____

3. Neck: Enlarged Glands, Yes_____No_____Stiff Neck: Yes_____No_____

4. Respiratory: Bronchitis, Yes_____No_____Pneumonia, Yes_____No_____Asthma, Yes_____No_____

5. Cardio-Vascular: High Blood Pressure, Yes_____No_____Heart Irregularity, Yes_____No_____

6. Gastro-Intestinal: Indigestion, Yes_____No_____Ulcers, Yes_____No_____If Yes, Type_____

    Unable to Eat Certain Foods, Yes_____No_____Bowels Regular, Yes_____No_____Cathartics_____

7. Genito-Urinary: Frequent Urination_____Burning Urination_____Blood in Urine_____

8. Locomotor: Weakness in Legs_____Dizziness_____

9. Blood: History of Anemia, Yes_____No_____Blood Type_____Rh Factor_____

10. Allergies: To Medicines, if yes, state which_____

        To Foods, if yes, state which_____

IMMUNIZATIONS (give last date of immunizations)

D.P.T. _____Tetanus Booster_____

Small Pox Vaccination_____Measles_____

Polio_____

HABITS

Drink (cups per day): Milk_____Coffee_____Tea_____Water_____Alcohol_____Carbonated Drinks_____

Smoke (amount per day): Cigarettes_____Cigars_____Pipe_____

Recreation: Bowling_____Tennis_____Fishing_____Hunting_____Other_____

MEDICATIONS (now being taken regularly)

1._____	8._____
2._____	9._____
3._____	10._____
4._____	11._____
5._____	12._____
6._____	13._____
7._____	14._____

Bibliography

Principles and Practice of Medicine   OSLER
Introduction to Medical Science   BOYD
Psychosomatic Medicine   WEISS AND ENGLISH
The Specialties in General Practice   CECIL AND CONN
The Neuroses   ALVAREZ
Baby and Child Care   SPOCK
The Prevention of Deformity in Childhood   RANEY
De Re Medica   LILLY
Gifford's Text Book of Ophthalmology   GIFFORD
Western Medicine   CALIFORNIA MEDICAL ASSOCIATION
California Medicine   CALIFORNIA MEDICAL ASSOCIATION
Medical Tribune   MEDICAL TRIBUNE INC.
Therapeutic Notes   PARKE DAVIS AND CO.
Medical World News   MEDICAL WORLD PUBLISHING CO.
Spectrum   PFIZER
Journal of the American Medical Assn.   AMERICAN MEDICAL ASSOCIATION
Archives of Internal Medicine   AMERICAN MEDICAL ASSOCIATION
Consultation   SMITH, KLINE AND FRENCH
A.M.A. News   AMERICAN MEDICAL ASSOCIATION
What's New   ABBOTT
Modern Medicine   PAGE AND ALVAREZ
Modern Drugs   R. H. DONNELLEY CORP.
Clinical Symposia   CIBA
Medical Economics   MEDICAL ECONOMICS, INC.
New Medical Materia
Image   ROCHE
Scope   UPJOHN
California G. P.   CALIFORNIA ACADEMY OF GENERAL PRACTICE
Current Therapy   CONN
Geriatrics   LANCET PUBLICATIONS, INC.
The Heart Bulletin   THE MEDICAL ARTS PUBLISHING FOUNDATION
A Textbook of Medicine   CECIL AND LOEB
General Practice Periodical   PICKERING AND KERR
General Practice Periodical   ARCARII AND WILSON
Medical Clinics of North America   BULL, CAMPBELL AND OWEN
Medical Clinics of North America   ROTH AND BOKUS
Todays Health   AMERICAN MEDICAL ASSOCIATION
General Practice Periodical   BROWN
Post Graduate Medicine Periodical   MAUR
Medical Clinics of North America   W. B. SAUNDERS & CO.
GP (Periodical)   AMERICAN ACADEMY OF GENERAL PRACTICE
Public Health Bulletin—Orange County

Index

503

REQUEST FOR FURTHER INFORMATION

The owner of this book may use this official blank to request free information on any problem of health or welfare. Dr. W. B. McKnight, author of *The Home Medical Encyclopedia*, will furnish the best available information, with the warning that you should see a doctor promptly for proper diagnosis and treatment of illness.

Your Question: _____

_____

_____

_____

_____

_____

_____

_____

_____

_____

_____

_____

_____

_____

Have you consulted a local doctor about this matter? ☐ YES ☐ NO

Address your inquiry to: DR. W. B. McKNIGHT
QUINCY, CALIFORNIA 95971

Please enclose a stamped, self-addressed envelope for the doctor's answer.

YOUR NAME _____

ADDRESS _____

CITY _____ STATE _____ ZIP CODE _____